ILLNESS AND SELF IN SOCIETY

Illness and Self in Society

CLAUDINE HERZLICH
and
JANINE PIERRET

Translated by Elborg Forster

The Johns Hopkins University Press
Baltimore and London

This book has been brought to publication with the generous assistance of the Ministère de la culture, France, and the Andrew W. Mellon Foundation.

Originally published as *Malades d'hier, malades d'aujourd'hui: De la mort collective au devoir de guérison*. Copyright © Payot, Paris, 1984

The Johns Hopkins University Press, 701 West 40th Street, Baltimore, Maryland 21211
The Johns Hopkins Press Ltd., London

Library of Congress Cataloging-in-Publication Data
Herzlich, Claudine.
  Illness and self in society.
  Translation of: Malades d'hier, malades d'aujourd'hui.
  Bibliography: p.
  Includes index.
  1. Sick—Psychology—History. 2. Sick—Social conditions. 3. Health behavior—History—20th century. 4. Sick—Interviews. I. Pierret, Janine. II. Title.
R726.5.H4613 1987   306.4   87-2893
ISBN 0-8018-3228-4

Contents

Translator's Preface

*T*he translator is a book's most attentive reader. It is on the strength of this claim that I venture to speak about *Illness and Self in Society*.

Written by two French sociologists, this book is in part a historical work, and historians will be sympathetic to the authors' forthright acknowledgment that it is well-nigh impossible to make the "ordinary people" of the past speak with their own voices. They will therefore all the more appreciate the wide range of well-known and not so well-known literary texts—from Herodotus to Huysmans, from Joinville to Jack London—that illustrate the place of illness and the sick in the societies of the past, the manner in which they were seen and in which they saw themselves. In Western societies these attitudes underwent a dramatic shift in the nineteenth century, and this development is compellingly described and astutely analyzed in chapter 2. A new twist of the story, the devastating AIDS epidemic that now raises the specter of the great epidemics of the past, is mentioned in one note only (chap. 4, n.1), for the simple reason that when this book was being written in 1981–82, the first reports of a "noncontagious but usually fatal illness hitherto unknown in the northern hemisphere" and affecting "hundreds of young American males" were just beginning to reach Paris. There could be no question of tacking on a chapter about this new development, and the absence of AIDS from a book on illness written only a few years ago serves as a poignant reminder of the suddenness with which a new scourge can befall humankind.

Sociologists will welcome the results of several in-depth studies of attitudes toward illness and health among different social groups, which the authors have conducted at different times over the last twenty years. Physicians will read in these pages of feelings that their patients do not often express in their presence, and I should think that future physicians especially would do well to pay attention to them.

If my own reaction, that of a nonspecialist, is any indication, many other "general readers" will be fascinated by what our own contemporaries, people of all walks of life (though all of them French, which may add a special dimension), have had to say in their everyday language about the body and its ills, about pain, fate, health, health care, the doctor/patient relationship, the role of the State, and indeed about the human condition.

Introduction

*A*t the outset, we wanted to write a book in which sick people speak, retrace their experience of illness, and tell us how they preceive their physical state and their social condition. This is not as easy as it may sound, for the individual who suffers biological disorder and pain feels that there is something inexpressible about them; it is hard to put illness and the body into words. Moreover, in our society the discourse of medicine about illness is so loud that it tends to drone out all the others. Caught between their undecipherable physical experience and the ordered and dominating language of science, today's sufferers are often at a loss to know whether they can speak, to whom they can speak, and how they can speak.

Does this mean that in our society there is silence about illness and the sick? Certainly not, and we could not begin to review all the works of different genres in which something essential is signified through an illness or a sick person. It has been said that illness is a "metaphor,"[1] a metaphor of society. The social scientists who some years ago began to explore this field, which was new for them, namely, the body and its ills, have shown that in all societies there is a correspondence between the biological and the social order. Everywhere and in all periods, it is the individual who is sick, but he is sick in the eyes of his society, in relation to it, and in keeping with the modalities fixed by it. The language of the sick thus takes shape within the language expressing the relations between the individual and society. This book therefore attempts to show, on the one hand, the reciprocal stimulation between the manner in which the sick experience their state, express it, and organize it, and on the other, the collective discourse that sets up the schema of biological misfortune and gives it meaning.

It has thus been our objective to assemble, on the basis of several empirical studies we have conducted ourselves and which we will present in detail further on, these personal experiences, all of which are nevertheless woven into the collective patterns of thought that form the social reality of illness and the sick.

The fact that our studies were conducted over a period of almost twenty years immediately suggested the need for a diachronic perspective. This seems all the more indicated since in the course of the last twenty years we have seen both an extraordinary growth of the medical establishment and an equally remarkable crisis of confidence with respect to it. Both of these developments had an impact on the sick, their self-image, and their behavior. We therefore obviously had to think about this evolution that took place between the 1960s and the early 1980s. But we very soon realized that we could not limit ourselves to so short a period and came to feel that we must place today's sick into a long-term history. That is why, though fully aware of the temerity of such an undertaking, we have attempted to place the experience of illness and the sick person into an historical perspective. In short, we want to make yesterday's sick speak along with those of today.

Before proceeding further, we must explain the limits of this undertaking and the approach we have taken. We have not tried to do original historical research. For the periods going back further than twenty years, we have not sought to discover or explore archival series or other as yet unexploited sources. We have essentially based our conclusions on the work of historians as well as on published documents—mainly chronicles, letters, and diaries—in which the sick speak of their illness or in which eyewitnesses describe them. Literary works, particularly novels, provided us with prodigious amounts of material. This we have sometimes used, not so much to find accounts of a sick person's experience—for this we have preferred to look, wherever possible, to documents other than novels—but because literary fiction obviously contributes to the making of the collective discourse of and about illness.

Being sociologists, our aim can only be to understand today's sick in the light of history. Our limited excursions into the past are meant above all to make us understand how the reality of what we call today "a sick person" and the notion of "the sick person" have come into being. We thus have not written a "history of the sick," which in any case would have been far beyond our powers or outside the scope of this book. Yet we have tried not to adopt a too strictly "genealogical" perspective, which would have looked to the past only to find the origins of the condition of today's sick and would thus have seized sick people of past ages by means of categories that are our own. And it is a fact that in doing our work we have been struck by both continuities and similarities and by differences and discontinuities. For nothing is more misleading than to consider the condition of today's sick as the result of a linear evolution that always deals with the same physical realities, the same notions, the same values, and the same institutions. The transformation of the very nature of the principal diseases over time, the development of medicine with its false starts, its periods of triumph, and its explosion in the last century, the sudden linking of illness and work in the legal framework brought about by industrialization—all of these are examples of a restructuring of illness and the sick which show us that each society has its own way of letting the sick exist, defining them, and taking charge of them.

This study, then, demands a constant back-and-forth from sociology to history and from history to sociology. Sociologists and anthropologists, at least in the English-speaking world, were the first to become aware that illness, health, and death could not be reduced to their "physical," "natural," or "objective" evidence, that they do not escape the impact of society. They have shown that illness is a human construct and that the sick person is a social being. And today historians are producing evidence for the "historicity" of the relationships and the institutions through which the condition or, as the sociologists say, the "status" of today's sick person has been structured. They make us aware of the relativity of the categories and the schemata of reference which we use to think about these matters.

This book also confronts the experiences of the sick and their own understanding of them with the discourse of medicine. This approach is similar to that of a certain number of recent studies by sociologists and historians who have attempted in various ways to hear those who usually do not speak. Looking at the hidden facet, the "other side,"[2] the anonymous reverse of legitimacy and institutional power, these are studies of "popular culture" and "traditional wisdom" as opposed to "learned cultures;" they examine the outsiders, the marginal, and the powerless in their relation with the insiders, the establishments, and the powerful. To some extent, our book is part of this trend. For what all these categories of individuals have in common is that they are "taken charge of" by systems of knowledge, established practices, and powerful institutions that "know" what is to be done, decide what is right and proper for their charges, and proceed to implement it. The sick are one of the groups that are "taken charge of," for the medical establishment speaks of them more than they themselves speak. Nonetheless, the notions that we will use for our analysis are neither those of "traditional" or "popular" as opposed to "learned," nor those of "powerless" as opposed to "powerful." Rather, we will contrast the concepts, the knowledge, and the patterns of behavior of the sick or lay people with those of the "professionals."[3]

These concepts and patterns of behavior are organized, as the sociologists who have used these notions say, according to different "perspectives."[4] For the professionals, in this case the physicians, the understanding of illness is fixed within the perspective of a set of practices organized in a space and upon a circumscribed object, for as medical knowledge came to be focused progressively on the body, the latter became the space and the material of medical work, the object of a set of rules over which the physician wants to keep total control, so that it has become the foundation of his power. For the lay person, whether sick or not, understanding the state of his body is more than a matter of recognizing physiological mechanisms and their reactions to outside agents. Anyone who is ill seeks an interpretation that goes beyond the individual body and its physical state. The sick person needs to give his illness a sense and to work out a new relationship with his society. However great his dependence on medical knowledge and practices, this "perspective" continues to be paramount.

To be sure, in our society—and we will see many examples of this in the present book—the "lay" perceptions of illness cannot be separated from the development of medicine, which at all times, and today more than ever before, contributes to shaping them. Nonetheless, we wanted to study them in their own formulations and their own logic, without reference to their medical "truth," and we hope that we have succeeded in showing that they do have their own logic. Moreover, and there will be many examples of this as well, this relation can go both ways, from the "professional" to the "lay person" but also from the "lay person" to the "professional." This was true in the past, when medical knowledge was uncertain; but even today, when medicine enjoys a secure position as a legitimate science, it is still embedded in society. After all, the physician's thinking and practices are dependent on the experiences of the sick, on the vision they have of their ailment, and on the collective discourse on illness.

In our attempt to recapture the past we have encountered the inevitable problem of the fragility and the unevenness of the sources depending on the period and on the social categories envisaged. For certain periods, that of the great epidemics for example, practically no testimony by a sick person has come down to us. For sociologists, moreover, it is particularly disappointing to see that those who did leave such testimony almost never belonged to the lower classes, but were nobles, bourgeois, and even more often intellectuals and writers, since writing was for centuries the patrimony of a minority. The largest part of society remained as silent on the subject of illness as on many others. We are well aware that such a situation is almost bound to produce a skewed image, but all we can do here is to refer the reader to the difficulties encountered by all historians, as well as to the special pitfalls inherent in the history of mentalities. Other authors have evoked these problems better than we could. We would only like to add that for the sociologist the effort at adopting a historical viewpoint, if it is genuine, seems to have a positive effect, whatever the hypothetical nature of its results, for it is a way of testing our analytical categories.

For the sick and the illnesses of today, we used several empirical studies that we conducted at different periods. The first study was undertaken in the early 1960s. It involved eighty middle-class men and women who were executives, intellectuals, technicians, and professionals. This study was designed to investigate the representations of illness and health in this group, one quarter of whom were ill at the time.[5] The second study, conducted in 1972 among sixty sick persons of both sexes who were hospitalized in Paris and the provinces, involved farmers, laborers, and white-collar workers. Half of these patients were hospitalized in wards of general and orthopedic surgery, pneumology, endocrinology, and intensive-care units. This study was designed to investigate the patients' behavior during illness and their attitude toward medicine.[6] Two years later a study of forty patients with chronic renal insufficiency treated by the kidney machine repeated the questions asked by the previous study. The group investigated consisted of men and women between the ages of nineteen and sixty-five, twenty-five of whom resided in Paris or in provincial towns.[7] Another study was conducted in 1979 among a group of 112 persons, executives, teachers, and middle-class people, but also white-collar workers, laborers, and farmers, living in Paris, the Parisian suburbs, and southeastern France. This study investigated the meaning of health.[8] Finally, since 1980, some twenty interviews with sick people enrolled in associations or health clubs were conducted to complete our materials. Altogether our work is based on more than three hundred interviews.

Each of these studies was made with a somewhat different objective, and retracing the patients' experience was not their main purpose. It is probable that this too is a source of bias. Moreover, our material could be criticized because the "repertory" of possible ailments is unevenly represented; in fact, it is almost exclusively limited to somatic illness.[9] Nevertheless, in all cases the analysis of individual patient's representations of illness, as well as that of their relations with the physician, with the hospital, or with a particular technique (such as hemolysis), is based on the patients' accounts of their illness, which form the common substratum on which this book is built. Here, then, we have "patient's histories," because they have indeed told us their stories and also because, as we pointed out, these piecemeal experiences, articulated though they may be after the fact in necessarily fragmentary accounts, are nonetheless part of the history of society, of the collective discourse about illness.

It is our purpose to analyze how the figure of the sick person as we know it today has been shaped by the sufferer's experience of illness and his dealings with medicine. Our work is organized around two complementary points of entry. The first starts with a consideration of illness, and the second with the sick person.

For in order to understand the sick it is necessary to analyze in a first section how in each age one illness among the many incarnations of physical suffering has dominated the reality of people's experience and the structure of their mental representations. In its turn this dominating illness refers back to the entire complex of the conditions of life, the values, and the meaning given to existence that obtained at the time. The sick person must be situated first of all within the context of these different configurations of physical suffering which are the great epidemics of the past, tuberculosis in the nineteenth century, and cancer today.

In parts 2 and 3 we will be looking at the attitudes and the discourse of the sick themselves. It should be stated from the outset that there are different ways of reading and interpreting physical suffering. In the second part we therefore examine the way in which the sick in different periods perceive the presence of illness in the body, integrate and retranslate the medical knowledge of their time, wonder about the causes of their suffering, and try to give their suffering a meaning.

The role of society in constructing the status of the sick and the structuring of their identity are at the core of the third part. From yesterday's *fatum* to to-day's self-help, we have analyzed how at different times the sick person's iden-tity is structured around different forms of pathology, in keeping not only with the state of medical knowledge and with the institutional system that takes charge of the sick, but also with society's dominant values and schemes of reference.

I·

DISEASES AND THEIR VICTIMS

1·

The Ancien Régime *of Disease: Epidemics*

*O*ne cannot speak about the sick without also, and first of all, speaking of *their illnesses*. It would not do to separate the sphere of representations and collective feelings from what one might call the events, meaning the diseases that in each era have constituted the specific experience of the sick and shaped their consciousness and their identity. Although many ills have existed from all eternity, every era has its own diseases. Studies in historical epidemiology show us that certain pathologies appear, spread, and become rare or even disappear because of a concatenation of complex reasons. This kind of event has an impact on people's representations. At different times one specific disease was seen by everyone as the embodiment of illness itself, not only because of its frequent recurrence and the danger it represented, but also because in various ways it was the material sign of the conditions of life, of the concepts of human existence and the values of the time. In the Middle Ages the plague mowed down millions of victims, but it also embodied, better than any other scourge, the fragility of every person's existence, and it crystallized — in the figures of the flagellants, for example — a conception of the world that was imbued with the notion of divine punishment. In the nineteenth century phthisis expressed both the Romantic myth of the personality marked by fate and the wretched condition of the working class in the early phase of industrialization.

Despite the scope of the task, one must therefore try to trace the broad outlines of this evolution and its impact on the collective consciousness. At the same time one must also attempt to determine the major features of the experiences of the sick and their actual status in society. Accepting the risk of extreme simplification, we will examine what one might call the *Ancien Régime of Disease*, a regime — one that essentially no longer exists — in which illness was marked by three characteristics: numbers, impotence and death, and exclusion. In this regime, disease — in all of its dreadful reality — was above all the *epidemic*, a collective and social phenomenon that, whatever form it took, was the very embodiment of evil.

Numbers are its first striking feature. In an epidemic, one was not ill and one did not die alone, but in great numbers: it was not the individual who was struck and succumbed; it was the family, the neighborhood, the province. How important was this fact in forming collective representations? Do we find in them any trace of an individual's status as a sick person or do they focus on the collective fate of individuals affected by the epidemic? Did "the sick person" exist at all when the main task at hand was counting the dead? In addition, *impotence* and almost inevitable *death* were also characteristics of the *Ancien Régime of Disease*. That is why, unlike today—when chronic illness is a way of life—the epidemic could hardly be considered as anything but a way of death. Most of the time that death was real and immediate, as in the plague; sometimes it was slow and symbolic, but also real and attended by all manner of ritual; this was the case with leprosy. There was only one way to forestall this threat, namely, *exclusion*. The response of society and the socialization of this disease thus took the form of confinement and isolation. We actually know a great deal more about these practices than about the individual experiences of those involved, for lepers have rarely spoken. But we do know that life eventually overcame death by means of these practices; little by little the epidemic was defeated. The struggle against epidemics has bequeathed to us a whole network of medical and hygienist practices and institutions.

The Putting Away

The three characteristics of the epidemic become visible in the two diseases that reached their apogee in the Middle Ages, leprosy and the plague. In some respects they were the opposite of each other, for one was slow and the other swift, but both were violent and fatal.

Appearing around the sixth century and in full expansion by the eleventh, leprosy is still present in our speech as the symbol for that which gnaws away. In leprosy the body slowly destroys itself, often over a period of years, until the stage of final mutilation, when the organs give way. It is a disease that remains invisible for a long time and then deploys itself in all of its horror to the eyes of the world; concealment is impossible.

To escape the leper's fate was quite impossible. We know almost nothing about lepers, about their suffering and about their attitude toward this invading evil. We do not know, for example, how much truth there is in the words that Paul Claudel lends the leper Pierre de Craon: "It is hard to be a leper, to bear this shameful wound, knowing that there is no cure and that there is no help for it . . . but that each day it spreads and bites deeper; and to be alone, and to suffer one's own poison, and to feel oneself alive in corruption."[1] But we do know about the exclusion and the social death that were meted out to the lepers. As early as the sixth century, various Church Councils, those of

Orléans, Arles, and Lyon, recommended the isolation of lepers. Even though the notion of contagion was not clearly perceived, the leper was considered dangerous; he was condemned, and death, death to the world, was the only sentence. The leper was removed from the community, deprived of all property, and made to live exclusively on public charity.

Leprosaria were created. Eventually there were as many as two thousand of them in France, the first one being located near Saint-Claude in the Jura. Henceforth the "denunciation" of the leper, his "separation" or "putting out of the world," was carried out according to strange rituals in which the Church played a major role and which always symbolized death: the church was draped in black, a mass for the dead was said, and handfuls of earth were thrown on the sick person's head. Thereupon the "*ladre*" was led to the sickhouse and handed the rattle with which he would have to warn the healthy to avoid meeting him. As the centuries passed, and perhaps with the abatement of the disease, the fate of the lepers improved somewhat. Certain leprosaria received sizable gifts and became rich and comfortable. In the fourteenth century even healthy persons sometimes came to live there. Gradually, as the number of lepers in Europe began to decline, a trend that was irreversible by the sixteenth century, the leprosaria lost their function and disappeared. The medical profession, incidentally, has thought a great deal about this decline, wondering whether it was brought about by the segregation of the lepers or whether it was, as some experts believe, the result of a competition between the leprosy bacillus and the more mobile tuberculosis bacillus.

At that point, leprosy became an exotic illness, a tropical disease by which Westerners no longer felt threatened. Moreover, and rather mysteriously, it ceased to be contagious. "The ostentatious kissing of a leper," says Marcel Sendrail, "is no longer a dangerous act."[2] Yet some texts suggest that brutal exclusion persisted for a long time. In *Michael, Brother of Jerry*, written around 1900, Jack London depicts the fate of Dag Daughtry, who had served for many years as steward on the Makombo and had, unbeknownst to himself, contracted leprosy from contact with his black servant, Kwaque. During a stopover in San Francisco, Dag and Kwaque go to see a doctor for what they believe to be a tumor of the servant and the rheumatism of the master. Having recognized leprosy in both men, the doctor immediately calls the police and states, pointing to the servant: " 'I should say ... that it is the finest, ripest, perforating ulcer of the *bacillus leprae* order, that any San Francisco doctor has had the honour of presenting to the board of health.' 'Leprosy!' exclaimed Doctor Masters. *And all started at his pronouncement of the word* [italics added].* The sergeant and the two policemen shied away from Kwaque; Miss Judson, with a smothered cry, clapped her two hands over her heart; and Dag Daughtry,

---

*[Throughout the text, all material in brackets has been added by the translator.]

shocked but sceptical, demanded: 'What are you givin' us, Doc?' 'Stand still! Don't move!' Walter Merritt Emory said peremptorily to Daughtry. 'I want you to take notice,' he added to the others, as he gently touched the live-end of his fresh cigar to the area of dark skin above and between the steward's eyes . . . And while Daughtry waited . . . the coal of fire burned his skin and flesh, till the smoke of it was apparent to all, as was the smell of it." Dag does not flinch. "With a sharp laugh of triumph, Doctor Emory stepped back. 'Gentlemen, you have seen,' [he] said. 'Two undoubted cases of it . . . Take them away. I strongly advise . . . a thorough disinfection of the ambulance afterward.'" Dag tries in vain to protest but his fate, along with his servant's, is sealed: both of them will be confined in the "pest-house." "Already visioning a column in the evening papers, with scare-heads, in which he would appear the hero, the St. George of San Francisco standing with poised lance between the people and the dragon of leprosy," the doctor concludes: " [you would] *continue to be a menace to the public health wherever you are* [italics added] . .' 'Ready! March!' commanded the sergeant. The two policemen advanced on Daughtry and Kwaque with extended clubs. 'Keep away, an' keep movin','' one of the policemen growled fiercely. 'An' do what we say, or get your head cracked.'"[3]

Much closer to us, in 1938, in a book dominated by the ancient notion of fate, Georges Simenon shows us another and surely gentler way of excluding the leper: exclusion from knowing. Like all the other heroes of *La Mauvaise Étoile*, the one whom Simenon calls "the Alsatian" has separated himself from society and gone to the South Seas to look for a paradise that he can never find. His fate is leprosy, but when the author meets him, he does not know it. Everyone around him knows it, but no one wants to speak. Such a truth is useless or taboo. For "the Alsatian," being dead to the world is a gentle fate, but for a long time he is unaware of its double and ineluctable character:

> I knew another fellow in Tahiti whom I will call the Alsatian, for he is from a family of Alsatian industrialists . . . Like the others, he took a native companion, a beautiful girl with whom he lived for two years. One morning, a doctor on inspection tour noticed the Tahitian girl, examined her in private and took her away that very day. "She needs some care," he told the Alsatian. After a little while, the latter wanted to find out about her. "She is still in the hospital. We will give her back to you when she is cured." "Nothing serious, at least?" "Nothing . ." Months have gone by since then. I met the Tahitian girl when I visited the leprosarium, and her body and face were a beautiful blue from the treatment with blue spirits of methylene. "But what about him?" I asked. The doctor shook his head: "*I don't have the right to tell him. Professional secret!* And besides, what good would it do?" "What do you mean?" "In the first place, it is not sure that he is contaminated, even though he has lived with her for quite some time. Secondly, the disease is not likely

to come out for another twenty years . . . then it will still be time. All the Kanakas of the peninsula know the story, but not one of them would permit himself to trouble the peace of mind of this big blond boy in radiant health, whom one sees every morning, half-naked, striding down to the lagoon where he will swim after the bonitas. He has twenty years ahead of him, for sure . . . He is waiting for his little native companion to come back, and he probably wouldn't recognize her if he saw her, all steeped in blue . . . Just like he will be some day."[4]

The Inescapable Scourge and Its Victims

The plague seems different from leprosy in every way. Despite the scope of the scourge during the Middle Ages, leprosy always had the image of a disease that attacks an individual; the plague, by contrast, was seen from the very beginning as a collective scourge. The plague is thus the quintessential Epidemic. We think of *a* leper, but we think of *the* plague and *its victims*. Any description of the plague, and later of cholera, which shares the same characteristics, is first and foremost an enumeration of the *number of dead*. Samuel Pepys, the London gentleman, notes under 20 July in the diary he kept during the London plague of 1665: "Walked to Redriffe, where I hear the sickness is, and indeed is scattered almost every where, there dying 1089 of the plague this week." On 27 July: "At home met the weekly Bill, where above 100 encreased in the Bill; and of them, in all, about 1700 of the plague." On 10 August: "above 3000 of the plague." On 20 September: "The Duke showed us the number of the plague this week . . . ; that it is increased about 600 more than last week, which is quite contrary to our hopes and expectations, from the coldness of the late season. For the whole general number is 8297, and of them the plague 7165."[5]

In these accounts one also finds, superimposed on images of deserted places — closed doors and windows, empty streets, pervasive silence — images of overcrowding. At the time of the 1832 cholera, Chateaubriand recalls the 1720 plague of Marseilles: "In the neighborhood where all the inhabitants had perished they were immured in their homes as if to prevent death from coming out. From these avenues of great family tombs, one reached squares whose pavement was covered with the sick and the dying, lying on mattresses and abandoned without help. Half-rotted corpses lay amidst mud-soaked rags; others stood leaning against the walls in the position in which they had expired."[6]

The picture of the 1832 cholera is also one of numbers and huge crowds: masses of the sick arrive in search of medical help; corpses are piled up because of lack of transportation and coffins. To this was added the throng of spectators. In *Le Juif errant*, Eugène Sue tells of the beginnings of the cholera epidemic in Paris: "A rather large crowd which, as we said, obstructed the entrances to the Hôtel-Dieu, was crushed against the iron gate that surrounds the peristyle of the hospice . . . At every moment new victims were brought in on litters and stretchers."[7] And, further on: "The number of cholera victims arriving at the Hôtel-Dieu increased from minute to minute; and since the normal means of transport were no longer available when litters and stretchers ran out, the sick were carried in on men's arms."[8]

Here the social space is thrown into confusion by this overload of dead bodies. Time also is shattered. Leprosy slowly eats away the leper's body, but the plague acts with lightning speed. Its outbreak already is of that nature; only a few hours after the arrival of the galley bearing plague victims in October 1347, the first inhabitants of Messina were felled by the epidemic. The course of the disease itself follows the same pattern. As Boccaccio writes in the *Decameron*: "How many valiant men, beautiful women, and charming young boys, who might have been pronounced very healthy by Galen, Hippocrates, and Aesculapius (not to mention lesser physicians), ate breakfast in the morning with their relatives, companions, and friends, and then in the evening dined with their ancestors in the other world!"[9] And Samuel Pepys in 1665: "The town growing so unhealthy, that a man cannot depend upon living two days."[10] Daniel Defoe, for his part, tells the anecdote of a man of the people who, voluntarily it seems, went to take the plague to a middle-class family: "I have got the sickness and shall die tomorrow night," the intruder tells the family sitting around the supper table.[11] Eugène Sue depicts the swiftness of death itself: "For a few moments one had been hearing from far away in the winding streets of the Cité the deep and measured sound of several drums . . . emerging from the arcade, the drummers crossed the square in front of Notre-Dame. Suddenly one of these soldiers, a gray and whiskered veteran, slowed the deep roll of his drum and fell back a step; his comrades looked back in surprise . . . he was green, his legs gave way, he stammered a few unintelligible words and fell to the pavement as if struck by lightning before the drummers of the first rows had stopped beating their drums."[12]

In leprosy, finally, the sick person was excluded; the leper was socially dead, but by this very fact society was preserved. Society abolished the contact, decreed the rules, and thereby remained intact, indeed was strengthened by the new rituals. When the plague struck, there was no immediate possibility of excluding the victims, even if lazarettos and quarantines eventually had some effect. Once the plague had entered the place, it was too late, and flight was the only hope. The town was emptied of the living, first of all the rich and the powerful, along with all the representatives of authority. Society was threatening to collapse; all rules were abolished. The plague brought looting, wild drinking bouts, and rioting.

The plague had struck since antiquity. But at that time the term designated all epidemics with high mortality. It seems certain, for example, that the famous "plague of Athens" in 430 B.C., narrated by Thucydides, was not the [bubonic] plague. On the other hand, the so-called Justinian plague is considered fairly well identified. For Western Europe, the first Great Plague or Black Death was the outbreak that started in October 1347 at Messina, where it was brought by the passengers of twelve galleys arriving from the Crimean port of Kaffa. Like many other epidemics, the plague is related to great shifts of populations, sea voyages, and wars. The panic-stricken population of Messina fled and dispersed, spreading the evil by that very action. All of Italy was affected, Florence with particular severity. The plague had arrived in Europe and was to claim twenty-six million victims in this outbreak alone. It was to remain for four centuries.

It would be difficult to enumerate all the outbreaks, even for one country. In France, according to P. Hillemand and E. Gilbrin,[13] there were seventy-six between 1600 and 1786. It is known that there were periods of respite, such as the sixteenth century. It is also known—as Daniel Panzac has shown for Smyrna in the eighteenth century[14]—that certain episodes of the plague were relatively mild and claimed few victims. But we all remember the dates of the great plagues, which are also those that found their chroniclers: Boccaccio for Florence in 1348; Manzoni for Milan in 1629; the great plague of London in 1665, which Samuel Pepys recorded day by day in his diary and which Daniel Defoe was to reconstruct with great care in 1722, when the evil raged once again in Provence and threatened to attack England. In 1799 it was still found in Egypt, where it struck Bonaparte's expeditionary force, and in 1812 it was in the Crimea. Thereafter it disappeared from the Western world.

But then, around 1830, there came an outbreak of a disease originating in the Near East that strangely resembled the great epidemics of the past and gave rise to descriptions sounding the same themes. This was cholera. The cholera epidemic that broke out in Paris in March 1832 is as famous as the greatest plagues. Maxime Ducamp wrote:

> Cholera had devastated Russia and Poland, but there was no reason to believe that it would attack us when on 13 March there was a rumor that a porter of the rue des Lombards had been fatally struck. The physicians were still reluctant to state a definite opinion when, on the 26th, the deaths of four persons were reported in short order. They were the cook of Marshal Lobau in the rue Mazarine, a girl of ten in the Cité, a woman green-grocer near the Arsenal, and an egg seller in the former rue de la Mortellerie, today rue de l'Hôtel de Ville. On the 31st, thirty-five of the forty-eight sections that make up the city's subdivisions were affected; *on the day of 12 April 1200 persons came down with the disease, and 814 perished. On the 14th, 13000 were sick, and 7000 died.* Paris lost its head. *The inhabitants were panic-stricken; they ran away from themselves, all business came to a standstill, and one only meets people wearing mourning.*[15]

Throughout the nineteenth century, cholera was to strike again and again; in France there were outbreaks in 1832, 1849, 1854, 1865, and so forth.

Panic and Disorder

What was it like to live through the plague or another epidemic? We know little about the sick themselves, their despair, their suffering, their resignation, or their revolt. Suddenly struck down by a virulent ill, they had little time to keep the diary or "account book" that the historian Bartolomé Benassar would hope to find.[16] Furthermore, those around them had little interest in observing them or listening to them. It is true that Thucydides, Procopius, and Gregory of Tours have furnished precise descriptions of the symptoms of the plague. But during all these centuries when a certain insensitivity toward the weak creature that a sick person represented was the rule, victims of the plague, more than anyone, were rejected. In their terror, people simply tried to run away from them. Boccaccio eloquently makes this point: "This disaster had struck such fear into the hearts of men and women that brother abandoned brother, uncle abandoned nephew, sister left brother, and very often wife abandoned husband, and—even worse, almost unbelievable—fathers and mothers neglected to tend and care for their children as if they were not their own." He also says: "they always managed to avoid the sick as best they could."[17] The accounts of the plague thus often describe the state of the corpses but say little about the suffering and feelings of the dying.[18]

In the testimony of the survivors, fear and panic are therefore the dominant theme. This fear continued throughout the ages. Erckmann-Chatrian tell us that on the eve of the French Revolution the peasants of Alsace still prayed to God to preserve them from "plague, famine, and war."[19] The very word *plague* inspired terror. B. Benassar notes that in Spain, as the plague approached a city, people began to use euphemisms to designate it. Thus documents concerning the plague of 1599 at Valladolid speak of the plague when referring to Santander or San Sebastian but use the expression "contagious ill" when Valladolid itself is affected.[20] Equally revealing is the fact that the word *plague* was used as a generic term designating not only all epidemics but all calamities. For Bartolomé de Las Casas, who in 1552 described the massacre of the American Indians by their conquerors, the arrival of the Spanish is a plague: "The Christians wrought strange and astounding ravages among the Indians, killed a multitude of people and burnt many great lords alive. They perpetrated acts of abominable tyranny in the city of Mexico, in the nearby towns and throughout the whole region . . . then the *plague of tyranny advanced* and came to reach, contaminate, and devastate the very populous province of Panuco where stupendous ravages and massacres took place."[21]

Yet, as many testimonies show, this fear was not always and everywhere equally great. According to Michel Vovelle, it became more intense in the course of the centuries, as a new attitude toward death began to take shape. When death was no longer closely associated with God's will, it was "no longer accepted without a murmur."[22] But by the same token, it became all the more frightening. At all times, however, certain individuals seemed untouched by fear. In reading Samuel Pepys, for example, one is struck by the casualness, almost the indifference, with which he intersperses the enumeration of plague deaths with the description of his daily activities and pleasures: "Walked to Redriffe, where I hear the sickness is . . . there dying 1089 of the plague this week. My Lady Carteret did this day give me a bottle of plague-water home with me. I received yesterday a letter from my Lord Sandwich, giving me thanks for my care about their marriage business, and desiring it to be dispatched, that no disappointment may happen therein. Lord! to see how the plague spreads!" he reports on 26 September. On 30 September he even writes: "I do end this month with the greatest content, and may say that these last three months, for joy, health, and profit, have been much the greatest that ever I received all my life in any twelve months, having nothing upon me but the consideration of the sickliness of the season to mortify me."[23]

Pepys saw London emptying itself around him, but he was so busy making money and enjoying himself that he remained in town almost to the end. The sight of the dying and the dead saddened him less than the spectacle of the empty and silent city, where all activities had come to a standstill. Almost two centuries later, Martin Nadaud, a mason from the Creuse, equally absorbed in his work (in his case it was a matter of making a living and repaying the debts of his family), shows a similar fearlessness in the face of the cholera of 1832: "One day we were sent to the rue de la Huchette to work on some rooms. Were we ever surprised! The cholera was raging in that neighborhood, and soon there was talk of nothing else in Paris. In the house where we were working, three or four persons died. The whole neighborhood was panic-stricken . . . Finally we were a bit disconcerted ourselves; but like sailors threatened by a storm, we laughed and placed ourselves under the wings of God, who did protect us, for nothing happened to us."[24]

Many testimonies indicate that the rich were especially frightened and that they were the first to flee. Daniel Defoe states: "The richer sort of people, especially the nobility and gentry, thronged out of town with their families and servants."[25] They had the same reaction in the face of cholera. Marshal de Castellane wrote in his diary: "Anyone with more than 200,000 livres income is dreadfully frightened."[26] And Louis Blanc: "Most of the rich people fled, the deputies fled, the peers of France fled."[27] Ordinary people, by contrast, were at first incredulous. "The people shrugged their shoulders and sneered," the historian René Baehrel states in his analysis of the relations among social classes in times of epidemics. Chateaubriand and others relate how in 1832 people drank to the health of the cholera. "I have seen drunkards at the city line, sitting outside the door of the tavern drinking at a little wooden table, who, raising their glass, called out: 'To your health, *Morbus!*' *Morbus*, who appreciated this, came running, and they dropped dead under the table. Children played cholera, which they called *Nicholas Morbus* and *Morbus the Bad*."[28] These acts of derision culminated in the "Cholera Mascarades" described by Eugène Sue.

But derision is also a form of exorcism. One must tame one's fear and, when there is nothing else to do, play games with the evil, put up a fight for the space it wants to appropriate and snatch from it its victims, foremost among them the poor. For at all times it was the poor who died in the greatest numbers. Maxime Ducamp notes that the records kept by the public welfare authorities of Paris make it possible to trace the path taken by the cholera and to identify its victims with considerable precision. These records show without ambiguity that the poor were affected first and most frequently. Direct testimonies confirm this: "In the first week the cholera took its victims only among the poor," wrote Comte de Pontmartin.[29] This is a feature common to all epidemics. Charles de Mertens wrote about the Moscow plague of 1771: "Among these many dead I know of only three noblemen who were affected by the disease, very few solid bourgeois, and only 300 foreigners of the lowest category; all the rest were of the little people of Russia."[30]

No wonder, then, that derision and panic easily turned into anger. Plague and cholera, the people thought, are not natural; someone must have triggered them. In the Middle Ages, it was usually the Jews and sometimes the lepers who were suspected. Throughout the Black Death the epidemic was accompanied by rumors accusing the Jews of strange plots. Again and again there were outbreaks of violence in which the homes of Jews were ransacked and the suspects massacred. Such disturbances took place in Provence, Languedoc, Catalonia and Aragon, Franche-Comté, Savoy, Germany, Brabant, Silesia, Austria, and elsewhere.

In the nineteenth century, a period when class hatred was at its height, the animosity was turned against the rich and the physicians, who were also accused of poisoning the people. "More than once I was called a poisoner," a Paris physician recalled. Comte de Pontmartin reports that the people of Paris "accused the rich, both noble and bourgeois, not only of failing to die but of poisoning the poor . . . It came to the point, Oh what a wretched thing!, that we wished for the death of a rich person."[31]

On several occasions there were near-riots. In the nineteenth century, when the authorities had set up rules and organizations in an attempt to deal rationally with the scourge, rioting appears as the counterpart of the anomie, the looting, and the bacchanalia of the Middle Ages. The plague abolishes the rules. It also uncovers the true nature of social relations.

The Collective Defense of Society

It seems clear that even in antiquity humanity tried to defend itself. Against such a formidable enemy people simultaneously availed themselves of every means at their disposal. In the ancient world sacrifices to the gods went hand in hand with attempts at disinfection and the enforcement of public hygiene. When the plague reappeared in Europe in the fourteenth century, in a world where the Church and the Christian faith held a position of paramount importance, the disease was seen by everyone as a disaster visited upon humankind by the wrath of God. It was therefore obvious that masses, penitence, pilgrimages, offerings, and the invocation of protective saints such as Saint Roch and Saint Sebastian would afford the most powerful help. Even the physicians felt, and continued to feel for many centuries, as we hear from David Jouysse, a physician in Rouen in the seventeenth century, that medical treatment must "begin with the purification of our souls."[32] The processions and penitences culminated in the strange paroxism of the flagellants who for several years moved through Europe with the plague. "In the year of grace of Our Lord 1349 the penitents started on their way. They first came out of Germany. They were people who did public penance by flogging themselves with sticks studded with iron spikes," wrote Froissart.[33] The flagellants expected to regain the purity of baptism through their suffering and to be spared by the disease because they were without sin.

But piety and the recourse to God did not prevent people from engaging in the most outlandish superstitious practices and circulating the most pagan rumors. Daniel Defoe, for example, gives us a list of the amulets and talismans used by the population of London in 1665. He reports the advertisements of charlatans who peddled "an universal remedy against the plague," and "never-failing preservatives against the infection."[34] He also describes the dreams, predictions, and retrospective interpretations of various presages, in particular the comet that had appeared a few months earlier.[35]

Yet one notion gradually came to be accepted—more firmly, incidentally, by ordinary people than by the physicians—namely, that of contagion. A theory of contagion was offered in the fifteenth century by Fracastor, who thought that it operated "through particles that our senses cannot perceive."[36] Official medicine opposed this notion for a long time, but the people, for whom the term *contagion* was synonymous with plague, instinctively believed in it. In fact, it was this notion that gave rise to action. The struggle was to last for centuries. Dealing with this contagion, which could be felt even if its mechanisms were not understood, was a matter of recognizing the evil and isolating it. As early as 1377, Ragusa imposed a quarantine on visiting ships. Venice, then Marseilles, and eventually all ports took the same measure. Whereas the immediate reflex, that of flight, contributed to the dissemination of the scourge, it was discovered that what had to be done was not to send the healthy away but, on the contrary, to confine the sick and to cut off all contact with them. But first one had to know who they were. Over the centuries expert investigative procedures were developed and brought into action at the first sign of an epidemic. Thus, travelers were required to present a bill of health or *patente* stating that they were not bringing the infection before they were permitted to enter a city or a port. Then, when the plague had arrived, isolation was practiced. Houses where the disease had struck were closed, the sick and their families confined within; ships and all persons who had been in contact with a plague victim were placed under a quarantine; lazarettos were built.

One is immediately struck by the authoritarian character of these measures. In the fourteenth century already, certain Italian cities promulgated "plague regulations," which were later found throughout Europe. Everywhere towns created police authorities charged with enforcing the regulations, and by the fifteenth century the institution of health boards and health officers with dictatorial powers was very widespread. These authorities did not hesitate to mete out severe punishment to those who broke the rules. In many cases, incidentally, riots and revolts were sparked by these measures, which in the short run aggravated the suffering of the population. Daniel Defoe tells us how the confining of the sick and their families was experienced: "[There] were so many prisons in the town as there were houses shut up; and as the people shut up or imprisoned so were guilty of no crime, only shut up because miserable, it was really the more intolerable to them."[37] He cites many instances of sick people starving to death while they were locked up in their homes. He also describes the thousand stratagems by which the shut-ins managed to escape.

Defensive action was deployed from every angle. In addition to isolating the sick, steps were taken to count the victims, bring help to starving populations, the poor, the beggars, and the unemployed, to recruit specialized personnel such as policemen, guards, physicians, and apothecaries, not to forget the famous gravediggers [called *corbeaux*, or "crows," in French] who had to bury the dead. In trying to deal with the plague, Europe gradually developed a true global health policy, traces of which still exist in our present policies and institutions concerning public hygiene. J. N. Biraben also points out that this policy gradually assumed an international character. By the seventeenth century cities and states informed one another of a threat of plague. Indeed, the epidemic was defeated by the continent as a whole. At the end of the seventeenth century the plague was eradicated from Europe, and in the nineteenth century Turkey expelled it from the Mediterranean basin in a single year.

Today, however, certain historians doubt the effectiveness of the hygienic measures in which they had believed for so long. They now think that the disappearance of the plague from Europe in the seventeenth century must be attributed to the complex system of equilibrium among humans, animals, and bacteria; in this case to an antagonism between the plague bacillus and other microorganisms, compounded by an acquired immunity of the animal vector, the rat.[38] But whatever the objective effectiveness of the defensive measures, they have served to change the representations of the disease, and the plague is no longer one of the symbols of human helplessness. In the nineteenth century cholera was to give new life to the theme of the epidemic, but this episode marked the end of the *Ancien Régime of Disease*: resignation gave way to action.

Recurrent Fevers

But at all times epidemic disease has found other forms besides leprosy, plague, or cholera with which to oppress an impotent and fragile humankind. Even the most cursory look at the past shows us the omnipresence, the itineraries, and the sudden explosions — often striking in conjunction with the development of trade routes, with voyages and wars — of what was then called *the fevers*. They were originally perceived as a single disease entity — for a long time the term *plague* indiscriminately designated all epidemics — but gradually medical investigation learned to distinguish among them. Thus smallpox, which was already present in the Roman Empire, received its name and was described by Gregory of Tours in the sixth century. Influenza also had existed in antiquity, for Hippocrates mentions it in the *Book of Epidemics*. Syphilis, by contrast, which was given its name by Fracastor in 1530, was not known, at least in its present form, until it appeared on the battlefields of the late fifteenth century, to be precise at the siege of Naples by Charles VIII in 1494. It was therefore called the "Neapolitan Disease" by the French and the "French Disease" by the Italians, but everyone agreed that it was a new scourge,[39] for it was believed to have been brought back from America by Christopher Columbus's sailors and spread throughout Europe by the Spanish mercenaries who served in the various warring armies. The German physician Joseph Grümpeck described it as early as 1496; in a second work, published in 1501, he explained that he himself had contracted the dread disease: "In the last years," he writes in his preface, "I have seen new scourges, horrible diseases, and a great many infirmities attacking the human race from every corner of the world. Among them there slipped over from the western shores of Gaul a disease more cruel, grievous, and foul than anything the world had ever seen before." He then describes his own lesion: "The first poisoned arrow of the hideous ill hit me in the Priapic gland, which as a result of that wound became so swollen that two hands would barely have fit around it."[40]

While certain diseases appeared, others disappeared. Thus we have now forgotten the English sweating sickness, which completely regressed in the sixteenth century. Yet at the siege of Saint-Jean de l'Acre in 1191 this epidemic raged and struck down both Richard the Lion-Hearted and Philip Augustus,

As for syphilis, it may have played a role in the decline of certain dynasties, such as the Valois at the end of the sixteenth century.[49] But there can be little doubt that infectious diseases have most profoundly and most intimately affected the course of history by causing sudden shifts in the demographic equilibrium that could be as devastating as those brought about by the great plagues. In his study of Anjou, François Lebrun analyzes those sinister steeples that tragically punctuate the curves of burials.[50] A variety of infectious diseases—epidemics of typhus, influenza, smallpox, dysentery, paludism—periodically caused a terrifying excess of deaths in a context where global mortality was very high to begin with. In 1707 in Anjou, dysentery claimed 15,000 lives. And as late as 1830 in Berlin influenza still killed as many people as cholera. Mortality was even higher among the poor because epidemics almost always came in conjunction with famine, and young children were always the most seriously affected. Of 410 children born at Challain in Anjou between 1671 and 1698, 73 died within one month, 144 before the age of one, and 218 before the age of twenty.[51] More generally, in this demography of the *Ancien Régime*, levels of infant mortality (before the age of one) of 20–30 percent do not seem exceptional and were to decline significantly only at the end of the nineteenth century, especially among the poor.[52]

This, then, was still the traditional configuration of disease: it was the epidemic, the curse that suddenly befalls a collectivity, disrupting and decimating it. It is therefore not surprising that in extreme cases one finds in the writings of eyewitnesses the classic images from the days of the plague, especially those of sick bodies invading the social space. In 1707 at Challain in Anjou, many dysentery sufferers "are lying along the haystacks, screaming with pain like raving madmen."[53] One also finds the very same terror, the flight, and the breakdown of social ties and moral restraints. It is striking indeed to read in the testimony about the dysentery epidemic in Anjou by the parish priest Maussion a statement that might have been penned by Boccaccio about the plague: "It was a dreadful thing to see the parishioners so distressed that fathers abandoned their children, children their fathers; and almost everyone fled because the disease was so dangerous."[54]

We now know from the work of several historians[55] how the practices and attitudes concerning death have evolved in our Western societies. They have shown us that we have moved from familiarity and resignation in the face of death as a spectacle—that of a soul about to meet its Creator—to the concealment of an event that has become unbearable in a society whose demography has been transformed.

As we have seen, the panic created by the epidemic—which immediately threatened everyone—periodically broke this resignation. Little by little, however, panic loosened its grip and fewer people took flight. As the role of religious practices and superstitions, which had often been closely associated, was reduced, as for example in the plague, a system of defenses was put into place. The disease now became a natural phenomenon that one could try to combat by means of hygiene, isolation, and the distribution of food and remedies. Lebrun places this turning point, for western France, at the second half of the eighteenth century.

A hundred years later, Pasteur's discoveries opened an entirely new perspective. Between 1878 and 1905, the discovery of the nature of the germs responsible for the principal infectious diseases transformed people's attitudes toward illness. In actual fact, therapeutics did not immediately achieve the expected results, and the decline of the infectious diseases owed as much to a rise in the standard of living as to medicine. But thanks to some spectacular successes, there was now hope that infectious disease could be defeated, and this hope henceforth became part of the practice of medicine. It created a combative attitude toward physical ills that was not to be discouraged by even the most daunting obstacles. Robert Debré, for example, reports in his memoirs his mother's memories of a group of Russian peasants in the throes of rabies. These "men of gigantic stature, wearing huge fur hats on their bearded and unkempt heads" had come from the fringes of Europe to ask Pasteur for help.[56] In 1980, shortly before his death, Maurice Genevoix told the story of his uncle, a country doctor, who as early as 1894 did not hesitate to use Dr. Roux's serum, discovered that same year, to save him, Genevoix, from diphtheria.[57] Yet, contrasting with this new activism, one can still find in texts of the early twentieth century the persistence of a resignation that is barely tinged with indignation, especially when it comes to child mortality among the poor. In *La Maternelle* by Léon Frapié, the narrator, a young woman of middle-class origin who works as a volunteer in a school at Ménilmontant [a poor section of Paris], evokes the epidemics that still struck every year without fail and thinned out the ranks of the school children:

> During recess the school physician and the delegate of the canton had a long conversation with the headmistress. I overheard that they were worried about the inevitable epidemics favored by the change of seasons. "Do you remember how last year we had a great many cases of mumps, scarlet fever, and smallpox?" The headmistress, who was very fond of her small charges, smiled sadly: "Yes, and after the month of April there are empty spaces, like after a war—we have lots of names that have to be crossed out . . . and then the municipality sends new forms, and the gaps are closed."[58]

The Illness That Disfigures

All of these diseases were murderous and thereby terrifying, yet it seems to us that one of them had a special place in the collective feelings, where it was the focal point of intense fear and particular horror. This was smallpox. Its high incidence is well known. In April 1754 La Condamine wrote in his memoir to the Académie des Sciences: "Of one hundred persons who have survived the dangers of early childhood, 13 or 14 are killed by this disease and an equal number will carry its grievous marks for the rest of their lives. Here then, out of every 100 persons, are 26 or 28 witnesses to prove that this scourge destroys or degrades a fourth of humanity."[59] To be sure, it was possible to survive smallpox; Chateaubriand's detached statement about his own case is there to prove it. In September 1792, when he was fighting against the revolutionary armies, he was wounded at the siege of Thionville: "I was racked with fever," he writes, "and could barely stand up on my swollen thigh. Then I felt myself being seized by another ill. After 24 hours of vomiting, my face and body were covered with a rash that turned out to be a case of confluent smallpox; the rash came and went with the changing effects of the air."[60]

Despite his illness, Chateaubriand wanted to go to Jersey, from where he would be able to join the royalists in Brittany. Having traveled as far as Brussels, he saw a physician: "The doctor could not get over his astonishment: he considered this case of smallpox that came and went without killing me and without reaching a natural crisis a phenomenon without precedent in medicine."[61] Chateaubriand did reach Jersey, where he collapsed from exhaustion:

> For four months I hovered between life and death. My uncle, his wife, his son, and his three daughters took turns at my bedside. I occupied an apartment in one of the houses that had recently been built along the port; the windows of my room reached all the way to the floor, and I could see the sea from my bed. The physician, Dr. Delattre, had forbidden everyone to speak to me about serious things, especially politics. In the last days of 1793 my uncle entered my room clad in deep mourning. I trembled at the sight, thinking that we had lost someone in the family, but the news he broke to me was the death of Louis XVI.

The writer continues:

> I was beginning to leave my bed; the smallpox had passed, but I had a chest complaint and a general weakness that stayed with me for a long time.[62]

But the laconic attitude of Chateaubriand, who was more concerned about the fate of the royal family than about his own illness, was rare. Usually smallpox gave rise to sheer terror. For it not only killed, it disfigured. History is full of these pockmarked figures who, like Danton or Mirabeau, bore the stigmata of the ill. Balzac, in *Le Curé de village*, vividly portrays the intense anxiety felt by the parents of Véronique Sauviat, who contracted the disease at the age of eleven. She was not to die, but her beauty would be destroyed.

During the two months when their daughter was in danger, the whole neigh-borhood became aware of the Sauviats' tender love for her. Sauviat no longer went to the sales; he stayed in his shop all the time, went up to his daughter's room every few minutes and kept watch by her bedside all night long, together with his wife. His silent grief seemed so deep that no one dared to speak to him; the neighbors looked on with compassion and only asked Sister Marthe for news about Véronique. During the days when the danger was at its height, the neighbors saw, this once in Sauviat's life, tears stream-ing from his eyes and running down his hollow cheeks; he did not wipe them away and remained as if stunned for hours on end, not daring to go up to his daughter's room and looking about without seeing: One could have robbed him then and there. Véronique was saved, but her beauty was gone.[63]

Despite periods of quiescence, smallpox still represented a considerable dan-ger in nineteenth-century France. In 1872, at a time that incidentally brought a flare-up of the disease, little Marie Bashkirtseff, then ten years old, noted in her diary a prayer that she said every night: "Dear God, make that I will never have smallpox, that I will be pretty, that I will have a beautiful voice, that I will be happily married, and that Mother will live for a long time."[64] Marie's first wish was to be granted: she never had smallpox, but she died young of tuberculosis.

But it is perhaps a late nineteenth-century novel by Erckmann-Chatrian which, though not a first-hand experience, most fully conveys the terror spread by the disease. Evoking the early days of inoculation in Alsace at the very end of the eighteenth century, the authors write: "You cannot understand the mag-nitude of this blessing unless you have an idea of the ravages wrought by small-pox before 1798. It was horrible! This disease could break out in one village, then in another; it spread like fire and everyone, especially fathers and mothers, would quake with fright. They said: 'It is here . . . It is coming . . . So many people have had it . . . this woman . . . that girl, have had a particularly bad case. So-and-so has lost his sight in one eye . . . another is unrecognizable . . . So many dead, so many deaf, so many blind. Oh, what fright!' "[65]

Despite their fear, people were hesitant to accept inoculation. After all, to let oneself be inoculated was to expose oneself deliberately to the disease, and bring it into one's body, whereas the traditional therapeutics—one only has to think of bleeding and leeches—were designed to remove it. One understands the Alsatian peasants:

"Where do you have this 'cowpox?' " Chauvel asked. "Here it is, in my bag." And right away the doctor showed us some still fresh vaccine in a little vial. We stood there as if stunned. The people in the shop, bending down around us, looked on in amazement. We went into the library with these strangers. The two other men were also doctors. They told us how the blisters come out, open, and dry up, that all this caused only a little fever, and that the children whom they had already vaccinated in their own families were very well; they said that for them everything had gone as Jenner, the English doctor, had said it would go. But despite that neither Marguerite nor I would have dared keep our promise to Dr. Schwan, if old man Chauvel had not exclaimed: "That's good enough for me. If you, Schwan, and these two gentlemen have tried it out, I have full confidence. Let's try it out on our own. What do you say?" The narrator still hesitates and wants to wait. "But Chauvel says: 'No, nothing could be worse than smallpox.' "[66]

In fact, inoculation had long been known in the Near East, and was introduced in England as early as 1721 by Lady Montagu after her return from Constantinople.[67] It then came to France, where the first inoculation was performed by Tenon in 1755. But despite some undeniable successes, criticism arose from many quarters. The Church, in particular, was opposed to inoculation. Even after 1796, when Jenner had developed the first vaccine made from cowpox, the opposition persisted, and society remained divided on this issue. However, the last decades of the nineteenth century brought a general change in attitude. Here again, there was a growing confidence that the evil could be eradicated. But in France this confidence developed later than in the other European countries; smallpox vaccination became compulsory only with the Public Health Law of 1902.

Throughout the centuries dominated by epidemic disease we see great numbers of the dying and the dead, but it is not certain that we already perceive those who today are called "the sick." An epidemic was the prelude to collective dying, the wages of sin, the trigger of social disorder; but it was not, as illness has become in our own time, the foundation of a special way of life and of social integration.

To be sure, there were other illnesses than epidemics. These were individual conditions of which one did not die and with which one had to live. The kidney stones of which Montaigne tells us so much in his *Essais* are a good example. One must also keep in mind that at that time most of humanity was beset by one kind or another of debilitating and crippling infirmity, as is indicated by the importance of pilgrimages to which the infirm flocked in great numbers. But these ills and ailments did not match the importance of epidemic disease and did not structure the image of "being sick." They delineated the figure of the "sufferer," which was consubstantial with the human condition, but they did not create a specific "status." It has even been said that until the end of the seventeenth century medicine was much more concerned with the suffering individual than it was to be after the advent of clinical medicine. Until Sydenham at least, the conception of illness tended to the particular, for it assumed an indissoluble link between the sufferer and his illness. But this presence of the "sick man" in the medical cosmology did not necessarily lead to the structuring of what we today call the "status" of being sick.[68] The appearance of today's "sick person" seems predicated on at least three conditions: first, disease must cease to be a mass phenomenon; second, illness must not be followed inevitably by death, so that it can be a form of life as well as of death; and third, it is probably also necessary that the diversity of suffering be reduced by a unifying general view, which is precisely that of clinical medicine. At that point the diversity of bodily ills will give birth to a common condition and a shared identity: that of the sick person.

2·

From Consumption to Tuberculosis

*A*fter the era of the great epidemics, another disease became, for more than a century, the embodiment of illness and gave rise to new representations. This was tuberculosis, above all pulmonary consumption. Long the focal point of unbounded public anxiety, consumption became for several decades the primary preoccupation of the medical profession. In the *Grand Larousse du XIXe Siècle* one can read: "Never at any time in history has a subject preoccupied the medical world to the same extent or produced in such short order so many studies, experiments, and discussions. It is true that this is the most widespread disease and that it claims the greatest number of victims."

The Romantic Illness

In the early nineteenth century, when the disease reached its epidemiological high point, first in England and a few decades later in France and on the rest of the Continent, the collective imagination seized on tuberculosis to elaborate a concept of illness that was of one piece with the dominant notions of Romanticism. To be sure, ancient Greek, Roman, and Asian texts show the previous existence of tuberculosis. Traces of the disease have also been identified in prehistoric skeletons, for example in a set of vertebrae marked by Pott's disease. Nonetheless, the nineteenth century was indeed the age of consumption.[1] In England rather precise statistics were kept from the 1850s onward; in France, this was not the case until the end of the century, but it is known that at the time of Laennec—that is, during the first quarter of the century—tuberculosis was responsible for 20 percent of all deaths. Around 1850, existing statistics show considerable death rates from tuberculosis in the great cities.[2]

Consumption was considered an inherited disease at the time; it was especially liable to befall the rich, the young, women, and the fragile beings consumed by "the passion of sadness" of whom Laennec speaks.[3] It was an ailment that was one with an inability to face life, with an existential trauma. The illness was but the expression of the deepest truth of the consumptive, a being "apart," threatened but all the more precious for it. Such beings were celebrated for their ethereal beauty, all slenderness, pallor, and transparency.[4] But they were also fascinating for the passion that devoured them. This passion expressed itself in amorous ardor and also in artistic sensitivity, in the love of beauty, and in creativity. Throughout the century a special relationship was assumed to exist between tuberculosis and art, tuberculosis and literary creation. Fever and consumption were thus seen as only the physical signs of an inner fire, whether it be of desire or of genius, which made the sufferer's pallor glow. The shining eyes, their "glow that matches the pink cheeks," as Thomas Mann has put it, came from the fire of a soul that was destroying itself: the consumptives "burned up their days."

They burned them, at least if they were rich, in comfortable circumstances. For them, tuberculosis was also a way of life full of luxury and leisure. It was an illness in which there was "much sweetness," as Kafka wrote to Milena around 1920.[5] In the bourgeois milieus of the early nineteenth century, the illness was for the most part experienced in the bosom of the family, enclosed in the intimacy of the bedroom and kept secret by a family that wanted to keep open the possibility of an advantageous marriage. But at the same time another, contrapunctual utopia began to take shape, namely the belief that travel would bring salvation. The journey to the south was in appearance the apotheosis of life and adventure, yet everyone knew that it was the privilege of the condemned. Later the illness moved into its own space, the sanatorium. The first of these were created in Silesia between 1854 and 1859, and in 1924 Thomas Mann described their unsurpassed archetype in the Berghof of the *Magic Mountain*.[6] Here the wealthy patient led a life filled with pleasures and refinement. In this place Death—as well as the distressing material aspects of illness, such as the spittoon—was both omnipresent and concealed. The inmates played the game of life and health, but even while doing so proclaimed it an illusion. They were excluded from the world, yet the "magnetism of the world of the sanatorium"[7] made them believe that theirs was the real world, and that they themselves had chosen to stay "up here."

The existence of this world apart, of this different way of life that shaped the image of the consumptive to such a great extent, is related to medical history in the narrow sense. The history of tuberculosis is marked by the work of illustrious physicians from Fracastor, Bayle, and Delsaut to Laennec, Villemin, Koch, and Calmette. These scientists provided increasingly exact descriptions of the disease and progressively refined the understanding of its etiology. Their work culminated with the discovery of Koch's bacillus in 1882, but therapeutic measures were not developed until much later. Long into the twentieth century, diet and hygiene, "fresh air," and the sanatorium remained the essential weapons against tuberculosis. Eventually, gold salts and the pneumothorax were added.[8] These weapons were of limited effectiveness. It was only in the 1950s, when specific antibiotics were developed, that the mortality curves were definitively "broken."[9] A. Boudard tells us that as late as 1952 streptomycin prolonged the life of all tuberculosis patients, but that the most serious cases could not be cured. In certain hospital wards one still found "all those left over from before strepto, patients already too far gone who still hung on, were kept alive, but could not really go any further."[10]

Yet in the course of the nineteenth century, even before the discovery of Koch's bacillus and before the development of any effective medical or hygienic measures, the disease had spontaneously begun to regress.[11]

However, the contemporaries were unaware of this fact. "Half of Western Europe has more or less defective lungs," Kafka stated, for example.[12] And indeed it was in the very early twentieth century, no doubt because the importance of the other infectious diseases and their impact on mortality had begun to wane, that the terror of tuberculosis was at its height. It was also at that time that the notion of this disease as a "social scourge" began to counteract the Romantic vision and that society "declared war" on tuberculosis.[13]

The Proletarian as Spreader of Germs

This war had its "campaigns," its weapons, propaganda, reconnaissance missions, and troops, namely the members of the antituberculosis societies. Above all, it had its enemies, not only the omnipresent Koch's bacillus—"that invisible monster, more dangerous than wolves, tigers, and lions"[14]—but also those who had just been found to be the germ carriers *par excellence*—the proletarians. What had happened was that irrefutable empiric evidence had shattered previous convictions: tuberculosis was not, as had been believed, an illness of the rich; it was above all—and precise statistics were now available to prove it—a disease of the working class. The question of how to deal with the evil of poor people and slums now took its place beside that of how to understand the inner self-destruction of the bourgeois and the artist.

But the preventive measures put into practice were of a moral and social as well as a medical nature. The identification of the sick, the razing of slums, and the efforts at inculcating habits of personal hygiene amounted to a vast campaign for the control and moralization of the lower classes, which, over the last half-century, had come to be considered dangerous both for their epidemics and their revolutions. The recent bacteriological discoveries gave a new content to these already well-established ideas. The danger had acquired a new auxiliary, the germ, and a new mode of action, contagion. But both of these were treated as social and not only biological realities. The microbes, after all, developed in dank and airless slums, but it was also thought that they were spawned by the detestable habits of the lower classes. Lack of hygiene was seen as one aspect of the deterioration of the "people." The writings of the period, whether they were administrative reports or medical treatises, unanimously condemned the way of life of the working class, which was criticized above all for its negligence of hygiene, but also for its indifference or passivity in the face of the terrible disease. "While the populace becomes very agitated as soon as there is talk of a single case of diphtheria or smallpox, it remains undisturbed about tuberculosis; people seem to have become accustomed to it, and although everyone recognizes and fears it, that is the end of it for most of them," one reads in a report produced by the Prefecture of the Seine.[15]

There were also many censorious accounts that depicted tuberculosis among the lower classes as caused or aggravated by alcohol. These can be found even in popular novels. In *Les Deux Gosses*, the poor fortuneteller, Rose Fouilloux, is consumptive, but she aggravates her illness with cognac and absinthe. On the occasion of a medical examination she becomes aware of the seriousness of her condition. "She admitted to herself that until that tragic instant when she had seemed to read her sentence in the book of destiny she had deluded herself, wanting to close her eyes to the light."[16] This new lucidity prompts her resolution to stop drinking. But that lasts only a few moments: "The expression on Rose Fouilloux's face changed; she lapsed back into the most dreadful despair . . . Her good intentions melted away. There in the cupboard was the fiery liquor that would warm her. Once again her suffering would be dulled, she would forget. She greedily seized the cognac bottle and set it to her lips, not even taking the time to find a glass."[17]

To these attacks on the working class some physicians and syndicalists, seconded by a number of investigative reporters, responded in different terms. They pointed out that the lack of hygiene, the slums, and the alcohol must be incriminated much less than insufficient wages and excessive working hours. Tuberculosis, they said, is a working-class disease mainly because it is caused by misery and overwork. Before these professionals, Victor Hugo in *Les Misérables* had already in 1862 depicted the progression of Fantine's illness in these terms: "Fantine was worn out by overwork," he tells us, "and the little dry cough she had became worse."[18] And, further on: "Her eyes shone very brightly, and she felt a pain in her shoulder around the left shoulder blade; she coughed a great deal . . . she was sewing seventeen hours a day."[19]

Forty years later the argument that misery and physical exhaustion from overwork are responsible for tuberculosis was explicitly developed to refute the spokesmen of the official epidemiology, especially those who blamed the disease on unhealthy conditions conceived in purely physical terms.[20] On the basis of a series of investigations on "the economic and moral condition of male and female factory workers" carried out in 1902, the Bonneff brothers wrote: "The four causes of tuberculosis that we have discovered among the working class at Lille are therefore the following: (1) physical overexertion, (2) inadequate diet, (3) and (4) unhealthy living and working conditions. No other cause needs to be added, not even alcoholism, which has been found in only 17 percent of the tubercular workers."[21] In reporting the words of a Lille textile worker's wife, the authors write: "It is a singularly distressing impression to see this young and still vigorous creature destined to meet a prompt death as surely as a condemned prisoner on the eve of his execution. 'To what do you attribute your illness?' 'To misery. I have worked since I was very little. I was a tulle worker at Calais. Since my marriage I have never eaten my fill.' And then this word, said without any irony: 'By God, if you earn 2 francs 50 a day and if you have eight to feed, you have to cut down if you are to make it.' "[22]

Fernand Pelloutier affirmed the same thing: "Tuberculosis is the most fatal enemy of the working class, which falls victim to this disease in proportion not only to the unhealthful nature of its work, but also to the inadequacy of its wages and the length of the working day."[23] Even more clearly he made a distinction between unhealthy living conditions and misery in discussing the respective mortality patterns in the neighborhood of the Temple and at Ménilmontant: "The neighborhood of the Temple, one of the unhealthiest areas of the center of Paris, is occupied both by rich merchants who have their homes there and by large numbers of workers who come down every day from the very healthful heights of Ménilmontant. And yet, where does one find the highest death rates? Around the Temple? No indeed, but at Ménilmontant. What can be the reason for this but that in one place good food and sufficient rest overcome the insalubrious surroundings, while in the other the purity of the air is powerless to counteract the effect of incredible deprivations."[24]

In the course of the nineteenth century, tuberculosis thus became bound up in two successive chains of signifiers: passion, the idleness and the luxury of the sanatorium, and a pleasure-filled life "apart" on the one hand; the bacillus, the dank and airless slum, and exhaustion leading to an atrocious agony on the other. The disease therefore gave rise to a twofold discourse that both celebrated the consumptive and stigmatized the germ-carrier.

But beyond the duality of the theme of tuberculosis, one is struck by the number, the diversity, and the prolixity of the writings that attempted to elucidate its deepest nature. The end of the century in particular saw the deployment of an immense discourse concerning not only tuberculosis but also syphilis, alcoholism, neurosis, and madness—indeed the entire complex of illness and life. This discourse testifies to a new way of looking at this complex, for illness and life were removed from the realm of moral and religious interpretation and inserted into that of science. Henceforth one had to look to science to explain the world. Illness and the body were the principal subject matter of science; they were now made to carry significations central to society as a whole. They constituted both the origin and the points of application of two notions crucial to the ideology of the time: one of these was "degeneracy," the investigation of the individual and his or her lineage; the other was the "social scourge," the investigation of social relations and their determinants.

From this perspective it is striking to note, for example, the predilection of the naturalist writers for "clinical" descriptions of illnesses and neuroses and their attraction to the body of knowledge held by the physicians. Flaubert, the Goncourt brothers, and Zola used to follow the rounds at the hospital.[25] Léon Daudet[26] and others had many conversations with such celebrated physicians as Charcot. The Goncourt brothers, for example, asked Dr. Robin for a description of consumption and its physical and moral effects before writing *Madame Gervaisais*. All of them diligently read medical textbooks and dictionaries. It should be added that for this reason their descriptions, being totally impregnated by the learned discourse, are of little use to those who seek to re-create the vision of the lay person and the experience of the sick. For instance, the famous description of Coupeau's *delirium tremens* at the end of *L'Assomoir* is, by the author's own admission, "the verbatim reproduction of an observation made by the head of St. Anne's clinic."[27] Most importantly, these writers' works are evidence for a conception in which illness—more perhaps than any other phenomenon—*signifies*. Until then, particularly in the face of the great epidemics, human beings had sought, as Pascal expressed it, "to put it to good use." Now it had become a matter of making it say something. The naturalist writers, to be sure, had the ambition to express a clinical reality clearly and precisely. The writers wanted to share in the scientist's work.[28] Nonetheless their entirely positivist description of illness is always also a vision of something else. Zola's novels, for example, treat the interaction between heredity and social conditions, while in J.-K. Huysman's *A rebours*, reality, art, and the fantastic can stand for one another. These are examples of what Susan Sontag calls the use of illness as "metaphor." Its most accomplished example was to be the use of tuberculosis in Thomas Mann's *Magic Mountain*.

The Emergence of the Sick Person

In this new configuration of illness, a figure that we were until now unable to perceive clearly stands out: the sick person. It is our hypothesis that in the nineteenth century, and particularly with the advent of tuberculosis, the figure of the sick person crystallized existentially and socially, assuming its modern form. This figure emerged as an individual with his or her concrete experience yet also, and by the same token, as a social phenomenon. Henceforth the sick person was to be defined by his or her place in society.

One can give several reasons for this development. At the end of the eighteenth and in the nineteenth century illness, as Michel Foucault has said, "became detached from the metaphysics of evil of which it had been part for centuries."[29] It now took the form of bodily states that could be "read" by science. One might be tempted to believe that such an objectification in the body is incompatible with the emergence of the sick person. But clinical medicine spelled the definitive end of both the religious and the individualizing conception of illness. Now that the symptoms became the means of determining the nature of the illness, they ceased to be the expression of an indissoluble and specific link between the sufferer and his illness. The "sick man" seemed to disappear from the medical cosmology as the clinical discourse began to take shape.[30] Nonetheless this new rationality, by diminishing the multiplicity of symptoms, provided the basis for the appearance of a homogeneous status that could arise from all kinds of failures of the body. However great the diversity of illnesses, they all refer to a fixed place in society and to a shared identity. Indeed, it is quite likely that the figure of the sick person could only take shape once the bewildering variety of illnesses had been reduced. In this development the specific characteristics of tuberculosis also played a role. For even though tuberculosis was a mass killer it did not, unlike the great epidemics, submerge its victims in a sudden and collective death. One died individually and rather slowly of tuberculosis, so that the victim was in a position to perceive his condition, to form a self-image, and to discern the way in which others saw him. First of all, the long-term nature of the disease gave the sufferer time to elaborate a vision of himself and his illness, but only if his condition was serious, for there is little need to seek the meaning of something that can be quickly and easily taken care of. For a very long time, however, this was not the case with tuberculosis, and the need to find a meaning could usually express itself over a span of several years. This need is clearly visible in the many intimate diaries where we hear the voices of the sick themselves and can read the evolution of their attitude toward their illness.

Above all, its very duration made this illness a form of life before becoming a form of death.[31] "Treatments," journeys, and stays in the sanatorium, which for so long constituted the only therapy for tuberculosis, gave a specific status to the sick: being sick was more than an existential state, it was also defined by a way of life and a special place in society. One might be tempted to see this as no more than a new form of the traditional exclusion, comparable to that of lepers and plague victims, to which indeed it harks back. Yet it was different, for the condition of the sick was no longer characterized by a radical cutting-off and no longer simply a matter of confinement that made the disease and its victims disappear from view. In the sanatorium the tubercular patients received visits and were permitted to leave. Unlike confinement in a leper colony, for example, a stay in the sanatorium did not spell "death to the world" but, rather, access to a "world unto itself" that had its own existence and indeed a fascinating attraction. The sick had "their own world" and were beginning to be perceived as a separate group.

It is precisely this specific condition, albeit perceived in different ways, that was the common ground of the antithetical discourse of the Romantic ill and the "social scourge." We can now see how each of these strands both continued and broke with the earlier set of themes. In the early nineteenth century the vision of tuberculosis focused on the Romantic hero, for the illness had entirely engulfed him and he expressed himself through it. This vision harked back to the old individualizing conception of illness that was about to disappear, but it also paved the way for the practice of modern pathology, which deals in disease entities affecting isolated individuals. And when patients were assembled in treatment centers, the notion of a "world of the sick" also began to emerge. In the discussions of tuberculosis among the lower classes — that "social scourge" — on the other hand, the main emphasis was placed from the outset on the number of poor people affected and on the scope of the damage inflicted on the social space, such as lower-class neighborhoods and factories, as well as on the identification of groups and places that were labeled dangerous and should therefore be eliminated.[32] Through this theme the "social scourge" is related to the epidemic of earlier days. But here again, a shift took place. The writings about the great epidemics showed us towns thrown into utter confusion, crowds, and corpses; in those about tuberculosis we see places for living and working and families inserted into social and therapeutic networks.

Yet these two sets of signifiers, far from being opposites, are but the two faces of a new reality, that is, illness in the modern sense. Moreover, along with the vision of Romantic suffering and the concept of the social scourge, one can also discern a break between two ways of practicing medicine and two types of doctor-patient relationship. The Romantic tuberculosis still reflects the individualizing, even "patron-client" relationship between a wealthy patient and a physician who is unsure both of his science and his social status. Their relationship is not predicated on curing the illness, but on negotiating an acceptable image of it and on working out a way of life that will satisfy the precious and condemned patient. A few decades later, when tuberculosis was seen as a social scourge, the physician appeared as a professional who, assured of his knowledge and of his social status, dealt with large numbers of socially inferior patients whom he faced with a scientifically worded diagnosis and etiology and to whom he dictated, on the strength of the new authority of science, appropriate forms of conduct.[33] New notions of *illness,* *the sick*, and *the physician* were thus formed in correlation with one another.

But there is one more set of questions: were the sick themselves aware of the emergence of what we now call their status? And, in a larger sense, how did they experience tuberculosis at a time when its incidence was so widespread? How indeed did those who had the disease feel about the multifaceted discourse that claimed to set forth the deepest truth about their condition? To what extent did this discourse shape the consciousness of the individual? Did the sick actually experience and perceive their illness in terms of these words and images?

The answer is not simple, for whereas an abundance of texts, such as letters and diaries, is available for the middle class, especially writers and artists, we have nothing for the proletarians. Traces of their situation can only be found in the views of physicians and bourgeois who constantly incriminate the negligence of the poor, their unconcern in the face of the dread disease. A passage in *La Maternelle* by Léon Frapié shows an example of this unconcern. "In fact," says a housewife in the neighborhood of Ménilmontant, "I have only one lung left . . . I have earned my living, I'm not complaining. *Everybody can't have two lungs, right?* I just want to tell you that kids today are really lucky . . . Take mine, now; the doctor claims that *he has a touch of tuberculosis.* Well, never mind, if that's true, he won't have to go into the army; at least he'll be ahead by that much."[34] But the book's context sheds light on this attitude and on the perception that informs it: disease is only one of the many ills that threaten the survival of the lower classes, indeed it is practically indistinguishable from poverty and from the exploitation that has spawned it.

This is the context that permits us to understand the resistance and the outright refusal to comply to which public health measures gave rise in the working class.[35] Poor people refused the unsolicited visits of public health nurses; they objected to the placing of their children in institutions; they left the sanatorium prematurely and even staged embryonic revolts.[36] All of this shows that to the poor, preventive measures against tuberculosis, especially the lower-class sanatoria, were but another form of regimentation, as ineffectual as it was dismal. They knew that for them, even more than for the rich, the final outcome could only be death.

The Experience of Illness: From Myth to Reality

We do not hear much from the poor, but the bourgeois, especially writers and artists, have left abundant testimony. Anton Tchekhov, Franz Kafka, Katherine Mansfield, and the very young Marie Bashkirtseff, for example, have noted from day to day, in their correspondence or in their diaries, the image of the illness from which all of them were to die. What a painful road they had to travel: within a few years it led them from the revelation of an affection that was almost abstract, being barely felt in their daily experience and barely discernible in their body, to a harsh and real ordeal, that of physical decline and impending death.

Initially the event seemed to them steeped in the Romantic myth with all the significations that emerge from it; their own discourse naturally partook of it and contributed to it. But over the months and years the sufferer somehow experienced the inversion of the myth. In the beginning these writers felt as if their illness had removed them from ordinary life and engaged them in an abstract confrontation with passion and with death, a confrontation in which the body was barely implicated. As time went on, each of them discovered the weight of the most material limitations—symptoms, the invasion of the self by the illness, the difficulty of maintaining relations with others, exclusion from the world. In this manner all of them gradually discovered that they were "sick."

At the time of the initial diagnosis, all of them stated that they were not afraid of the illness. Katherine Mansfield was at first delighted that after a pleurisy in the autumn of 1917 her physician sent her to the south of France. In a letter to his publisher, written on the very day after the medical examination in which his condition was revealed to him, Franz Kafka wrote: "The illness that had been drawn to me for years by headaches and insomnia has finally broken out. It is almost a relief."[37] Marie Bashkirtseff at first adopted an attitude of complete bravado. She wrote in her diary under 10 September 1880, on the day when she had learned that her "bronchial tubes were affected": "I would be glad to have something serious and be done with it. My aunt is terribly upset; I am elated. Death does not frighten me; I would not have the courage to kill myself, but I would like to be done with it. I will not put on flannels, and I will not dirty myself with iodine. *I don't have to get well.* Even without it I will have enough health and enough life for what I want to make of it."[38]

At least in the beginning and for long periods, the illness barely made itself felt: it was nothing or almost nothing. "My illness?" wrote Kafka to Max Brod, "I will tell you confidentially that I barely feel it. I have no fever, I do not cough much, I do not have any pain. My breath is short, that is true, but when lying down or sitting I don't feel it, and when I walk or do any kind of work it is easy to bear; I simply breathe twice as fast, it is not much of a burden."[39] The description of the life Kafka led in the countryside in September 1917, right after the discovery of his illness—rest, siestas in the sun, a great deal of cold milk—sounds positively idyllic: his illness remained "slight."[40] In fact he still wrote in 1923, a year before his death, "I will never understand from my own experience, indeed I will never even have the possibility to understand that someone who is otherwise cheerful and essentially unworried can perish of the lung disease alone."[41]

Marie Bashkirtseff played with the idea of death. "You see, I find this position of being condemned or almost condemned entertaining. It is a pose, a special feeling to know that I contain a mystery, that the finger of death has touched me; there is a certain charm in that. First of all, it's new. To speak *in all seriousness* of my own death is interesting and, I repeat, I find it entertaining."[42]

Yet, paradoxically, each of these authors felt this almost abstract illness to be profoundly his or her own. Kafka and Marie Bashkirtseff stated that they had felt it coming. The young girl wrote, also on 10 September 1880: "I have suspected that something is wrong for a long time; I coughed all the time and am still coughing and choking. The only thing that would have surprised me would have been if I had nothing."[43] And Kafka to Max Brod, following his diagnosis: "But I am not complaining, today less than usually. Besides, I predicted it myself."[44] The reason is that these authors, as soon as they found out about it, felt that their illness was a very different matter from a bodily ailment brought about by material causes. They were convinced from the outset, totally in agreement with the Romantic vision in this respect, that it came from the soul, from themselves. Over the years, Kafka especially expressed this conviction in various ways. "There is also this wound, of which that of the lungs is only the symbol,"[45] he wrote in September 1917. In March 1918: "The physical illness is only the overflow of the spiritual illness."[46] In March 1920: "It is not a real illness, but it is not health either; it is part of this group of ailments that do not have their cause in the place where they seem to be lodged."[47] The development of the illness and the cure were also related to the sufferer's psyche. "In order to get well . . ., one must above all have the desire to get well. I have it, but if it is possible to say such a thing without seeming affected, I also have the opposite desire," Kafka wrote to Felix Weltsch.[48] Katherine Mansfield also felt that the illness of the soul made it difficult to get well. "*I must heal my Self* before I will be well . . . This must be done alone and at once. It is at the root of my not getting better."[49]

But as time went on, the very register of discourse would change for all these authors: little by little their illness ceased to be an abstract threat, a wound of the soul, or the mark of destiny's finger. In its "simplicity," as Kafka put it,[50] it turned into an accumulation of painful symptoms, of more and more narrow limitations brought about by the insidious decay of the body.

For Tchekhov, Kafka, and Katherine Mansfield, the first manifestation of the illness was blood-spitting. All of them affirmed that this did not unduly upset them. Kafka wrote to Milena: "For me this thing began about three years ago with a hemorrhage. I got up, excited as one is by all new things . . ., a bit frightened too, of course, went to the window, leaned out, went to the washstand, walked around in the room, sat down on the bed—the blood kept coming. But I was not unhappy at all."[51]

The experience of constant coughing and difficult breathing proved much more trying. "I cough and cough and at each breath a dragging, boiling, bubbling sound is heard. I feel that my whole chest is boiling. I sip water, spit, sip, spit. I feel I must break my heart. And I can't expand my chest; it's as though the chest had collapsed. *Life is—getting a new breath: nothing else counts*," wrote Katherine Mansfield.[52] Like Kafka, she spoke with a forced humor of the concerts of nightly coughing that echoed through the small hotels of southern France as well as the sanatoria of central Europe. "The man in the room next to mine has the same complaint as I. When I wake in the night I hear him turning. And then he coughs. And I cough. And after a silence I cough. And he coughs again. This goes on for a long time. Until I feel we are like two roosters calling to each other at false dawn."[53]

All of them eventually had to face the reality of their decline, first only in the physical sense. "I am in bed; I feel very sick. Queer, altogether—decomposing a bit," wrote Katherine Mansfield.[54] Elsewhere she analyzed her feeling of being reduced to the state of an insect crushed between the pages of a book; there was no longer any space to live. "The pains in my back and so on make my prison almost unendurable. I manage to get up, to dress, to make a show of getting to the restaurant and back without being discovered. But that is literally all. The rest is rather like being *a beetle shut in a book*, so shackled that one can do nothing but lie down. And even to lie down becomes a kind of agony."[55] In May 1884, when Marie Bashkirtseff's condition had worsened considerably, she sounded a note of anguish in which there was no longer any room for playfulness: "Dying is a word that is easy to say and to write; but to think, to *believe* that one will die soon? Do I believe it? I do not, but I *fear* it."[56]

Kafka remained for a long time stoic in the face of his symptoms, refusing to attach any importance to them. As we have seen, he still refused to believe that tuberculosis was dangerous a year before his death. Yet in May 1921, on the occasion of a stay in the sanatorium during which he felt particularly unwell, he wrote to Max Brod: "It was a mistake that until now I have not lived among people with lung disease and that I have not yet really looked the disease in the face. This I have done only here."[57] In his case, as in those of Katherine Mansfield and Marie Bashkirtseff, the reality of the illness was finally brought home through confrontation with the Other. Kafka now perceived the effect of the work that had been slowly accomplished: *he had become a sick person.* At this point the Romantic vision broke down: he had believed that the illness expressed him, yet it had changed him. All these authors eventually came to face the problem of their identity, which was threatened by the illness. They were, after all, creative artists, and so their deterioration was more than physical. The impairment of their ability to work and to create was for all of them the most distressing aspect of the illness. They constantly envisaged the agonizing interrelation between illness and creation: illness prevented them from working. Katherine Mansfield wrote: "But although I've an armchair and a fire and little table all drawn up comfortable I feel too ill to write. I could dictate I think pr'aps—but write—no. Trop Malade."[58] In her case, not being able to write implied the threat of leaving her life's work unfinished, of nonexistence as an artist in addition to physical death. "And I shan't have my work written. *That's what matters.* How unbearable it would be to die—leave 'scraps,' 'bits' . . . nothing real finished."[59] Marie Bashkirtseff expressed her bitterness at being incapacitated by comparison with her active and productive fellow art students.

Not being able to paint while the others, the healthy ones, were working and learning was unbearable: "I am deeply distressed. I am doing nothing, and what about my painting? But above all, don't do any work! Do you understand my despair? I just stand there without lifting a finger while the others work, make progress, prepare their paintings!"[60] It was in this same context that Marie Bashkirtseff, comparing herself to one of her fellow art students who made a brilliant career, yielded and admitted to her "chest complaint." The other girls who worked with her in the workshop had become painters; all she had was her illness. Being ill had taken the place of art and of a career. "Breslau has gotten her prize. She has commissions. Mme X . . ., who has been very helpful to her and at whose house she has met the most important artists, has commissioned her to paint her portrait for the next *salon*. She has already sold three or four things. And I? *I have a chest complaint!*"[61]

This recognition of all-encompassing illness as the individual's final identity now appears as the tragic end point of the painful road that all these authors have traveled. This awareness was particularly keen for Katherine Mansfield, who almost always expressed it in relation to others who were well. Love in particular had become impossible, because the very being of the sick person had changed. She frequently expressed this feeling: "I am an absolutely hopeless invalid. What is my life? It is the existence of a parasite. And five years have passed now, and I am in straiter bonds than ever."[62] She continued, speaking of her life with the man she loved: "Yet there is a deep, sweet, tender flooding of feeling in my heart which is love for him and longing for him. But what is the good of it as things stand? Life together, with me ill, is simply torture with happy moments. But it's not life."[63] Again and again she returned to the theme of her incapacity to communicate with others: "But perhaps to people who are not ill, all this is nonsense. They have never traveled this road. How can they see where I am?"[64] She also wondered: "Do they treat me as posthumous already?"[65]

By way of compensation, Katherine Mansfield intently read the letters of Keats and Tchekhov who, like herself, had been ill with tuberculosis. She sadly identified with them, especially with the suffering of Keats, who also found that he was not understood by the woman he loved: "These letters written during his fatal illness are terrible to one in my situation. It is frightening that he too should have known this mental anguish. And to read his letter to Fanny . . .;—nay worse, that in which he says that she has no *right* to that kind of happiness if she loves him . . . My God, does another soul on earth understand his torment as I do?"[66] She felt in herself the anguish of Tchekhov, saying, "There is no more Tchekhov. Illness has swallowed him."[67]

In the course of their illness and their slow advance toward death, then, tuberculosis sufferers entirely abandoned the Romantic vision of their illness.

They had not believed in its material nature, yet it turned out to be *all* matter. They had believed that it was their creation, yet they were profoundly changed by it. They had believed that it concerned them alone, yet it assigned to them a place in society and sometimes even in history.

3.

Registers of Memory and Forgetting

*I*t is tempting to contrast the images of epidemics and collective dying — disease taking over and destroying the public space as well as the human body, tuberculosis encapsulated in specific places — with those of today's illness, which, totally turned inward upon the individual, is not discernible in the public space. Perhaps Jean Reverzy's novel *Le Passage* (1954)[1] depicts one of the models of today's sick. At any rate it is the model many physicians would no doubt like to see. Palabaud, the protagonist, goes through his illness without hope and without dread, in solitary and tranquil discretion. Having contracted cirrhosis in Tahiti, where he has been living for years, he returns to his native city of Lyon in order to revisit the sites of his youth before he dies. His agony lasts for six months, and during this time he walks the streets of the city, alone and unknown. No one notices his presence, and his illness passes unnoticed. Palabaud knows that he is no longer part of the world, but his exclusion is altogether interior, invisible to anyone. Moreover, Palabaud will never rebel, nor will he embarrass others. He does not want to burden anyone with the weight of his agony. Being extremely polite, considerate, and genteel, he knows that nowadays it is proper to let the doctors handle such things and that the correct way to die is under their care. A model consumer, yet a man of moderation, he regularly goes to the doctor and conscientiously, though without any illusion, follows his orders. An exemplary patient, he even knows how to lie on the examining table in the position best suited for his checkup. With equal docility he agrees to go to the hospital to die. There he is rewarded with becoming the "personal patient" of the "chief" and with his own room. In the end his body is autopsied.

Memories of Yesterday's Ills?

Despite the very different realities of our time, have we preserved some memory of the *Ancien Régime of Disease*? Do our representations still bear the trace of the many centuries when illness was above all the epidemic? Its persistent presence is still noticeable in the metaphors of our speech. We still say, for example, "I avoid him like the plague." One can also observe how easily the age-old patterns of behavior are revived at every recurrence of such calamities.[2] In 1973 in Italy, a cholera epidemic broke out at Naples and at Torre del Greco. Almost immediately the population panicked; people locked themselves into their homes and avoided contact with others. The mayor of Torre del Greco said a few years later: "I remember that on the very next day all the Italian newspapers reported this event with large headlines, whereupon the population was taken by collective terror; and the first thing people did was to lock themselves up in their homes."[3] A physician reports: "At that time everyone tried to avoid people who had relatives in the hospital because they were afraid of contagion that could spread even through speaking. I remember that at the time people wouldn't even shake hands from fear of the disease." Those who could left town: "All those who had the means took their families away." "A lot of citizens went away, preferring to leave the center of infection."[4] Very quickly too, as in the Middle Ages, the blame was put on "outsiders." One cholera victim made this accusation: "We have been infected with this disease, which has come from the outside; we think it has come from Africa." The parish priest of Torre del Greco voiced the same opinion: "I personally think that this microbe was brought in by persons who came from abroad."[5]

Above all, however, one notices the importance of the theme of the plague in our culture. As we have seen, there are many descriptions of it, from Boccaccio to Chateaubriand; from Thucydides to Manzoni or Daniel Defoe. In our own time, far from any reality, plague and cholera continue to fascinate such writers as Giono, Camus, Thomas Mann, and Pagnol,[6] to cite only a few. The plague is indeed one of our essential signifiers, which at its paroxysm is used to express the disintegration of the individual and society. No one has formulated this better than Artaud. In *Le Théâtre et son double*, he says that the plague, like the theater, "takes us all the way." Both are "the revelation, the bringing forth, the exteriorization of a depth of latent cruelty by means of which all the perverse possibilities of the mind, whether of an individual or a people, are localized. Like the plague, the theater is the time of evil, the triumph of dark powers that are nourished by a power even more profound until extinction."[7] The plague is also "a superior evil because it is a complete crisis after which there is only death or extreme purification."[8]

But in reading these works dealing with epidemics one is also struck by their repetitive character. Every author repeats and cites another. Nor could it be otherwise, for in order to describe and understand a present epidemic it is indispensable to refer to another, to all the others. Artaud's extraordinary picture of the symptoms of the plague condenses all the descriptions we already know.[9] In describing the cholera of 1832 Chateaubriand successively evokes the plague of Athens, the Black Death, the plague of Milan depicted by Manzoni, and, finally, the accounts of the plague in Provence of 1720. It was from fear that this last epidemic might reach London that Daniel Defoe in 1722 painstakingly reconstructed the history of the London plague of 1665.

This series of plague chronicles thus seems comparable to one of these bodies of myths whose variants can be traced in many places, although the full significance of each one of them is revealed only in comparison with all the others. This is because the plague, in its multiple manifestations, was a single entity, the very embodiment of disease. It is also because the recurrence of epidemics—a sign of the fate that always threatens humankind, of the eternal return of evil—was one of the most striking aspects of that fate. One could always count on the eternal recurrence of the scourge, however quiescent it was. In fact, Camus ends *The Plague* with a reference to this threat, to the perennial character of this evil:

> And, indeed, as he listened to the cries of joy rising from the town, Rieux remembered that such joy is always imperiled. He knew what those jubilant crowds did not know but could have learned from books: that the plague bacillus never dies and disappears for good; that it can lie dormant for years and years in furniture and linen-chests; that it bides its time in bedrooms, cellars, trunks, and bookshelves; and that perhaps the day would come when, for the bane and the enlightening of men, it would rouse up its rats again and send them forth to die in a happy city.[10]

Yet, and this is paradoxical, the plague and the great epidemics, though entrenched in the culture as deeply as any myth, are no longer part of individual consciousness. People no longer refer to them when speaking of illness, or even when trying to evoke their own past. The very fear of the scourge has vanished. Already in 1960, when a group of informants was asked to compare the past and present faces of illness, epidemics, plague, and cholera were mentioned only once, namely by a postal employee, who spoke in an extremely detached manner: "History is full of these calamities, cholera, plague, and such, diseases that must be as old as the world and which for a long time were, I wouldn't say unknown, but ... people's ignorance and their fatalistic temperament made them accept this in their daily lives as something quite ordinary ... There were populations, entire cities, that were decimated by cholera in the old days, among the primitives. They just didn't realize, these poor people."

By contrast, leprosy, which does not play nearly as central a role in our culture,[11] still has a certain place in the individual consciousness or, rather, fantasies. It is true that there are still about eleven million lepers in the world today, including in several Western European countries.[12] But it is not only because of this permanence that leprosy remains somewhat present in our minds. It is because of its very nature, which lends itself to the work of the imagination, for leprosy is the illness of an individual and therefore closer to our present-day experiences and conceptions; it is also the slow and then suddenly visible destruction of a body that is eaten away. To our thinking, leprosy is thus similar to the ultimate illness, cancer, the other ill that eats away. Witness what a young speech therapist of 24 said in 1960: "As long as I don't see the external damages caused by the disease, I am not scared, but as soon as I see the damages . . . one disease, for example, that would scare me would be leprosy, because it would eat up parts of one's body."

The Age of Fevers Is Over

Very different again is the case of the other infectious diseases. If smallpox has disappeared today, and if typhus has become rare, we still know influenza, whooping cough, and measles. But none of these affections is evoked when people think about real threats to health. They are part of our discourse only in a residual form: the flu, experienced as a seasonal incident, or the "childhood diseases," which no longer give rise to any anxiety, now appear as "normal" stages of development. "I have never had any serious illness; I mean I had childhood diseases, measles, mumps, scarlet fever, but that was only normal; it was kid stuff," said a 66-year-old housewife in 1972. In 1979 a 48-year-old cleaning woman was not particularly worried about her children's health, for "they are never sick. Like all kids they have had measles, whooping cough, chicken pox, but other than that they have never been sick." In such a statement there is no longer the slightest connotation of tragedy. In his memoirs published in 1980, Maurice Genevoix, at the age of 90, evokes the attack of "croup" that he suffered as a very young child. "Today's young mothers," he remarks, "would find it difficult to imagine the dread of parents when they had to hear in their children's throats 'the dark morning song of the dread sepulchral rooster.'"[13] Today the age of the fevers, like that of the epidemics, is over. And that not only in actual fact but equally in our representations. Illness no longer bears their face.

But this is a recent development. Even yesterday, and by that we mean in 1960, these ailments spontaneously appeared in every discourse on illness, and people still knew that they had been dangerous. Some informants, among them an elderly lady of 71, evoked tragic cases that happened not so long ago: "No question about it, when I was young I knew of many deaths from scarlet fever, many deaths from typhoid fever, and many even from measles. At the time I knew of cases of children my age; when I was 5 or 6, I knew a little boy of 5 who died of measles."

Several informants talked about a personal experience that has left lasting traces. Typhoid, for example: "I was sick when I was very young; I caught typhoid fever. Now at that time typhoid fever was not treated as it is today, and I have kept an intestinal weakness from this typhoid fever ever since . . . I had to be on a diet of course, and then the war came, so a diet was no longer possible, and so it just became chronic," recalled a 36-year-old housewife.

Above all, however, one disease remained terrifyingly present in 1960. A "disease of today," a "modern disease," poliomyelitis was frightening, even terrifying. It was present in everyone's consciousness as much as cancer, and sometimes even more than cancer in the minds of mothers, especially this one, 47 years old: "For the children . . . everyone today thinks of polio right away . . . It's the worst disease I think, and there are an awful lot of handicapped young people because of it. It is horrible, *and I think it is the one that scares people most*, with cancer coming right behind it." Poliomyelitis evokes the image of an exclusion reminiscent, *mutatis mutandis*, of the exclusion that was meted out to the victims of the great scourges of the past. A young professor said: "Polio diminishes the individual. One feels that one has had it . . . It's the problem of putting an individual back into a world where he no longer has a place, of being someone who is rejected or pitied." As in all the great scourges, the very word arouses fear, as for example in this 31-year-old businessman: "For years now there has been so much talk of polio . . . and one sees so many children paralyzed for life that there are words that evoke memories in us or make us grimace with horror."

At the time of our study the disease was in fact on the wane and the polio vaccine had been in existence for several years. Some people were aware of this and had had their children vaccinated. These people felt that "polio," however frightening, was about to be vanquished. Others, some of whom were highly educated, like one young architect, the father of two children, did not know anything about it. For them poliomyelitis remained one of those scourges that we can hope to overcome only in the distant future. It still had the aura of an irremediable calamity. "Polio scares me a lot . . . , and besides one feels that one must not have any illusions, and one knows that someday this disease will be better known and that there will be more effective remedies, but . . . for the moment there is no hope." This disease is particularly frightening because it strikes mainly children. It was not very long ago, after all, that it seriously threatened children and put their very lives in jeopardy. Yesterday's fear had not completely disappeared from the memory of the persons interviewed in 1960, even though at that time infant mortality was clearly declining. This fear is probably also the manifestation of an age-old social preoccupation, the desire to ensure offspring and the continuity of the lineage.

The other infectious diseases, however, no longer frighten us; for we know that they can be cured. A retired army officer, in speaking of the bouts of malaria to which he is subject, immediately went on to say: "But malaria can be taken care of, it's not too serious if one gets the proper treatment; after that it's over, it stops." The connection between the possibility of a cure and the disappearance of fear is quite explicit: "When I was young," says a 50-year-old teacher, "I remember reading medical books, accounts of syphilis; syphilis scared me, but from the day when it was classified among the curable diseases – today it can be cured perfectly well – I no longer worried about it."

The fear of tuberculosis also was already gone by 1960. Indeed, at that time, a number of our informants believed that the disease no longer existed at all. Thus a 47-year-old mother of several children asserted without any hesitation: "Tuberculosis, that's a thing of the past. What with x-rays in the schools, they can screen it out right away. No sir, tuberculosis doesn't exist any more." For others it had become an illness "like any other." One elementary school teacher evoked his own case: "I have had a lot of minor troubles, for example a white tumor when I was young . . . of tubercular origin." He immediately added: "But that sort of thing can be taken care of, it's curable, I didn't get upset about it." Sometimes tuberculosis was considered less troublesome or less frightening than other diseases. Thus a postal employee suffering from gastritis said: "I always tell myself: if someday they find out that you have the TB bacillus, well, you'd be all right, you could take care of that . . . I even think that if they found that I have the TB bacillus I would worry about it less than I have worried about my stomach."

But if, by 1960, all fears about the present had been exorcised, the memory of the terrors of the past remained astonishingly vivid. Several persons of different ages and sociocultural levels evoked the anguish, the "haunting fear," they had suffered, often for years on end. A 79-year-old retired printer was speaking, to be sure, of an already distant past: "I used to be afraid of the chest complaint, because my intestine was in bad shape from the enteritis I had contracted; I was very thin around the age of 40 and so I felt I might be consumptive. This stayed with me for a long time: I was terribly afraid of chest complaints." But a much younger executive, 37 years old, also said: "Around the age of 19–20, I had a rather severe pulmonary congestion and a kind of obsession with tuberculosis that haunted me for a long time . . . and when I was young, every time I had a chest x-ray I would get into a terrific sweat . . . that haunting fear . . . and then I would go home, reassured until the next year."

Nor had people forgotten the feeling of impotence in the face of this illness, the "label" of consumptive that inevitably meant a death sentence for the person to whom it was attached. A 55-year-old taxi driver remembered: "If you heard 'they are consumptive,' well, that was it, *you expected them to pass away.* It used to be, when they said about a guy, 'he has it in the chest,' well, you just expected him to quietly pass away . . . Someone with chest troubles, why, all he could do was to wait till his time had come, that's all there was to it."

In the 1960s, then, tuberculosis had a twofold image: the benign reality of the present, though recognized by everyone, was powerless to overcome the horror of yesterday's scourge. For some, the memory of the anguish it used to elicit was still stronger than any more recent fear. In the mind of the engineer quoted above, his present feelings about lung cancer did not even come close to the intense terror of tuberculosis that had held him in its grip in his youth: "Tuberculosis was *the* dread disease, the one that brought physical decrepitude, and besides, one was condemned . . . If I compare lung cancer, I wouldn't like to have it, but I don't think that it is . . . that I would become neurotic about it, or even have feelings that would upset me as much." A disease that had become benign in reality and its representations in 1960, tuberculosis nonetheless remained one of the references to illness as such.

The Persistence of the Myth

Even today, persons who actually have tuberculosis can experience it in this twofold manner. Tuberculosis, nothing to it . . . and yet "tuberculosis is like a headache except that the treatment takes longer," as a student from Cameroon living in Paris, who had recently contracted it, said in 1980. Nonetheless, he showed an ambivalence that reflects the double reality of the illness, which bears very different faces in Africa and in the Western countries. "I have experienced tuberculosis," the student said, "in two different ways, on the one hand in connection with some of my African friends and my family in Africa, on the other hand as someone living in France who knows that there is absolutely nothing to tuberculosis." "In France," he also said, "tuberculosis is banal, but when you think of Africa, it's a different matter . . . In Africa, when the man in the street talks of tuberculosis, it's something horrendous." But his discourse also shows that although today the disease has lost all reality for the population at large, it can still evoke thoughts of death for the individual who is affected by it: "I know that at times I saw a lot of clichés, death and the whole thing."

For a 32-year-old musician interviewed in 1979, who had contracted it two years earlier, tuberculosis is an illness "no more and no less dangerous than any other," which is "not serious, but used to be." Nonetheless, he said, "it is an illness that has to do with death," and also, "one becomes much more sensitive to things that die, and one can't escape the fact that one subconsciously has the impression that, perhaps, one is decaying inside." The double register of his discourse once again shows us the continuing presence of the Romantic image of tuberculosis. It is clear evidence of the symbolic work that has grown up around it for at least a century and still expresses itself in identical terms, even though the objective reality has undergone a radical change. For this man the illness, in the purest Romantic tradition, is more than only an organic state that can be reduced to its physical determinants. It is not extraneous to the individual who is affected by it: "It is an illness, and it is physical at a certain level; it is that, no question about it; one can see it when one looks at the x-rays, one can see perfectly well that one is ill . . . yet it is an intellectual illness." He also said: "It is always said that tuberculosis is an illness that one wants to get, *that is a form of self-destruction* . . . perhaps there is something to this . . . I mean that one puts oneself in a position to get it, and especially not to defend oneself . . . I believe that this is true in my case."

For this young musician, tuberculosis represented an ultimate experience that permitted him to change and redefine his self-perception. It was, he said, a "key period" that "marked a dividing line": "It is a moment when nothing goes on except being sick, *so it is a moment when one is bound to think about things*, and this is bound to bring change, it's sort of like . . . a dividing line." He subsequently did cross that dividing line: he was divorced, moved to a new location, changed his relationships with others, and sought out new experiences. Immediately following the period "when one is really ill, when one is in bed," his life changed radically: "There sure was a change in my life; I came to Paris, that's when I left Lille, where I used to live, and here I led a life that I found interesting . . . I felt like discovering things, I wanted to visit with a lot of people, not stop anywhere, play music all over France, be really open to all kinds of experiences and look for them wherever they were."

Throughout this period, he said, his intelligence was "sharpened," his potential for musical creation was replenished: "In this period I came to Paris to play a certain kind of very extreme music, and I have said ever since that this music had something to do with it [the illness]." Yet at the same time the illness represented a form of disintegration: "I have experienced moments of disintegration in different areas, disintegration of the personality, of the body." But he felt that the best image to express the experience of tuberculosis was that of the "no man's land." In that "not very livable" space, he said, which has no structure because it lies outside of society, the individual, stripped of all trappings, reveals his truth. "When I first became ill, I remember, I coughed . . . there was a record called 'No Man's Land' . . . and, at one point, I used to take the car, drive off, and I would find myself at airports, Roissy and so forth. These are really weird places, at the edge of town . . . places where some people say that nothing goes on and others that everything goes on . . . There are also places where one has to run through open spaces, where one can't hide, like a guy who crosses a border under machine-gun fire. This is still with me from that time of my illness."

The individual who expresses himself in this manner is fully aware that he is reactivating a more than century-old vision and that he partakes of a perfectly encoded literary tradition. In fact, he makes this explicit when he compares tuberculosis and cancer: "Cancer has not yet transformed our cultural and artistic life. It is still raw in people's heads, it has not yet been worked over and prettied up, that's just beginning . . . , tuberculosis is more than a raw illness; it has so many references to a lot of things in literature, history, politics

. . . it is an illness that is still tremendously dramatized." But awareness of the existence of this myth does not mean that it is no longer effective. Isabelle Grellet and Caroline Kruse[14] have found the same theme expressed by young students in recent years. The "consumptive," a blend of reality and popular imagery, remains one of the significant embodiments of the sick person. The symbol has preserved its impact.

The Victories of Modern Medicine

In our collective representations of biological misfortune, the past thus appears in an uneven and diverse manner. Nonetheless one point seems certain: In France at least, 1960 represents a turning point, a pivot between a past dominated by infectious disease – poliomyelitis was its last embodiment, and tuberculosis is its symbol to this day – and a present in which illness has definitely assumed a different face. It should be added that in 1960 people not only preserved the memory of the threat formerly posed by infectious diseases but also were very much aware of the "victories" that their cure has represented.

In 1960, like twenty years later and like centuries earlier – for "antimedicine" is a timeless phenomenon – physicians and medicine were often targets of the protests and criticisms that we will frequently encounter in these pages. Yet the matter of infectious diseases was different. In this area a triumphant discourse unfolded; it was that of the "victories of medicine," which has since come in for its share of criticism.

Because the memory of yesterday's ills was still so fresh, their disappearance was seen as an unqualified success. Moreover, it was attributed without hesitation – since nothing was known about the spontaneous regression of infectious diseases – to the effectiveness of medical action: "There are diseases that are notoriously regressing, particularly in children; twenty years ago, meningitis in little children was usually fatal. *Today, because of the progress of medicine, this can be handled, after all . . .* Typhoid, that used to be very serious, and if someone got out of typhoid, that was considered a miracle," a 47-year-old postal employee acknowledged.

In this struggle, two stages are commemorated. First that of the vaccines: in 1960 Pasteur's discoveries and the techniques that were derived from them were welcomed without any reserve. As one young woman put it: "The vaccines also play a very important role in the retreat of the diseases; smallpox, diphtheria, all that is pretty well gone by now, there are very few cases." Then came the stage of antibiotics, which, although severely criticized in other cases, were seen as absolutely positive by many, including a 36-year-old female hotel manager: "After all, we do have medications now, look at typhoid fever, look at all these diseases, in the past, when a woman in childbirth got puerperal fever, she wouldn't recover . . . Now we don't see this any more, *for they did find antibiotics,* and they do give results when it comes to infection."

Sometimes, in a curious foreshortening of time, as in the conversation with a 40-year-old bookbinder-artisan, the discourse melds yesterday's terms, still impregnated with age-old terrors, with the reassuring reference to today's therapeutics: "*Personally, I always think that a cure is possible,* even if I saw a baby that would be blue because it had croup or something like that .. typhus even, I would always think that it is possible to cure it. I would say to myself, 'Okay, they have what it takes, we'll call the doctor, and then there are antibiotics . . . there is no reason why he shouldn't be all right.'"

These traditional illnesses, although they had become benign, were thus still part of the image of illness in 1960. Some even stated that they were "real illness." A 47-year-old mother spoke of "illness, bronchitis, bronchopneumonia, pleurisy, scarlet fever, or typhoid. This is what I call a real illness: you have it, and then it is cured." One chemical engineer asserted: "What I call real illnesses, these seem about to disappear, and therefore have become less and less frightening . . . the real illnesses of the past, which were very serious, do seem to be disappearing little by little, all that is left are a certain number of heart conditions, and cancer, but viral or infectious diseases do seem to have a tendency to disappear just about completely."

We understand the meaning of this characterization: in mentioning recovery and in marking the contrast with the illnesses "that are not properly understood," it intimates one and the same idea. To proclaim infectious diseases the "real illnesses" is not only to refer to an image of the past but also to express the desire to put a reassuring face on all illness, to believe that it can be understood and mastered. Here we are dealing with an instrumental discourse that wants to bring about the happy outcome, virtually certain recovery, and our triumph over nature and over death. By designating infectious disease as *"real illness,"* we may hope to experience henceforth, as Courteline has put it, "only the pleasant feeling of no longer being threatened by it."[15] This is in sharp contrast with the fearful image of one illness whose "reality" we so desperately wish to deny: that, of course, is cancer.

In 1960, then, there was a twofold discourse about illness and medicine. Their twofold face was this: that of an anguishing threat but also that of possible victory. This was indeed a turning point; our informants easily slipped from one register into the other. At times they said that infectious disease, the kind that can be cured, is "real illness" and saw the other kind, cancer, as but a fortuitous accident that medical progress would soon bring under control. But very quickly the other register emerged: was cancer, perhaps, the only "real" disease, the only one worth talking about? Now, in the 1980s, the second theme has won out. The very success of the struggle against infectious diseases has made us forget this fight. Despite the development of therapeutics, there is a certain disenchantment, and more and more voices critical of medicine are being raised. Henceforth the collective consciousness is haunted by the fear of cancer.

4.

The Illnesses of Modern Life

*T*oday the chronic and degenerative illnesses from which industrial societies suffer have little in common with tuberculosis and even less with the great epidemics, those collective scourges that used to decimate our ancestors. For us, "being sick" evokes the image of a person staying in bed for a few days with the flu, of another living with a heart pacemaker for the last five years, or perhaps a third whose checkup has just revealed a malignancy. In all of these cases the reality and the image of the illness have ceased to be collective and have become those of an individual ailment. It is a *specific individual* who is sick, and this does not in any way imply that his neighbor will be sick as well. This individual's illness is neither a warning nor a threat to others. Its physical reality concerns only the person who is affected.

Individualization and Socialization of Illness

The individual character of illness intensifies the solitude of the sick person and gives it a new meaning. For if sufferers have always had to face their illness alone, the great epidemics had nonetheless spawned a social mechanism for the defense and protection of the community. The ill was collective, and the only way to protect oneself was to keep away from those who had been struck by isolating and confining them. At the core of this mechanism was the notion of contagion: the illness was born out of contact with the Other, it was born out of a relationship, to the point that mononucleosis was called the "kissing disease." Today the sick are alone because the Others, no longer being in danger of becoming like them, are not affected by their state. The bacterial diseases have been brought under control, contagion is no longer feared, and certain new etiological models have individualized illness even further by stressing the involvement of genetic mechanisms or complex immunological processes.

The individual character of illness is also reinforced by the fact that the great diseases of the past, leprosy, cholera, smallpox, and tuberculosis—some of which continue to affect certain areas of the world in epidemic or endemic form—no longer constitute a threat for humanity as a whole. Indeed, they are no longer part of the collective imagery of the Western world as a present reality, for scientific and technological advances have made it possible to control and limit them. Yet even now certain atypical phenomena that are not yet completely understood by medicine can assume epidemic proportions by dint of their scope and seriousness, and they always serve to reawaken age-old anxieties. The media have not failed to report the hundreds of deaths caused in Spain between spring and winter of 1981 by the atypical pneumonia contracted by persons who had ingested an adulterated oil, or the many cases of "Legionnaires' disease" which occurred in Parisian hospitals in the summer of 1981. Some papers even spoke of a "cancer epidemic" in connection with the hundreds of young American males who came down with a noncontagious but usually fatal disease that was generally unknown in the Northern Hemisphere.[1] Even if these phenomena are very far from the epidemics of the past, they do preserve certain of their traits: they are mysterious diseases, not understood by science, and their outcome is usually fatal, especially for the young. Today, in a society dominated by science and technology, it is the failure of medicine to control the disease, rather than its contagious nature, that causes the deepest anxiety.

At the very time when illness assumed an individual character, it also became a social phenomenon. From the nineteenth century onward, illness assumed its meaning in relation to work. As modern industry developed, it became important to have a labor force capable of meeting the needs of production. Health came to mean the capacity to work, and illness the incapacity, to the point that "being ill" and "to stop working" are equivalent to this day. This is indeed a social rather than a natural equivalence, and it still exists in sectors of activity where "work governs everything," as a sheep breeder of Hérault put it: "We need to have our health, that's all that health means to us." For farmers, health is an indispensable capital that permits them to meet the demands of their work. But this equivalence is also found in the urban working-class milieu. For a 48-year-old welder living in a large development in the Paris area, "this is the basis of everything, and without health one is hamstrung in every way. If one is in good health, on the other hand, one tries to give more, one can do anything, go in for bigger things, bite off a big chunk." For a 40-year-old cleaning woman living in Paris, "when you have your health, everything is possible for you; I'm not saying that everything is open to you, but you can work and do something." For her, then, health is "a great fortune, the true wealth."

In taking its meaning from its relation to work, illness has become the inability to work, and health a condition of production. In this context it was imperative to find the means of preserving the health of the work force and restoring it when it was threatened. This is what was at stake in the development of the social legislation that came into being during the Third Republic. The labor movement collectively stated this problem when it demanded healthful working conditions and compensation in case of work-related accidents, as well as in its campaign to have tuberculosis recognized as an illness caused by the wear and tear of hard work.[2] This was indeed a major stake, as one can see by the long time that elapsed between the first debates in the National Assembly and the definitive passing of the legislation: it took eighteen years from the time the first bill was introduced by Martin Nadaud in 1880 to the adoption of the law concerning work-related accidents; similarly, twenty years passed between the introduction of the Laisant Bill and the passing of the law concerning workers' and peasants' pensions in 1910.[3] The Social Security Law had to wait for almost a quarter-century before it was passed in the wake of the liberation in 1945, having been introduced as a Social Insurance Bill in 1921.

Henceforth, all wage earners are insured in connection with their occupational activity. They are "entitled" to social coverage, and in case of illness they have access to medical care and sick leave. Social Security guarantees their right to be sick. The security that this public health care affords the wage earner greatly impressed a young woman from Argentina who has lived in France since 1971: "Here all the people who work are covered, they have Social Security." But this was not always the case. As late as 1960, the 47-year-old wife of an artisan and the mother of four children found it difficult to accept that she had no rights, except that of being afraid to seek treatment, for she "didn't have Social Security." "Being artisans we don't have Social Security, but I think that if people were fully reimbursed they would be less afraid to seek treatment. Because if you have to have an operation, it's just terrible. I can tell you that for our youngest it cost us more than 100,000 francs both times, and then we were reimbursed 40,000, that's all. Operations are just terrible, this should be revised, for we artisans get the short end of the stick in all of this because *we don't get anything out of it* . . . Last year I was afraid that I had a fibroma, this scared me, and I said: 'So I don't have a right to anything, do I, being the wife of an artisan.'" Since 1960, however, Social Security coverage has been universalized and today illness has ceased, in France at least, to be associated with financial ruin. By the same token it is now perceived as part of a relationship of being provided for that involves such things as sick leave, reimbursements by Social Security, or limited-payment insurances.

Illness Has Become a Medical Matter

At the same time that illness was financially provided for, it also became medicalized. The last quarter of the nineteenth century simultaneously brought the maturation of medicine as a scientific discipline, the professionalization of the physicians, who became organized in professional organizations for their common purposes, and the promulgation of the first social legislation. Although the majority of physicians took a dim view of the proposals for social insurance, the most enlightened segment of the profession understood that it was in its interest to help the poor gain access to the medical market. It was the means to enlarge their clientele and to be paid for taking care of those whom they had hitherto treated free of charge.

Henceforth, being sick and being treated became synonymous, and illness could no longer be conceived of without recourse to the physician and treatment. This goes so far that for some persons the memory of past illnesses only consists of visits to the doctor, examinations, and the taking of medications and "shots." Already in 1960 an electronics technician in his thirties said: "I have been sick several times already; it started when I was very little, at the age of 2. I don't recall the details very well, but I do remember that it annoyed me to have to stay in bed and that I was very upset with the nurse who gave me shots; I wanted to run away." A 36-year-old woman hospitalized in Paris in July 1972 did not tell the history of her illnesses but that of her treatments. She began by saying: "I took care of myself as everyone does, went to see a doctor when I had a cough, and he gave me antibiotics." A garment worker also "was lucky to have changed doctors" just before his heart attack in 1976.

Being sick today thus amounts to dealing with one of the most important institutions of our society — medicine. Starting out as an institution that provided diagnosis and treatment, it has become a norm-setting institution: being sick means to submit to its rules, obey its prescriptions, and carry out its orders, for "one must be a good patient" in order to get well. The physician, being the depository of a system of knowledge and technical know-how, identifies the problem, and by deploying the means necessary for a diagnosis legitimizes the patient's inactivity. The physician signs an attestation and starts patients on their way to recovery or cure by prescribing treatments. Medical care has become the obligatory response to illness: one must seek treatment if one is ill, and the anticipated cure is actual "work" because everyone has the duty to get well.

Secure in its legitimacy and founded upon science and technology, medicine has gradually extended its jurisdiction to other fields than illness alone. It increasingly tends to prescribe a personal hygiene and to dictate the adoption of healthful and rational behavior as a means to remain healthy. Since the 1970s its principal preoccupation has been the protection of that collective patrimony, the health of the population, by developing preventive measures and training the citizens to take care of their capital of health. In this manner the "right to health" tends to assume a different meaning. In the 1960s it implied the development of a medical infrastructure and the reduction of inequalities in the access to the health-care system; in the 1980s it is a matter of making all individuals responsible for their health and motivating them to modify their behavior and habits. Medicine is playing an instrumental role in this movement, which tends to make health into a supervalue, an end in itself. This means, according to the American sociologist I. K. Zola, that health is becoming life itself and that medical science now indicates the meaning of life.[4] It therefore becomes necessary, as medicine recommends, to do everything to avoid becoming ill. This demands eating a proper diet by following the recommendations of the nutritionists, abstaining from certain substances that are labeled unnecessary and above all dangerous, such as alcohol and tobacco, leading a healthy and hygienic life by exercising, and adopting a balanced rhythm of life. In this manner, according to Marc Renaud, the "right to be sick and to receive adequate treatment" has been replaced by the "duty to be healthy."[5]

In the course of this double movement toward the individualization and socialization of illness, one new category has definitively emerged: *the sick*. To be *sick* in today's society has ceased to designate a purely biological state and come to define a status, or even a group identity. It is becoming more and more evident that we perceive the reality of illness in these terms, for we tend to identify our neighbor as "a diabetic," almost in the same manner as we identify him as "a professor," or "a mason." To be "sick" henceforth constitutes one of the central categories of social perception. Its importance, moreover, is becoming ever greater because the most frequent ailments today are chronic illnesses and because it is possible to live with a handicap or an illness for many years. This reality was already clearly perceived in 1960. "You see people living for 10 or 15 years with a heart condition," said a 40-year-old housewife, "they are doing quite well, they are not in good health but they live a fairly normal life just the same; they live like that, just like there are people who live with one leg or one arm, they do have something missing but they get used to it." This perception has been considerably strengthened in recent years by developments that make it possible to prolong the life of patients who formerly would have been condemned, owing to the successful use of new therapeutic means, such as chemical substances, prostheses to replace failing organs, and safer operating techniques.

To be sick, then, more and more frequently means to live with an illness or a handicap, and illness tends to become an identity for the sufferer, and a category of social perception for the others. But the sick person has to master this identity, accept it, and make others accept it. This process of identification is full of pitfalls and ambiguities, because illness still carries a stigma. To be ill still means to be marked in one's body, even if no trace is directly visible, if nothing "shows": "Being in dialysis is not written on one's face," a 36-year-old man who had been receiving these treatments for six years said in 1975. The fact remains, however, that if one is ill, one is not like everyone else, one is different. Today some chronically ill persons feel that the quest for a positive identity must pass through a stage of standing back and objectifying their illness: I am not my illness, and there is more to me than my illness. The sociologist I. K. Zola, having himself suffered a case of polio that has left sequela, puts it this way: "Why cannot others see me as someone who *has* a handicap rather than as someone who *is* handicapped?"[6] This is also the position taken in 1975 by a technical expert with respect to his chronic renal insufficiency: "I do not consider myself sick, I have an organ that is not working; there are blind people whose eyes are not working, and they don't consider themselves sick, although they may perhaps at first feel handicapped in their way of life. All right, let me put it this way: the kidney is a pumping station. Three times a week I have the pumping station cleaned out, and that's all. Aside from that, I am in very good health."

Henceforth, illness is signified by time off from work, a medical diagnosis, the taking of medications that punctuates the day or, perhaps, dialysis sessions three times a week or daily injections of insulin. Outside of these moments, one is, or tries to be, "just like everyone else." But "is one really?" wonders a young man of nineteen with chronic renal insufficiency, who has been in treatment for three years. He is struggling with a painful search for identity; he feels "like everyone else," yet "at other times one is not, and then one says to oneself: 'Who am I, and what the hell am I doing here?'" The way others look at the sick person is a painful reminder of reality. The sick or the handicapped person is afraid of being stigmatized, but also of being pitied. The young man with the kidney trouble "does not want to be a monstrous creature that people point out to each other and for whom they feel sorry." He also refuses to be "THE sick person who can get away with anything."

Caught between what they have and what they are, what they would like to be and the way in which others see them, today's sick are concerned not so much with *being* like everyone else as with *living* like everyone else. "How will I manage to get back to living a normal life?" The answer to this question, which is asked by many sick and handicapped persons, cannot be found by rejecting and denying the illness, any more than by marginalizing and confining the individual in a ghetto of the sick. It implies *living with* one's illness, with all of its constraints and limitations, and succeeding in making illness into a form of life.

The New Scourge: Cancer

Yet this new reality of illness as a form of life is not paramount in the collective imagination, and, despite all the transformations of pathology, a phenomenon of the past is still with us, for the anxieties of our industrialized societies still crystallize around one scourge of illness, which is totally associated with death. In our representations cancer is the specific illness of our society, the prototype of the "modern illness" that has become the very embodiment of physical suffering for us. It occupies such a central place that it tends to overshadow the diversity of ills from which we suffer and is often seen as the *only* illness. The most diverse and sometimes the most contradictory phantasms have grown up around it.

For us, cancer is THE illness of our time. Some persons go so far as to deny it any existence at all in the past; thus a 76-year-old woman asserted in 1976: "Illnesses like cancer were much less developed at the time than they are now ... I don't seem to recall that in my younger days cancer wrought as much havoc in our milieu as I see now in my children's milieu." It is true that others have a more nuanced opinion. In 1980 a farmer's wife of the Dordogne said:

> Don't you think cancer has always been with us? The country people used to say that they were dying of a bellyache, but what kind of a bellyache was that, I'd like to know. At the time there was no name for it and they didn't know yet what it was, and then, too, people did not take care of themselves as they do now. My mother-in-law, who died ten years ago, had known in her village cases of cancer of the face. People used to buy meat at the butcher's and lay it on their face so that the cancer would not eat into the skin and eat into the meat instead. So you see, it was with us even then, but it wasn't called cancer.

Indeed, many facts and testimonies are there to attest to the antiquity of this evil and to show that human beings have suffered and died from cancer for a very long time. Anne of Austria, for example, died of breast cancer in 1666,[7] as did the dowager Duchess of Orléans in 1820, as a result of a blow from a falling book.[8] Napoleon's autopsy report includes the words *scirrhus* and *cancerous mass*. Alfred de Vigny died of stomach cancer in 1863, and Rimbaud died of a bone tumor in 1891.

By the same token, cancer has been studied and known for a long time.[9] It is true that until the nineteenth century cancer and tuberculosis were not very well distinguished from each other and that the notion of "consumption" was used indiscriminately for both diseases. It was thanks to Virchow and the development of cell pathology in the years around 1850 that the role of the cell in the cancerous tumor was recognized. Yet Galen had already described a disease—*karkinos* in Greek and *cancer* in Latin, meaning *crab*—that is characterized by a growth or protuberance, and whose name is derived from the resemblance of the swollen veins caused by the tumor with the legs of the crab. The *Oxford English Dictionary* gives as the first definition of cancer: "Anything that frets, corrodes, corrupts, or consumes slowly and secretly." In 1528 Thomas Paynell wrote that "a canker is a melancholye impostume, eatynge partes of the bodye."[10] Until the end of the nineteenth century, the description and differentiation of the various cancerous affections remained imprecise; yet as early as 1775 Sir Percival Pott had perfectly described cancer of the scrotum in chimney sweeps and presented clear evidence for a causal chain that linked together an occupational group, the chimney sweeps, an agent, soot, and the resulting pathological state.

Even in the heyday of the obsession with "social scourges" the physicians did not completely lose interest in cancer. J. Jacquemet's study of the "lower-class diseases" in Paris at the end of the last century clearly shows their interest. Of the 22,400 theses in medicine defended in Paris between 1860 and 1913, there were 908 on tuberculosis, 586 on syphilis, and 301 on cancer.[11] The public at large was also preoccupied with the disease, as one can see from the medical works "for the layman" written by physicians. In 1822, for example, Dr. Constantin James published a book entitled *Médecine pratique des familles: Premiers soins à donner avant l'arrivée du médecin* [*Practical Family Medicine: What to Do before the Doctor Arrives*]. Its third part is called "Of the Radical Cure of Cancer."

Yet whereas in their discussions of the other major diseases—smallpox, syphilis, tuberculosis—the encyclopedias and scientific works usually devote ample space to the history of the disease, it is difficult to find a historical account of cancer. It is as if in the thinking of scholars and the general public, cancer had appeared only recently, at the very moment when the threat of the other ills was no longer as great. Everyone seems to feel that cancer is the illness without a past, entirely of our own time, a metaphor for present-day society and its conflicts. Yet, paradoxically, yesterday's ill comes to life again in today's: the representations and the phantasms that are associated with it make it the modern equivalent of the age-old scourges. The expressions used by many people to speak of it have roots in the distant past, the days of the great epidemics, and revive the archaic representations of illness, such as the suddenness and severity of the disease, its unpredictable and incurable nature, and sudden death: "You can be as healthy as you please; without knowing how and why you suddenly have an operation, and three months later they take you to the cemetery," said a farmer from Hérault in 1980. Another archaic notion is the large number of victims who "drop like flies"; it is said that cancer "strikes" without distinction of age, sex, or class: "It affects all levels of society, that is quite certain," one person said in 1960. Like the diseases of the past, cancer is also fraught with phantasms of rot invading the body, animals that gnaw and destroy it.

In this context it is not surprising that the fear it arouses today, a fear shared by everyone, bears some resemblance to the great obsessive fears of the past. It was manifestly present in the collective consciousness in 1960. A 56-year-old taxi driver spoke of "having cancer on one's mind, being steeped in anxiety about cancer." A housewife said: "Cancer is the obsession of our century, just as tuberculosis was in the past, so now it's cancer." A house painter hospitalized in July 1974 for nephritic colics, and who had "a spot on the head that keeps growing all the time," hoped that "it isn't cancer, because right now that is all everybody talks about." Any suspicious symptom brings up the idea of cancer. In 1974, as in 1960, the mother of several children said: "If you have a child who is anemic *you immediately think of leukemia*, cancer of the blood, whereas in the old days, a strengthening medicine . . . when a woman has a lump in her breast, she will be operated on, and she'll be told that it must be analyzed, *to find out if it is cancerous*. When you go to the doctor, if you have an x-ray, he will often tell you himself: 'You don't have to worry, it's not cancerous.' " One female teacher in the Dordogne, interviewed in 1980, even feels that the absence of fear of cancer is the very definition of feeling in good health: "Good health is not to be psychotic about illness, for example not to think of cancer right away if one has a lump somewhere."

Cancer is so frightening that one often does not dare to speak of it, not even to utter the word. The very name of the disease seems endowed with magic powers, and to utter it, as was the case with tuberculosis in the nineteenth century, amounts to condemning the sufferer. Karl Menninger has written: "The very word 'cancer' is said to kill some patients who would not have succumbed (so quickly) to the malignancy from which they suffer."[12] The fear of having it spoken of and named is reflected in this conversation reported by a 61-year-old woman hospitalized in 1974: "Last year when the swelling in my abdomen began, I met a lady whom I knew quite well, and she said: 'Oh dear, oh dear! Would I worry about this; I would say to myself: this is it.' So I said to her, 'Listen, you are really demoralizing, because *one must never say this to anybody*, and besides, I am not thinking of it. Of course I may have it, and one does think of it without meaning to. Just because you see these illnesses all around you, cancer is what everybody thinks of. Just because you see it all around you, that still is no reason to say, that's it, I have it.' "

Suffering and death are hidden behind cancer, but frequently the illness is also hidden from the victim and from others. Indeed the victims often want to hide it from themselves. In this case they may even avoid seeing a physician. A passage of André Gide's *Journal*, dating from 1934, shows that at that time he both feared that he might have cancer and wished "not to know it." From time to time the writer would accidentally bite his tongue, always in the same place. The small wound was painful; one day he began to worry about it and evoked the idea of cancer. He tried to imagine what his reaction would be and realized that he would wait as long as possible before consulting a doctor: "This little wound, however insignificant, which keeps recurring, always in the same spot, might well end up providing the opportunity for a cancerous growth . . . I must find the courage to consider this coldly. It would begin with an almost painless kind of callosity, but even for this I would not dare to consult a doctor, and by the time I would finally decide to do it, the doctor might well give me to understand: too late."[13] Today, some people consider it most important to have regular medical checkups so that they can be treated in time, if necessary, for "one never knows;" others by contrast consider checkups useless: "Might as well wait until there is trouble."

It is only in very recent years that, in France, the silence about cancer is beginning to be broken. It is still rare for a family to announce that a person has died of cancer, rather than of a "long and painful illness." It is also rare for cancer victims to speak about their own illness. But in 1980 the singer Pia Colombo spoke and sang about it, and the minister Norbert Ségard gave witness on television. An article published at the time of his death described his last public appearance; he was brought in in a wheelchair, he had lost his hair, and his face was bloated from cortisone: "A moment of horror, of cringing, seized the hall," and the journalist continues, "Norbert Ségard was upsetting. One does not exhibit one's illness, such suffering, and one's death in this manner. It is indecent. But this sick man is a minister, and he knows it. He uses it to impose the spectacle of his illness on the world of the living. Not so much as a defiance as to give witness."[14]

The Diversity of Today's Pathologies

In our representations, cancer is associated only with death and indeed has become the only face of death. When someone evokes cases of recovery from cancer or of people who are still alive 10 or 15 years after an operation for cancer, it is usually done by way of conjuring fate. Thus a waitress hospitalized for a cancer of the rectum in 1974 never uttered the name of the disease but in the course of the conversation reviewed all the cases of *recovery* from cancer in her family. This one, for example: "I have a brother-in-law in Loir-et-Cher who was operated on for a cancer of the jaw five years ago. He no longer had any teeth, top or bottom; he had a hole in his throat through which he was fed, and in his nose he had little tubes to make him breathe. My husband and I saw him about three weeks after the operation; one could hardly believe that he was alive. And today he laughs and says to me: 'Look at me, it's been five years and I am not in the hole yet, so above all don't give up.' "

Here again, the reality is different. Cancer is not the illness from which the greatest number of people suffer and die. It is only the second cause of death after the cardiovascular diseases (37.1 percent). It is true that the death rate from cancer has risen steeply since 1930, having increased from 8.8 percent to 23 percent in 1978, but this is in part due to profound changes in the structure of mortality during this period: the role of infectious diseases (17.4 percent in 1930) has disappeared, and that of diseases of the respiratory system has declined by almost two-thirds (from 18.2 to 6.7 percent).[15]

As for the number of persons suffering from cancer, it is very difficult to establish precisely, given the heterogeneity and especially the partial character of the available data.[16] Nonetheless, we do know that in 1977 malignant tumors came in sixth place among the discharge diagnoses in public hospitals (including those of deceased patients) for men (6.6 percent), and in seventh place for women (5.0 percent), after injuries (22.9 and 15.8 percent), cardiovascular diseases (12.3 and 12.4 percent), senility and undetermined causes (10.1 and 10.2 percent), complications of pregnancy and childbirth for women (10.3 percent), and digestive (8.9 and 8.7 percent) and respiratory (8.4 and 5.8 percent) problems.[17] However, the methodological problem involved in estimating the prevalence of cancer is by no means solved.[18]

Moreover, cancer is not *one* disease, but a congeries of different affections that present the common characteristic of uncontrolled proliferation of cells in the organism. This cell disorder can affect various parts of the body and give rise to *different kinds* of cancer. It is also true that the young and the old, men and women, workers and managers do not suffer from the same kinds of cancer and do not have the same chances of developing it and dying of it. G. Desplanques has shown that in a male population between the ages of 45 and 54 the probability of death from cancer of schoolteachers and manual workers varied as 1 to 2.5.[19] M. H. Bouvier and N. Varnoux have produced evidence for different localizations of cancer according to the social hierarchy. In 1974, among men between the ages of 25 and 64, agricultural wage laborers, low-level employees, and blue-collar workers were those who died most frequently of cancer, particularly of the digestive tract (mouth, esophagus, pharynx, and stomach), a finding that can be related to the high incidence of alcoholism observed in these socio-occupational categories. The highest level of mortality in this group was due to cancer of the respiratory apparatus (trachea, bronchi, lungs), but its variation by socio-occupational category was slight, whereas cancer of the prostate, which was relatively rare, was observed mainly in mid-level employees. As for women executives, artisans, and shopkeepers, they were most likely to die of breast cancer, whereas cancer of the uterus more often struck women in the "service occupations." These findings point to the importance of the different "risk factors" involved in these two categories of tumors: late childbearing and few children for the former; a large number of children and early sexual activity for the second.[20]

The epidemiological data thus add up to a complex picture of the cancerous affections; illness today can no longer be reduced to cancer alone. Yet the fear aroused by cardiovascular conditions—which after all are at the core of the Western societies' pathology, considering that they are the most frequent cause of death—is not even comparable to the fear of cancer. "Heart conditions," to be sure, have long been associated with the possibility of rapid death. Thus, in 1849, Balzac's mother, writing to her son, worried: "You do not tell me enough about how your heart feels ... I am in a dreadful state so far away from you, my dear! I know how nervous you are and how badly you must feel, for any heart condition makes one feel that one will soon be dead."[21]

But today, heart conditions can be treated, and one can hope to survive; as a young female hotel manager of 36 said in 1960: "My aunt died at the age of 78, of everything and nothing, if I may put it this way. She had had a heart attack a few years ago, and that was pretty serious. Well, she picked herself up and *she was treated for it*, she was at the Hôpital Broussais, and *she managed to get better*, because that is not what she died of." Cardiovascular illness is conceived of as at least partly controllable, while everyone believes that cancer, despite the intense efforts expended on it, has checkmated medical science. The same hotel manager also evoked the case of a young relative of 11, a girl suffering from a "heart murmur," "who was cured even though this was a real heart condition ... there just simply are better results in this area than when it comes to cancer."

Nor do occupational illnesses or work-related accidents occupy an important position in today's collective consciousness. Informants do tell us that "work makes us sick," but this is usually a stereotyped statement that they rarely apply concretely to their own case.[22] Thus, in 1960, a 60-year-old railroad employee associated his recent heart attack with the excitement he felt at the birth of his granddaughter and did not relate it in any way to his working conditions, even though he had spoken at great length about his irregular schedules, his meals eaten in canteens, his unsettled family life, and the heavy responsibility of driving a passenger train. Yet, every year, one in fourteen wage earners suffers a work-related accident, and [in France] 1,600 deaths per year must be attributed to this cause.[23]

These dry figures, however, do not immediately make it clear that all wage earners are not equally at risk in their work. In fact "manual workers,"[24] representing 55.8 percent of all wage earners, suffer 82.2 percent of the work-related accidents, and among them, in the year 1979 for example, specialized workers, representing 19.8 percent of the wage earners, suffered 30.1 percent of the accidents and 25.7 percent of the accidents resulting in permanent disability compensation; skilled laborers, representing a similar proportion of the work force (21.1 percent) accounted for 42.3 percent of the accidents and 42 percent of the disability payments.[25]

The definition of the categories "work-related accidents and occupational illnesses" thus represents a real economic stake and is shaped by an economic, political, and social power-relation. And, incidentally, these categories still do not by any means account for all work-related difficulties. To cite only one example: the sixty-six illnesses categorized as "work-related" correspond to well-defined criteria and are for the most part varieties of pneumoconiosis and dermatosis. On the other hand, there is no recognition of the sleep disorders of night workers, and even of ulcers and gastrointestinal problems related to certain activities. Yet the labor unions find it very difficult to use the relation between health and work as an issue in negotiations with companies. Except in the case of Penaroya, where between 1972 and 1975 the unions, in collaboration with certain physicians' groups, led the fight for a more comprehensive approach to lead poisoning, there are few social conflicts in which health and illness have been major issues.

By contrast, "overwork," "fatigue," "nervousness," "depression," "asthenia," and "mental problems" are integral parts of our representations. Not as frightening as cancer, these problems are also considered "illnesses of modern life," related to living in an urban society where the combination of working conditions, commuting, housing, and food adds up to a pathogenic environment that spawns a new *"mal du siècle."* In 1960 already, one of our informants, a judge, stated that "neurosis is to the twentieth century what tuberculosis was to the nineteenth, it is the illness of our century." At the end of the 1970s the whole area of the so-called "mental problems" brought on by modern living conditions dominated the discourse: "Mental health is jeopardized by the way of life in the megalopolis," said a woman journalist in 1979, "of course, it is not what you would call madness, but if one were to investigate the use of tranquilizers, 'uppers,' and sleeping pills, it would be pretty impressive. People are nervous and aggressive, they have to deal with obviously stressful phenomena and they increasingly make use of pills to help them cope with daily life, which is very tough in the big cities." Others, among them a 40-year-old teacher, bring up the idea that "many illnesses today are of nervous origin; working conditions, and also housing conditions, all of this adds up, commuting time, too. At some point, people crack up. They keep going, I don't know how, on nervous energy, and they are completely overworked. Nervous tension, anxiety, and stress are a real problem." Cardiovascular disease is also frequently placed within this context. Spawned by "overwork," "agitation," "anxiety," "annoyances," and the "stress" of life in our time, heart conditions have also become "illnesses of modern life," and thereby alarming. "Heart attacks," said a postal employee in 1960, "hit people who lead a particularly hectic life, who are overworked all the time." A 46-year-old technical expert was of the same opinion, also in 1960: "All those very busy and very emotional people, they are the first to succumb. It [heart trouble] is an illness of our time, and it has a lot to do, precisely, with this overactive life that human beings cannot take."

The Representation of the Illnesses Produced by Modern Life

This last idea—illness as a product of a "life that human beings cannot take"—touches on one of the paramount aspects of the representation of the "illnesses of modern life." Certain illnesses are considered typical of our time, widespread, and, above all, produced by modern life. At this point certain of the themes sounded in connection with cancer also become clear, and we begin to understand how cancer has come to combine the images of yesterday's scourge with those of today's illness. By dint of its association with death, by the fear it arouses, and by the reactions to which it gives rise, cancer is like yesterday's scourge, but it is altogether modern because of the meaning attached to it and the causal theories to which it is related. Although its etiology is not yet clear, two conceptions of cancer have developed side by side since the end of the last century and circulate in medical as well as lay circles. One of them sees it as an illness of the individual, the other as a disorder of our way of life and of society. In fact—and this concept ties together the entire set of significations that make cancer the prototype of illness in our time—*cancer is the illness of individuals in their relations with society*. It is indeed an illness of the individual, but this individual can only be conceived of in relation with society as a whole. At the same time cancer is also an illness produced by society, but one that manifests the flaws of the present-day individual.

Certain psychologists and psychoanalysts believe that cancer has its origin in the individual history and the psychological characteristics of the subject. This conception is not altogether new, for we have already seen its widespread application to tuberculosis, but it has now assumed a different form: cancer, it is said, is caused by the repression of feelings and vital energy. Groddeck claims that the human being himself manufactures his illnesses; their "causes" should not be sought outside himself. "The cancer victim," he writes, "experiences an ebbing of his vital strength and his courage for life."[26] Most notoriously, Wilhelm Reich developed the theory that accounts for cancer as an illness of repression. The illness, he claims, is triggered by the inhibition of sexual energy, that vital energy *par excellence*, and the repression of the "orgastic power." "Persons who fall victim to cancer," he writes "are for the most part personalities of moderate emotivity, given to resignation by temperament."[27] He analyzes, for example, the case of one woman suffering from cancer as an "eloquent illustration of the functional unity in which psychic resignation and loss of vital energy go together." "Resignation as a character trait," he asserts, "always precedes the atrophy of the vital powers."[28]

In fact, even before the psychoanalysts, Tolstoy in 1886 had already related Ivan Ilyich's cancer to his resignation in the face of life and his withdrawal into himself.[29] In our own time, the Japanese filmmaker A. Kurosawa showed us, in his 1952 film *Ikiru*, a humble civil servant, a conscientious, meticulous, submissive, and resigned man who discovers the pleasures of life and starts living when he learns that he has a stomach cancer. Even more recently Fritz Zorn, pseudonym for a young Swiss bourgeois who died in 1976 at the age of 32, wrote that when he saw a tumor growing on his neck he immediately thought that "these were swallowed tears. What this phrase suggested to me was that all the tears I had not wept and had not wanted to weep in my lifetime had gathered in my neck and formed this tumor because they had not been able to fulfill their true function, which was to be wept." And he continued: "All the suffering I had swallowed and dammed up could no longer be compressed inside me. The pressure became too great, and the resulting explosion destroyed the body containing all that compressed pain."

This explanation of cancer, totally convincing to Mars, had little to do in his mind with the medical diagnosis, for, as he wrote: "The doctors know a great deal about cancer, but they don't know what it really is. I think that *cancer is a psychic illness. If a person swallows down all his suffering, he will eventually be eaten up in turn by the suffering buried inside him.* And since a person like this is destroying himself, standard medical treatments will usually do not the least bit of good."[30] This search for the meaning of the illness makes it quite clear that it is a matter of resignation in the face of life, for if one wants to conform too much, one will die of it, as Fritz Zorn writes a few pages later: "I have been unhappy all my life, but since my good breeding told me that it was 'not nice' to complain about unhappiness, I never said a word about it. In the world I lived in tradition demanded that I not create a disturbance or call attention to myself, no matter what the cost to me. I knew that I had to be correct and to conform; above all I had to be normal. But normality as I understood it meant that I shouldn't tell the truth but should be polite instead. I was a good boy all my life and that's why I got cancer."[31]

Here the illness is both the consequence of an exemplary life spent being "well-bred" in order not to "create a disturbance" and the price paid for it, the punishment that for Fritz Zorn was "the only thing that was capable of freeing me from the misery of resignation."[32]

Here we touch upon the difference from the Romantic conception of tuberculosis. In that case the illness was the tell-tale sign of character, the expression of the individual's soul, especially lust for life and untamed passions. Cancer, on the other hand, is seen as the individual's failure to express and live these passions. Some years ago Susan Sontag, herself stricken with cancer, rejected this interpretation and showed its "moralizing and penalizing" resonances[33] for the sick person living in a society that values the pursuit of pleasure and free expression for everyone.

However, it seems to us that, for the population as a whole, this is not the schema that expresses the concept of cancer as an individual disease. In the course of a television program presented in the early summer of 1982, a group of cancer patients were asked if they were able to give a meaning to the illness that affected them. "Why," did they feel, did they have cancer? One person, who had cancer of the colon, did make a connection between his illness and himself. Yet, contrary to the explanation issued from psychoanalysis, he related it not to resignation and fear of living but, on the contrary, to excessive passion and dynamism: "I thought," he said, "that it might come from this passionate involvement I have with everything, and that in the last twenty years I have perhaps overworked the machinery. I felt that I was big and strong, when in fact I am like everyone else. Perhaps that is something to look for. Perhaps that is it. I don't really know, but that surely has something to do with it."[34]

The persons whom we have questioned over the last twenty years, whether suffering from cancer or not, attach a great deal of importance to the notions of "favorable terrain" or "predisposition"; these "contributing factors" give rise to intense concern. In 1960 a taxi driver whose mother had recently died of cancer did not hesitate to say: "For me personally, cancer is the thing that really worries me; it is my constant anxiety since the death of my mother. Every time I have something, like a pain that keeps coming back in a certain place in my body, I quite obviously not only worry about it, I also buy illustrated magazines and medical reviews, which I devour." The same anxiety was recently expressed by a 51-year-old woman whose mother and grandmother had died of breast cancer: "I am very sensitized to this problem because *I carry a very heavy heredity in this area*. Whenever you listen to the radio or when you see an oncologist on television, they don't dismiss the risk of a favorable terrain. They say that cancer is much more frequent in women whose mother and grandmother have had the same disease. So, you see, I have more chances or more risks of getting cancer than someone else."

The concept of cancer as an illness of the individual, of the individual as responsible for his or her condition, also crops up whenever one evokes—whether to agree or to take one's distance—the various educational campaigns designed to denounce the pathogenic effects of certain kinds of behavior, such as drinking, smoking, and sunbathing. The relation between tobacco and cancer was already known and present in the discourse in 1960. A 33-year-old technical expert felt that "heavy smokers can get lung cancer." A postal employee who smoked "a pack a day" showed more ambivalence toward this information: "I keep seeing in the papers that all the people who have lung cancer are smokers. Lung cancer is attributed to tobacco . . . but, would you believe it, that doesn't scare me. I love to smoke, especially my after-dinner cigarette . . . But I don't think that the amount I smoke can do me any harm. I see people around me smoking much more, and they are not sick, so there is no reason why tobacco should make me sick."

Most people feel, however, that our individual behavior is more or less dictated by the milieu, conditioned by our physical and social environment. "Nowadays the milieu influences a guy much more than a guy influences the milieu," a journalist said in 1960. In 1979, a young postal employee also said: "Of course, individuals as such have a responsibility for their health, but there are much higher, much more important responsibilities. It seems to me, for example, that the people who are responsible for pollution have a much greater responsibility than we as individuals." Thus there is no split between a concept of cancer as issued from the individual and another that sees it as an illness brought about by modern society. Cancer is widely seen as an illness caused by pollution and an increasingly unhealthy environment; by the pollution of air and water through industrial waste and exhaust fumes from automobiles and factories; and by toxic substances contained in foodstuffs. In 1960 a teacher in his fifties was convinced that diet was responsible for the rise in the incidence of cancer. He accused "the hormones": "It is amazing, the number of people I have seen pop off from cancer, and I believe it has to do with what we eat. All these plants they grow with hormones . . . in fact, ever since they have been using these hormones there are species in nature that are disappearing . . . ever since they have started applying these so-called harmless products, which in fact are dangerous to animals, though I don't know to what extent they are dangerous to people if they get them through the plant." For the previously cited taxi driver who called himself "obsessed" with cancer, all the elements of modern urban life come together to account for the increased incidence of cancer: "There is the physical and nervous fatigue with which we have to contend in the cities, and then, especially, breathing in the atmosphere in which we live, full of CO_2 and sulfurous gases. And so, right? cancer in my opinion must be caused, especially in the big cities, by people's fatigue for one thing. Besides, I do believe that *fatigue is the condition sine qua non of cancer*, this fatigue, this running on one cylinder if you will, of the individual permits these cancers to come into being, and then, what with this polluted atmosphere in which we live in the big cities, and with all this chemical food, all of that makes for the arithmetical or geometric growth of these cancers."

For this man, cancer is part of a complex configuration of threats: the "predisposition" revealed by his mother's cancer—"I have the feeling that I am in a precancerous state, in the condition that favors its hatching," he confesses—is compounded by the harmful effects of his way of life on both his psyche and his body. The anxiety he feels about urban life, which he qualifies as "industrial," "chemical," and "adulterated," further weakens his resistance. Significantly, he says: "I think that cancer is due to a loss of speed, a constant and accelerating loss of speed that I personally feel, to a lack of vitality, and I know that cancer usually strikes at a time when one undergoes this loss of physiological speed." The solution would be a change of life style: "If I could get away from Paris, I have the feeling that I could recover my natural health, and that by eating natural, nonchemical and nonadulterated things, I would regain a certain vitality, above all a nervous equilibrium that would allow me to fight back effectively and not to get this cancer."

Are we dealing with an illness of the individual or with an illness of society? Is cancer part of myself, or does it come to me from the outside world? the sick person wonders. In this manner the two interpretations, far from being contradictory, are joined together, just as in the representation of cancer the threat of death, that sign of the symbolic permanence of the timeless scourge, comes together with the dangers of modern life as vectors of today's illness. If cancer, like all the great diseases whose impact on the collective consciousness we have tried to retrace, is indeed a metaphor, it is infinitely richer than Susan Sontag would lead us to believe: it is a metaphor that merges the archaic with the modern vision of illness; a metaphor that uncovers our relationship with today's world and at the same time brings us face to face with our fragility as individuals.

II·

READING AND INTERPRETING DISEASE

5.

From the Body Horrible to the Space of Disease

Before proceeding with our investigation of the status of the sick—from ancient times to today—we must ask ourselves what goes into the perception and interpretation of that status. It appears that illness was first perceived and interpreted at the level *of the body.* Reflection and mirror that shows and expresses its condition, seat of being and appearance which reveals social customs and bears the marks of its time, the body is involved all at once in work, pleasure, and attraction, as well as in illness, pain, and death. What can be read upon the sick body, and how has the sick body been read in the past? But also, how can we speak of it, and what can we know about it? For there is always something inexpressible about the body; there are cries and whispers that cannot be put into words. We are always overcome and mute in the face of our bodies' cataclysms. This is precisely one of the reasons why the observation of our own body, if it is to reach the point of understanding and speech, must proceed from a distance, must select and serialize the body's manifestations and convert them into signs. The reading of the body can only be a construction, that of the body itself and its relation to illness. Historically also, as the slow maturation of the discourse of medicine shows, the reading of the body has become more circumscribed, because the suffering flesh, the shapeless body of the sick person, has now become the object of knowledge and the space of disease.

There is, to be sure, one objective reality in the historical evolution of the vision of the sick body: the reality of morbidity. Regardless of the perspective from which they are viewed, all diseases do not convey the same signs; in the era of epidemics the body presented a different aspect than it does in that of chronic illness. But the ability to read the body is also, and most importantly, derived from the manner in which medicine has gradually learned to understand and express its afflictions. In this area, more than in any other, medicine has indeed shaped our representations. Little by little our vision of the body has espoused the categories of anatomo-physiology and has structured itself in accordance with medical perceptions and concepts. Yet this is a recent development: for centuries, medical knowledge – uncertain, fluctuating, and unstructured as it was – did not always carry the same weight or affect everyone in the same manner; for much of the past it left a great deal of room for systems of knowledge of a different kind. Above all, the way in which a society, including its physicians, perceives the sick body also reflects a set of much larger cultural significances which informs the approach to this phenomenon. The vision of human beings and of the world expressed in the notion of the body as a microcosm attuned to the macrocosm of the universe and the collective attitudes toward uncontrollable misfortune and sin that illness represented have most certainly structured our ancestors' perception of the sick body as the locus of exteriorized horror. Today the modern conception of the body as machine helps to make the body into the silent and somewhat neutralized space of disease that can be controlled by medicine.[1]

The Horror of the Signs

In the many chronicles of epidemics, those of the plague in particular – from Procopius to Boccaccio, from Gregory of Tours to Daniel Defoe by way of accounts by anonymous witnesses – bodily suffering is not the most important object: the descriptions of piled-up corpses, collective behavior, panic, debauchery, and rioting, as well as those of the multiple practices by which individuals attempted to protect themselves from the epidemic, are more numerous than those of suffering bodies. But then, the plague was too quick; one barely had time to notice the sick person before he or she died. Later, the same thing was true in cholera epidemics: one barely suspected that a body had been affected before it turned green and collapsed. Yet all these different accounts soon yielded a set symptomatology: high fever, coughing, vomiting, spots, buboes, irregular pulse, palpitations . . . The buboes and the spots, for example, are clearly described by Boccaccio for the Black Death of 1348:

> It showed its first signs in men and women alike by means of swellings either in the groin or under the armpits, some of which grew to the size of an ordinary apple and others to the size of an egg (more or less), and the people called them *gavoccioli* [plague buboes]. And from the two parts of the body already mentioned, in very little time, the said deadly *gavoccioli* began to spread indiscriminately over every part of the body – then, after this, the symptoms of the illness changed to black or livid spots appearing on the arms and thighs, and on every part of the body – sometimes there were large ones and other times a number of little ones scattered all around. And just as the *gavoccioli* were originally, and still are, a very definite indication of impending death, in like manner these spots came to mean the same thing for

whoever contracted them. Neither a doctor's advice nor the strength of medicine could do anything to cure this illness ...; and *almost all died* within three days after the appearance of the previously described symptoms (some sooner, others later), and most of them died without fever or any other side effects.[2]

In 1720 the devastating plague of Marseilles struck horror into the beholders, especially by its sudden onset. Its description is particularly terrifying, but it contains the same elements:

All of a sudden *one saw death painted on a hundred different faces and in a hundred different colors.* One had a pale and cadaverous face, the other was red and burning, some were pale and livid, others bluish-violet, or marked with a hundred other disfiguring hues. In some, the eyes were dulled, in others they shone brightly; some looked languid, others wild-eyed, and all looked so troubled and frightened that they became unrecognizable ... One heard all kinds of wailing, caused by pain in the head and in all parts of the body, cruel vomiting, colics in the belly, burning carbuncles, and all the other effects of this terrible ill: Some languished in wordless silence, others in their delirium talked ceaselessly; in short it was an assemblage of every kind of ill, which became even more cruel because of the cold that the people suffered at night.[3]

As we pointed out earlier, each of these accounts, like the variants of a myth, repeats all the others. The reason is that all of them had to find a way to make such misfortune thinkable. That is why in the course of the ages such accounts have come to espouse an existing form to which they must adhere, for repetition seems to convey a fixed meaning and thereby to appease anxiety. Even in the twentieth century Antonin Artaud presented an astonishingly precise inventory of the symptoms of the plague. His is a literary composition of a haunting formal beauty, a masterful synthesis of all the earlier descriptions, embedded in a tradition and yet going far beyond it, for here the plague becomes the myth of absolute and suddenly incarnated Evil. In depicting the tumultuous disorder of the body, Artaud wants to take stock of all the "perverse potentialities of the spirit," the multiple embodiments of Evil:

Before the onset of any very marked physical or psychological discomfort, the body is covered with red spots, which the victim suddenly notices only when they turn blackish. The victim scarcely hesitates to become alarmed before his head begins to boil and to grow overpoweringly heavy, and he collapses. Then he is seized by a terrible fatigue, the fatigue of a centralized magnetic suction, of his molecules divided and drawn toward their annihilation. His crazed body fluids, unsettled and commingled, seem to be flowing through his flesh. His gorge rises, the inside of his stomach seems as if it were trying to gush out between his teeth. His pulse, which at times slows down to a shadow of itself, a mere virtuality of a pulse, at others races after the boiling of the fever within, consonant with the streaming aberration of his mind, beating in hurried strokes like his heart, which grows intense, heavy, loud; his eyes, first inflamed, then glazed; his swollen gasping tongue, first white, then red, then black, as if charred and split—everything proclaims an unprecedented organic upheaval. Soon the body fluids, furrowed like the earth struck by lightning, like lava kneaded by subterranean forces, search for an outlet. The fieriest point is formed at the center of each spot; around these points the skin rises in blisters like air bubbles under the surface of lava, and these blisters are surrounded by circles, of which the outermost, like Saturn's ring around the incandescent planet, indicates the extreme limit of a bubo.

The body is furrowed with them. But just as volcanoes have their elected spots upon the earth, so bubos make their preferred appearance on the surface of the human body. Around the anus, in the armpits, in the precious places where the active glands faithfully perform their functions, the bubos appear, wherever the organism discharges either its internal rottenness or, according to the case, its life. In most cases a violent burning sensation, localized in one spot, indicates that the organism's life has lost nothing of its force and that a remission of the disease or even its cure is possible. Like silent rage, the most terrible plague is the one that does not reveal its symptoms.[4]

The Tortured and Transformed Body

The old descriptions thus do show the body and the symptoms, but it is quite rare to see suffering, which was certainly always perceptible in the foreground of a statement, as it is in this passage from Defoe: "The swellings, which were generally in the neck or groin, when they grew hard and would not break, grew so painful that it was equal to the most exquisite torture; and some, not able to bear the torment, threw themselves out at windows or shot themselves, or otherwise made themselves away, and I saw several dismal objects of that kind. Others, unable to contain themselves, vented their pain by incessant roarings, and such loud and lamentable cries that would pierce the very heart to think of."[5]

Owing to the very nature of epidemics, the testimony comes from the outside: it is not the sick person who speaks. Usually, however, the observer wants to keep a certain distance and is not interested so much in the sick person's suffering as in the illness—the evil—that he carries. In 430 B.C. Thucydides in his account of the "plague of Athens"—which is no longer thought to have been the plague—speaks of pain between the lines or, one might say, between the symptoms: we hear about bile, coughing, fever, and diarrhea, which matter because they are the signs of the ill that must be recognized. Nonetheless, one finds in this text—which is among the earliest descriptions of an epidemic—one of the characteristic traits of the perception of the sick body in the past, namely, its total and radical transformation. Nothing escapes the disease, which is thorough in its destruction. Thucydides painstakingly describes the impact of the disease on the extremities but also emphasizes that the memory and the personality are destroyed, even if the victim escapes death:

> Many who were in perfect health, all in a moment, and without any apparent reason, were seized with violent heats in the head and with redness and inflammation of the eyes. Internally the throat and the tongue were quickly suffused with blood, and the breath became unnatural and fetid. There followed sneezing and hoarseness; in a short time the disorder, accompanied by a violent cough, reached the chest; then fastening lower down, it would move the stomach and bring on all the vomits of bile to which physicians have ever given names; and they were very distressing. An ineffectual retching producing violent convulsions attacked most of the sufferers; some as soon as the previous symptoms had abated, others not long afterwards. The body externally was not so very hot to the touch, nor yet pale; it was of a livid color inclining to red, and breaking out in pustules and ulcers. But the internal fever was intense; the sufferers could not bear to have on them even the finest linen garment; they insisted on being naked, and there was nothing which they longed for more eagerly than to throw themselves into cold water. And many of those who had no one to look after them actually plunged into the cisterns, for they were tormented by unceasing thirst, which was not in the least assuaged whether they drank little or much. They could not sleep; a restlessness which was intolerable never left them. While the disease was at its height the body, instead of wasting away, held out amid these sufferings in a marvelous manner, and either they died on the seventh or ninth day, not of weakness, for their strength was not exhausted, but of internal fever, which was the end of most; or, if they survived, then the disease descended into the bowels and there produced violent ulceration; severe diarrhea at the same time set in, and at a later stage caused exhaustion, which finally with few exceptions carried them off. For the disorder which had originally settled in the head passed gradually through the whole body, and, if a person got over the worst, would often seize the extremities and leave its mark, attacking the privy parts and the fingers and the toes; and some escaped with the loss of these, some with the loss of their eyes. Some again had no sooner recovered than they were seized with a forgetfulness of all things and knew neither themselves nor their friends.[6]

Illness is thus seen as the visible, externalized horror of this transformed body. In the accounts that have come down to us, yesterday's sick body was above all an object that had become, for the sufferer and for others, a horrible, even monstrous, sight. In such a body disease became immediately visible, and its end was a foregone conclusion, as in the case told by Defoe, where a mother discovers the plague spots on her daughter:

> While the bed was airing the mother undressed the young woman, and just as she was laid down in the bed, she, looking upon her body with a candle, immediately discovered the fatal tokens inside her thighs. Her mother, not being able to contain herself, threw down her candle and shrieked out in such a frightful manner that it was enough to place horror upon the stoutest heart in the world . . . As for the young maiden, she was a dead corpse from that moment, for the gangrene which occasions the spots had spread over her whole body, and she died in less than two hours.[7]

The horrible condition of the body could take many forms, such as the shriveling and blackening of the flesh in the "horrible epidemic" reported by Joinville in the thirteenth century, which was the scurvy that decimated the camp of the crusaders accompanying Saint Louis. "A disease spread through the army, of such a sort that the flesh on our legs dried up and the skin became covered with black spots and turned a brown earthy colour like an old boot. With those who had this disease the flesh on the gums became gangrened; and no one who fell a victim to it could hope to recover, but was sure to die. An infallible sign of death was bleeding from the nose."[8] Then there are the gnawed-away faces of the lepers, consumed by the ardent pain that, "slipping its poison beneath the livid and swollen skin, separates the flesh from the bones and consumes it";[9] or the face reduced to the state of a purulent mass of the "*honcreuse*" nursed by Saint Jeanne de Chantal. The canker from which she suffers has "eaten away her lips until the teeth are left uncovered, it has reached the ears and moved to the chin, so that only her eyeballs and her teeth have been left unharmed in a globe of purulent flesh."[10]

On the occasion of the miracles—which the Church did not recognize—experienced by the convulsionaries of Saint-Médard in the eighteenth century, a series of testimonies mention the state of the sick who came to seek help for their troubles. These testimonies, to be sure, had an interest in overstating the ills from which these people suffered, for in order to attest to a miracle it was necessary that the miraculously cured be indeed, like one 34-year-old woman, Madame Brochet de Saint-Prest, "the despair of medicine."[11] But if these descriptions tended to accentuate the horror that had struck these bodies, at least they can show us what at the time was considered the quintessence of biological misfortune. One kind of body whose illness could be read was the swollen body; Madame Brochet de Saint-Prest has "an extraordinarily bloated belly, her neck, shoulders, arms, and all her members are extraordinarily swollen up to the knees."[12] Or, on the contrary, the body emaciated to the point of resembling a corpse: "Her whole body was of such livid pallor and so

excessively thin that one might have taken her for a corpse,"[13] we read of a little girl of 11. The body can be deformed: another woman is described as having "a monstrous and contracted body, with twisted legs."[14] Then there is the
body that changes color, like that of one young girl who reports: "I suddenly
found my face and hands disfigured by a yellowish green color that spread over
these parts."[15]

One must of course relate these descriptions of the exteriorized horror of illness to the actual realities of the pathologies of the past: plague, leprosy,
syphilis, and smallpox were indeed diseases that marked the outer body. But
such descriptions were also produced by society's way of looking at illness,
namely as a mysterious scourge against which humanity is powerless, and as
the wages of sin. Moreover, one must probably also read them as the effect of
the state of medicine and surgery, which could do little to reduce these symptoms by other than the most brutal means. These, far from attenuating the
suffering, often added to its atrocity and its frightful appearance. Joinville, for
example, tells us how the barbers treated the scurvy epidemic that had befallen
the crusaders: "The sickness that had stricken the army now began to increase
to such an alarming extent, and so many people suffered from mortification of
the gums that the barber surgeons had to remove the gangrenous flesh before
they could either chew their food or swallow it. It was pitiful to hear around
the camp the cries of those whose dead flesh was being cut away; *it was just like
the cry of a woman in labor*."[16] In the case of the plague as well, the medical
treatments only served to make the suffering more atrocious: "The physicians
and surgeons may be said to have tortured many poor creatures even to death.
The swellings in some grew hard, and they applied violent drawing-plaisters
or poultices to break them, and if these did not do they cut and scarified them
in a terrible manner. In some those swellings were made hard partly by the
force of the distemper and partly by their being too violently drawn, and were
so hard that no instrument could cut them, and then they burnt them with
caustics, so that *many died raving mad with the torment*, and some in the very
operation."[17]

Moreover, from the end of the Middle Ages to the era of clinical medicine,
the reading of the body and therapeutic action were divided between two cor-
porations, the physicians and the surgeons. The former were called upon to
understand the inner body by means of theories in which the movement of the
humors long played an essential role; the latter were charged with the active intervention upon the outer body. However, given the dearth of means of investigation, the interpretation of the functioning of the inner body was based on
little more than a knowledge of the outward signs and remained precarious. As
late as at the beginning of the seventeenth century, dissections were rare and
difficult to carry out. It is true that Pierre de L'Estoile tells us that on 15 May
1610 the body of King Henri IV was autopsied following his assassination by

Ravaillac: "On Saturday the 15th of the month of May the King's body was opened in the presence of twenty-six physicians or surgeons who found all his parts in such good condition that according to the course of nature he could have lived for another thirty years."[18] In 1605 L'Estoile had already described the autopsy of two stillborn Siamese sisters at the Paris Medical School. His description of the different organs is fairly precise:

> The dissection of the inner parts, which was performed at the medical schools of Paris, revealed only one liver, one heart, two stomachs and all the other natural parts separated by a dividing membrane. The liver was very large; situated in the center, it was in one piece above and continued below divided into four lobes, to which two umbilical veins were attached. The heart likewise was very large, situated in the middle of the chest, and had four ears, four ventricles and eight vessels, four veins and four arteries, as if nature had intended to make two hearts; and even though there were two lower abdomens there was only one chest, separated from the lower abdomens by a single diaphragm.[19]

The Body as Envelope: Decomposition and Exhalations

Nonetheless the apprehension of the inner body remained essentially syncretic, a fact that should perhaps be related to the image that underlies so many of the descriptions, that of the "body as envelope." In such a vision, that which comes out of the body is the externalized horror of the ill. The body—that "discreet reservoir of our ills," as the Rouen physician David Jouysse put it[20]—is filled with some invisible and mysterious matter in which all kinds of ills develop in an unspeakable combustion, finally emerging not only in the form of spots, buboes, and ulcers but also as liquids and serosities, blood and pus, and even odors and exhalations of every kind. In her account of the death of Anne of Austria, Madame de Motteville mentioned the bad smells that emanated from the sick body: "In the last few days, when her wounds were dressed, perfumed sachets were held under her nose to relieve her of the bad smell that came out of the sores."[21] The same descriptions appear in connection with the miraculous cures at Saint-Médard: "Her mouth, where the cancer had originated, had become a filthy sewer from which the most stinking odor emanated at all times, corrupting all the surrounding air for ten feet around her,"[22] we are told about the little girl mentioned above. Loathsome fluids also come out of the body: "Great quantities of corrupted blood would spew forth from my mouth," we read in the testimony of the 37-year-old Catherine Chartier, the daughter of the head clerk of the general admiralty.[23] Another testimony mentions that a 64-year-old woman's wounds "continually discharge reddish-brown fluids."[24]

These images must also be related to the concept of the body as a microcosm attuned to the great macrocosm of the universe, a concept that prevailed in Western societies until the Renaissance at least and only slowly yielded to our vision of the organism as machine. Illness proceeds from the breakdown of the established harmony, and such a breakdown will simultaneously affect both the order of the body and that of nature. These ideas still have their repercussions in today's collective consciousness. In her study of a Burgundian village, Yvonne Verdier reports that the Burgundian peasants consider the flow of menstrual blood as the sign of a disturbance affecting the entire inner body. Even today they say of menstruating women: "It seems that if one could look inside a woman's body at that time, it is awful, complete disorder, all upset, an unspeakable mess."[25] Like people in other rural areas, they also continue to believe that the mere presence of a menstruating woman causes mayonnaise to curdle and fatback to spoil in the brine. The biological disorder of the woman has its counterpart in the putrefaction of the animal product. There is an intimate correspondence between biological ill and the order of nature.

Related to these kinds of representations, notions of decay and putrefaction have long dominated the descriptions of internal corporal ills: the body oozes, putrefies, and dissolves into purulence, its organs fall off, it gives off stench. These themes were already present in the *Miracles of the Holy Virgin*, where we are told that the Virgin healed the ardent pain of the lepers of Soissons in the twelfth century.[26] They were still found in the eighteenth century—Catherine Chartier, cited above, said: "What little food I took immediately turned into decay and corruption"[27]—and continued their reign in the nineteenth century in connection with syphilis: in the collective imagination, the syphilitic was "rotten." In 1861 in their *Journal*, the Goncourt brothers described the death of their fellow writer Henri de Murger from that disease: "Murger is dying of a disease in which one rots away alive; he has a senile gangrene compounded by a carbuncle, something awful in which one falls to pieces. The other day, when they wanted to clip his mustaches, his lip came off with the hair."[28] In 1905 the novel *Bubu de Montparnasse* by Charles-Louis Philippe appeared: the hero, the pimp Maurice, called Bubu, is afraid that his mistress, the prostitute Berthe, has given him the pox. He is haunted by fantasies of rotting away: "The pox! He remembered a story from his youth. He was fourteen years old when one of his neighbors died at twenty-two. The women in the neighborhood said: 'He was like a real manure heap when he died. *They say that he was completely rotten*' . . . To be completely rotten . . . he imagined red and oozing wounds, bandages and dressings and saw himself lying in a hospital bed with a green and completely rotten body."[29]

In this respect, then, syphilis was a direct prolongation of yesterday's disease. Smallpox, however—at least beginning in the nineteenth century, and perhaps because it had become somewhat less life-threatening—expressed a dimension of bodily horror that differed from the attitudes elicited by an immediately destructive epidemic. The horror that befalls the body no longer portends death, but it marks the sufferer for life and presages permanent exclusion, even to those who recover. Its victims are forever disfigured, like all those women of the eighteenth century for whom, as the Goncourt brothers wrote, the only place was the convent.[30] Balzac in *Le Curé de village* describes the face of Véronique Sauviat after her illness. Before she came down with it, Véronique, he tells us, was as beautiful as Titian's little virgin in his great painting of the presentation in the Temple. But now:

> That face with its smooth, evenly blended brown and red complexion, was marked with innumerable pits, which roughened the skin, playing havoc with its fair, smooth surface. The brow could not escape the ravages of the scourge, it became discolored and looked as if it had been dented with a hammer. Nothing can be more discordant than that brick-red skin against fair hair, it puts an end to preexisting harmony. Those deep, capricious ruptures of the tissue marred the purity of the profile, of the nose, whose Grecian shape could hardly be distinguished, and of the chin, once as delicate as the rim of a porcelain vase. The disease respected only what it could not reach, the eyes and the teeth.[31]

In the nineteenth century the epidemics were in regression, and with them a certain immediate apprehension of bodily ill faded away or changed its meaning. Yet, paradoxically, the horror of the sick body was expressed more and more frequently in literary works. In Balzac's novels already, and especially in those of the naturalists, physical illness, abundantly and minutely described, reflects the torments, the passions, and the vices of the soul. For these writers, says Jean Starobinski, the body is "the fragile stage where the destiny of the passions plays out its last act."[32] This is how one must understand, for example, the description of the state of Baron de Maulincour in *Ferragus*, and the horror to which it gives rise: the elegant young man has become

> a thing without name in any language, to cite Bossuet's word. He was in fact a white-haired corpse; his bones were barely covered with creased, withered, and parched skin, his eyes were white and motionless; his mouth was hideously half-open, like that of madmen or debauchees killed by their excesses. Not a glimmer of intelligence was left on his brow or in any of his features, just as there was no color or sign of blood circulation left in his flabby flesh. In short, he was a wizened, dissolved human being who had reached the state of those monsters that are preserved at the Museum, where they float in alcohol-filled jars.[33]

The fact that Maulincour is reduced to this monstrous state must be seen not only as the effect of the poisoning that is killing him but also as the bodily sign of the vileness of his soul and his conduct, especially his attempt to black-mail Madame Desmarets, whose secret he has discovered. In the same manner Zola's minute description of Nana's death is inspired by J. J. Barthélémy's *Recherches sur la variole*, for Zola, like all the naturalist writers, wanted to come as close as possible to a scientific description; yet, especially for him, purulence was not only the best way to depict debauchery but indeed its embodiment in the strict sense of the word:

> Nana remained alone, her face turned up, in the light of the candle. She was a heap of bones, a pile of fluids and blood, a shovelful of decayed flesh, thrown down there, on a pillow. The pustules had run all over her face, one pimple touching the other. Faded, collapsed, and muddy gray in appearance, they already seemed to be an earth mold growing on the shapeless pulp where the traits were no longer discernible. One eye, the left one, had been completely engulfed in the boiling mass of the purulence; the other, half-open, was deeply sunken, like a black and rotten hole. The nose was still oozing. A reddish crust started at one cheek and took over the mouth, which she drew open in a hideous laugh. And over this horrible and grotesque mask of nothingness, her hair, the beautiful hair that kept its hue of flaming sunshine, flowed down in golden ripples. Venus was disintegrating. It was as if the virus she had taken from brooks and from dead bodies that no one cared to remove, the ferment with which she had poisoned a whole people, had risen up to her face and caused it to rot.[34]

The Invisible Ill

Precisely perhaps because the threat had become less real, the visible horror, the apparent monstrosity of the sick body, could now become a metaphor. Yet this was the time when tuberculosis, the one illness that was to dominate the late nineteenth century in fact and in popular mythology, was no longer – or at least not to the same degree – outwardly visible. Hans Castorp, the hero of the *Magic Mountain*, at first finds his cousin Joachim, whom he comes to visit at the Berghof, "looking more robust than ever in his life before."[35] We have seen that in its early stages tuberculosis, as Franz Kafka put it, "can hardly be felt."[36] To be sure, symptoms do manifest themselves, and they can be frightening and evoke the thought of death. Katherine Mansfield was frightened in February 1919, when she spat blood for the first time: "I woke up early this morning and when I opened the shutters the full round sun was just risen. I began to repeat the verse of Shakespeare's: 'Lo, here the gentle lark of rest,' and bounded back into bed. The bound made me cough – I spat – it tasted strange – it was bright red blood. Since then I've gone on spitting each time I cough a little more. Oh, yes, of course I'm frightened. But for two reasons only.

I don't want to be ill, I mean 'seriously', away from Jack. Jack is the first thought. 2nd, *I don't want to find this is real consumption*, perhaps it's going to gallop—who knows?"[37]

Three months before his death, fever, fatigue, coughing, and blood-spitting brought it home to Kafka that he had lost his freedom and must return to the sanatorium.

> I should hate to leave here, but I cannot totally reject the idea of the sanatorium, for I have not left the house for many weeks because of the fever; and although I still feel strong enough lying down, any kind of walk assumes the character of a grandiose undertaking even before I have taken the first step, and therefore the thought of peacefully burying myself alive in a sanatorium is sometimes not all that disagreeable. And yet it is very awful too, to think that in these few warm months made for freedom one is to lose one's freedom. But then there are those coughing spells that go on for hours in the morning and at night, and the vial that is full almost every day.[38]

The symptoms frighten those around the sufferer and sometimes make them flee. Balzac shows us the kind of "curse" that suddenly becomes attached to Raphaël, the consumptive hero of *La Peau de chagrin* [*The Wild Ass's Skin*], when he has a violent coughing fit.

> Just then a violent fit of coughing seized him. Far from receiving one single word—indifferent, and meaningless, it is true, but still containing, among well-bred people brought together by chance, at least some pretence of civil commiseration—he now heard hostile ejaculations and muttered complaints. Society there assembled disdained any pantomime on his account, perhaps because he had gauged its real nature too well. "His complaint is contagious." "The president of the club ought to forbid him to enter the salon." "It is contrary to all rules and regulations to cough in that way!" "When a man is as ill as that, he ought not to come to take the waters—" "He will drive me away from the place."[39]

But such symptoms are intermittent; between spells the sufferer seems to return to health. Moreover, the body's appearance is not irremediably marked. Kafka, for example, considered "the contradiction between the looks of the face and those of the lungs" characteristic of tuberculosis.[40] The sick do not become unrecognizable and may continue to be beautiful. Indeed, tuberculars were often credited with a special kind of beauty, that for example of Raphaël in *La Peau de chagrin*, which appeared in his sleep a few hours before his death:

> It was about midnight. At this hour Raphaël, by one of those physiological caprices that are the wonder and the despair of medicine, shone with

resplendent beauty in his sleep. His white cheeks were suffused with bright pink. His brow, graceful like that of a girl, expressed genius. Life was blossoming on this tranquil face at rest. *He looked like a young child sleeping under his mother's protection.* His sleep was a good sleep, a pure and regular breath passed through his vermilion mouth. He was smiling, no doubt because a dream had transported him to a beautiful life. Perhaps he was a centenarian, perhaps his grandchildren were wishing him a long life; perhaps from his rustic bench under the sun, where he was sitting in the shade of a tree, he saw, like the prophet, the promised land high up in the mountains, in the blessed distance.[41]

Sometimes the sufferers themselves were convinced of their beauty. A few months after she had learned that she was consumptive, Marie Bashkirtseff wrote in her diary that she was delighted with her looks: "Since yesterday I am white and fresh and amazingly pretty. My eyes are spirited and shining, and even the contours of my face seem prettier and more delicate. It's too bad that this is happening at a time when I am not seeing anyone. It's foolish to tell, but I spent a half-hour looking at myself in the mirror with pleasure; this had not happened to me for some time."[42]

Indeed, the popular mythology associated the theme of beauty with Romantic tuberculosis. One cannot help being struck by the recurrence of portraits of consumptives in literature: languid creatures with long-limbed and frail bodies, soon burnt out but graceful to see, with emaciated faces whose skin is transparent but suffused with diaphanous hues, and with hollow but high-colored cheeks. This decadent beauty of condemned beings engulfed in ennui, watching their allotted time slip by, still moves us today.

On the other hand, also in the late nineteenth century, the proletarian's body was irremediably marked by illness. In the case of working-class tuberculosis, the "condemned" person was frightening by his or her very appearance, like the woman worker described by the Bonneff brothers in their report on the slum dwellers of Lille: "How old would you think the woman you see there is?— Forty-five to fifty.— She is twenty-six. Sitting on a broken-down chair, a woman in rags coughs and spits without stopping. She is so thin that her shoulder blades stick out under her shawl and her spinal column shows under her shirt. She is leaning against a table covered with pharmaceutical bottles and jars. She cannot stand up."[43] But in the case of working-class tuberculosis, one has the impression that the appearance of the sick body is overlaid with significations other than illness alone. Misery and the dangers with which the ideology of the time associated them can be decoded in this image of physical deterioration, which evokes the ideas of promiscuity, contamination—for the tubercular worker is a "spreader of germs"—alcoholism, immorality, and crime.

Integrity of the Outer Body
versus Impairment of Its Motor Capacity

In our own day, the sick body is only rarely the object of dread; illness has ceased to stamp the body brutally with the seal of externalized horror. The most hideous symptoms have disappeared or become rare. It is true that certain illnesses remain, as a technical expert said in 1960 in connection with his son's asthma, "spectacular": "Asthma is spectacular, very, very much so ... I don't know what the child feels, but to see him taking a breath and not getting it, because it's a matter of air that can't get through ... that is really spectacular ... one has the impression that the child is choking ... one sees him out of breath, turning blue, he can't breathe, one has the impression that he has something else than asthma, that he is going to die any moment." In 1960 as well, a young woman expressed her fear of "what can be seen on the outside": "To the extent that I cannot see the external damage of the disease, I am not scared, but as soon as I see the damage ... for example, a cancer on the inside does not scare me, but an external cancer would upset me terribly. When I see people with a cheek missing, and I have seen several in the Métro, I am sure they have a cancer ... I am sure that if I had that, *I would suffer much more if I had something on the outside* that can be seen, not so much because I would be afraid that I couldn't survive it, but much more because it would be on me, that I would carry it on the outside."

For this young woman, a disease of the past, leprosy,[44] is the symbol of a frightening illness because it attacks the integrity of the outer body. But her reaction has become exceptional. The persons we interviewed over the last twenty years did not express fear of an externalized ill: the ailments from which we suffer today cannot be seen, and it is precisely this absence of outward reality, this apparent unreality of illness, that gives rise to today's anxieties. This was made very clear, for example, in the uneasiness of an artisan, interviewed in 1960, in the face of the leukemia of a little girl who continued to look perfectly healthy:

> I have a little cousin who has leukemia, a cruel disease, it is cancer of the blood ... the kid was a picture of health that made all the Parisian relatives feel badly, the little country girl with big red cheeks, and six months later we learn that this kid has leukemia. So now with a lot of blood transfusions they have managed to keep the kid alive for a year and a half, but of course this can't go on forever ... It sure is a cruel thing because it's such a beautiful kid ... and all of a sudden, bingo, one thought that she was a picture of health, but she wasn't.

The character of modern pathology—for cardiovascular diseases as well as many kinds of cancer and chronic illnesses only carry discreet outward signs—

is reinforced by recent developments in medical techniques. Over the last decades medicine, even if it has not been able to cure, has learned to reduce many symptoms. This is the case, for example, for many kidney conditions, and this is a recent victory. Between February and July 1942, when he died, Dr. René Allendy, a prominent psychoanalyst, kept a diary about his illness, which indicates that at that time renal insufficiency was fatal and that it cruelly marked the body. In February Allendy described "these ankles puffed up with edema, fingers made shapeless by the swelling when I try to move them . . . this face in which I no longer quite recognize myself."[45] Some time later he noted with horror the radical transformation of his organism, which he felt with particular intensity when he was awakened by his pain:

> Gradually my ribs are becoming more painful, my limbs more battered, my legs heavier. In my mouth I perceive a taste of ashes and my cough brings up whiffs of ammoniacal odors, which I know to be the manifestation of the urea that is poisoning me inside. I am torn between the urge to escape from this coma, which will no doubt be fatal to me, and the horror of experiencing the battering and rending of this tattered physical raiment, *my body, which disgusts me.* To get back into this hurting, damp, diseased skin seems to me as horrible as it is for the exhausted soldier to get back into wet, dirty, stinking clothes that have become so stiff and tight that it hurts to wear them.[46]

Thirty years later, in 1974, when we interviewed a group of people suffering from chronic renal insufficiency and receiving hemodialysis treatments, they did not suffer in the same way, and the illness transformed their bodies only discreetly.[47] Many said with great satisfaction that thanks to the treatment "it didn't show," and that the treatment itself did not leave any traces. The dialysis patients even invoked this unchanged physical appearance as proof of their normality, and many of them refused to consider themselves "sick." One 37-year-old worker said:

> I think in fact that all my acquaintances feel the same way, you can't notice that I am getting dialysis. It doesn't show, and that I have something only shows if I still have my dressing on mornings when I have had my treatment, that's all, and at that only in the summer, because in the winter I wear a sweater, *it doesn't show, and so one isn't sick* . . . there is nothing wrong with one if other people don't really know, and they can't find out . . . In fact, that is what fools so many people . . . Well, let's say that three-quarters were yellow in the beginning, their complexion has turned kind of yellow, but I am not one of them, I have nothing to show that I am in dialysis . . . and if it's like that, one isn't sick.

This evidence of an intact body does correspond to a reality, but also to what we all want to see, namely a "positive image" of today's illness. None of us, whether sick or well, wants the body to change, even if we know that it is impaired.

Impairment of motor and functional capacities, on the other hand, reduced ability or incapacity to "perform," and the resulting enforced inactivity have today become the essential perceptions of the sick body. Several major affections against which medicine, despite its strides, is practically powerless manifest themselves in this manner today. In 1972 a young man of 18, paralyzed since the age of 4 following an attack of poliomyelitis, and living ever since with an artificial lung in an intensive care unit, described his motor incapacity to the interviewer in the following terms: "I feel everything . . . I do . . . if anyone pinched or pricked me, they'd see that I would yell all right . . . I sure would . . . no problem, like everyone else, I mean! But one can't move, one is stuck, one is . . . as if one had no strength, wiped out, I mean! If you try to make a move, it's heavy, you can't do it, you have the impression that you are trying to pick up tons and tons . . . no reaction out of the muscles." One woman described the slow progression of her husband's illness, multiple sclerosis, in terms of the successive cutbacks in his activities, contrasting them with his sound appearance:

> Beginning in 1947, my husband suffered all kinds of discomforts, in the liver, in the bladder, in the back, he had days of intense fatigue and he thought it had to do with his work (heating and plumbing contractor). In 1973 he was so worn out that he decided to give up his work, thinking that it was too tough for him. He bought a school-bus company, he liked to drive. Both his legs became very numb, and in 1973 he stopped going hunting because he could no longer walk as fast as his friends. He said, "One of my legs drags," and everyone knew that one of his legs was dragging. When we were invited out, it was always like that, he couldn't dance, but it was intermittent. *People didn't believe that my husband was sick, apparently he was in very good health, he was muscular, big and strong* . . . And every day he had to make an effort to get out of bed, go about his day's work . . . Then, all of a sudden, on 14 January 1980, he lost his sight in one eye.

A former taxi driver of 48, also suffering from multiple sclerosis and also obliged to give up his job, made a very sensitive analysis of the limitations with which he is faced:

> You will see me walk as far as the door, I will take two steps, and then stop to catch up with myself . . . if I walk with someone in the street I take his arm; I don't need a cane, but I must hang on to someone . . . When I am by myself I have a cane; I don't really limp, but I lurch along because I don't have my balance. Well, you see, I have always been active, I loved to dance, I loved to ski, I loved to go all over the place. The other day there was a party

to which I went, I danced a slow, two slows . . . I can still dance the slow but, you know, that's not a whole lot.

Arthritics are the perfect illustrations of motor impairment. The following two examples also show that, depending on the case, the limitations they face do not have the same meaning and that they can be more or less easily overcome. For a 56-year-old mason, hospitalized in 1972, they signify the end of his working capacity: "I first found out about this in '58 or '59, I couldn't work any more . . . In our work, you know, we have to climb up ladders a lot, and masons often have to kneel to reach small pipe openings, to do casings; to do masonry, period . . . But after a while I couldn't climb up the ladder any more, I had to do it 'the chicken way,' as it's called, one leg at a time. So it became impossible for me to work, even if I tried my hardest . . . I couldn't walk any more except with two canes, couldn't work, nothing, not even bend over." An elderly lady of 82 is resigned to the limitations imposed by her illness. Nonetheless she makes every effort to preserve a minimal mobility:

> At home I have had lower steps put in so that I can get down more easily . . . I certainly also mean to go out into the street sometimes . . . I can't do much with my arms, because I have arthritis in my arms, I have had crutches for ten years now, but I always went for walks anyway, I used to go out to the countryside. I could no longer get into trains and buses, but then I would take a taxi to go; to travel 8 kilometers, I would just take a taxi. I have been handicapped, no question about it, but if one is not completely bedridden— and I can get up, go to bed, walk around the house, even get a little fresh air outside—well, what more does one want? Of course, at 82, goodness me, one can't ask for the impossible.

The impairment of the body's motor and functional capacities is more than a symptom like any other. In a society in which we define ourselves as producers, illness and inactivity have become equivalents. That is why today we have come to perceive the sick body essentially through its incapacity to "perform," rather than through the alteration of its appearance. For many people this incapacity is the true signal of illness. This was the case, for example, for a nurse hospitalized for observation in 1972: "I noticed one day that my right breast was very tender . . . it was hard for me to iron, for example, or to do things with my right hand . . . So I palpated my breasts and I found small and rather painful nodules . . . It was very bothersome, because sometimes, at the peak of the menstrual cycle, when my breasts were enlarged, they hurt, and I could not do any manual work, it really bothered me a lot." Motor and functional impairment and forced inactivity mark the threshold, the passage from health to illness: "Being sick? Why, that's when you can't do anything," said an artisan in 1960. This, then, is where illness really begins, just as, conversely, many of the chronically ill today, people who are undergoing dialysis for example, attempt to derive a positive identity from the fact that they can continue to "perform," to keep up their activities. "Dialysis permits me to live a normal life," said a 45-year-old railroad employee in 1974, "this means that I am working, working normally; I go to work from 7:30 in the morning until noon and from 2:00 to 5:30."

Suffering and the Casualties of Medicine

Nonetheless, some of the examples we have cited show that, even if the body's appearance remains intact, anxiety is not always absent; and it is difficult to gauge whether the silence of today's sick body engenders more or less fear than the spectacular horror of yesterday's. In any event, these two kinds of fear are not of the same nature, and they do not take the same form: panic and fright in the face of an unbearable spectacle have turned into muted anxiety in the presence of a body that does not show anything. It would, of course, be a mistake to believe that all of modern pathology is marked by this discretion and that medicine knows how to control all of our symptoms; cruel mishaps still do occur and can reawaken fears that are not different from those of the past. Particularly frightening are accidents that involve blood, because blood has kept its symbolic value as the synonym of life; its sudden loss through a hemorrhage is directly associated with death. This is shown in an identical manner by three persons whom we interviewed. The first was a female white-collar worker, interviewed in 1960. She had cancer and revealed her anxiety through the violent image of murder:

> After they did the biopsy I went home, and suddenly I got a hematoma, my breast became three times as big as it was and I was crying with pain . . . it was horrible . . . and in the night . . . the whole dressing was full of blood and then all of a sudden the blood flowed from my breast . . . gushing out . . . and this went on for several hours . . . My whole bed was red . . . *It looked as if somebody in the house had been murdered* . . . It was terribly scary . . . at that point, really, I couldn't handle it, the hemorrhage frightened me so much . . . finally I had to send my little girl for help and I thought that when she came back fifteen minutes later, don't you see, I would be out of blood . . . If you have a very heavy dressing and if you see regular little jets of water, except they are not jets of water but jets of blood, inundating your bed and if it . . . it gushes like that, and if you can't do anything about it, because I had taken all the materials to stop it . . . Nothing could stop that hemorrhage, well, I really thought . . . I mean, I do know a hemorrhage is very serious when it's like that.

The same panic seized a 41-year-old woman who tried to communicate to us that perhaps inexpressible impression of "feeling oneself die": "I had a hemorrhage at the end of my pregnancy, one of those enormous hemorrhages that come on all of a sudden. When that happens one loses strength so fast, one loses blood so fast, even though one keeps all one's faculties, that . . . one sees it, one feels it, and so I had . . . I remember . . . *a horrendous panic, a feeling that I was dying* . . . And yet you see that it wasn't true, because I didn't die. But feeling all one's blood go, feeling such a hemorrhage, one really has the impression that one is dying." A cabinetmaker who suffered a work accident in 1972 expressed his anxiety by repeating the words "the blood was flowing." The speech pattern of all three of these persons, incidentally, became broken or repetitive at certain points and more halting than usual.

> The blood, the blood was flowing pretty hard, one of my arteries was cut, and so the blood, the blood was flowing. Because it was an artery, a venous artery, but an artery just the same, a rather big one, here under the thumb. The blood was flowing pretty hard. So then . . . when I arrived at the emergency room they took some blood samples, and then they cut off my wedding ring, because I was wearing a wedding ring, and they put on a dressing . . . You might say I lost a good bit of blood because I felt the dressing getting bigger, and when I lifted up my hand it was running down to the wrist, a flow the size of my little finger was running down, like my little finger it was running . . . One sure finds the time long because one is losing a lot of blood and one does feel that one is getting a bit weak. When one loses so much blood one can't help but think that one is going, that one has had it.

In the same manner pain continues to be a reality that medicine is still unable to control entirely. And pain, today as in the past, remains one of the things that is very difficult to express. This is precisely what persons who have undergone very painful diseases or treatments say about it. "It is impossible to define physical pain, one cannot describe it, and it is only a matter of experience," we were told in 1960 by a 41-year-old woman who had suffered a serious and painful automobile accident that has left her crippled. "One cannot speak of pain with a capital P," she added, "it is a succession of seconds, a succession of minutes, and this is what makes it so hard to withstand."

Testimonies of the past in which sufferers attempt to retrace their experience of pain are rather hard to find. But we do have the diary[48] in which Alphonse Daudet kept track over several years of the inexorable evolution of his illness, a tabes of syphilitic origin that eventually left him virtually paralyzed. The writer attempts to describe physical pain, which for him, as for the accident victim of 1960, was not a single phenomenon but rather made up of a juxtaposition of multiple ills: "Sometimes under my foot a very, very fine cut, like a hair, or else knife stabs under the nail of my big toe. The torture of the boot at the ankles. *Very sharp rat's teeth nibbling at my toes.* And in every one of these pains the impression of a rocket that rises, rises and then breaks apart in my head."[49] This image of an animal gnawing away at the bones is also found in the statements of certain of today's sick trying to describe their pain. Hospitalized in 1972, an elderly lady of 82 suffering from arthrosis said: "I have it in the palms, I have it in the shoulders, I have it in the elbows, I have it in the back, it hurts, it hurts ... In my shoulders, you see, sometimes it is as if I had a little stove going. It burns me, it burns me, *as if dogs were gnawing at my bones*." In 1981 a woman executive of 52, who was also diabetic, used almost the same words to speak of her rheumatoid polyarthritis: "Polyarthritis is very painful, it hurts a lot. I can recall nights spent in my bedroom, turning round and round crying, whimpering because I was suffering too much. And then this impression *that one's bones are being gnawed away*, it is too awful."

Most importantly, Daudet notes from day to day how his life is being invaded by pain: "Pain that slips into my entire vision, my sensations, my judgments; I am being infiltrated."[50] Further on he shows us how pain dominates his entire life, creating an empty space in which there is room for nothing else: "In my poor hollow carcass, left empty by anemia, pain echoes like a voice in a house without furniture or wall coverings. Days, long days, in which nothing within me is alive but this suffering."[51] Today's sick do not speak with the same lyricism, but they all assert one thing: one does not get used to pain. The woman cited above, for example, said: "One absolutely does not get used to pain in my opinion; in fact, after several months or several years exactly the opposite occurs: the more one is in pain the more one is afraid of pain ... there is a kind of panic, the fear of pain becomes worse, and the more the body is made to suffer, the more it objects, the less it accepts its suffering." Today as in the past, pain dominates us, and in its presence medicine all too often shows its impotence.

But in our day illness presents yet another paradoxical and particularly distressing aspect: that of the casualties of medicine. Today, when medicine frequently reduces the symptoms even where it cannot cure, it also often happens—and we know that this is the other face of its effectiveness—that it marks and mutilates those of whom it has taken charge. In Alexander Solzhenitsyn's *Cancer Ward*, the patient Kostoglotov would like to stop undergoing radiotherapy sessions, even though they have improved his condition, because he fears their long-run effects. "Extra treatment means extra torment,"[52] he tells the physician who, imbued with the logic of medicine, wants to continue the treatment. Among the persons whom we interviewed, several cancer patients unhappily evoked the stigmata left by the "rays." In 1960, an employee who, having refused to have an operation for breast cancer, had undergone many radiotherapy sessions said:

> I think my fatigue comes from the rays ... because it's really a weird thing about these rays, it is really something terrible. *I am completely changed, I*

have aged 20 years in the last 3 years. Physically, not morally at all, but physically, yes . . . They certainly are a terrible and very dangerous weapon, these rays; the radiologist who burned me didn't handle it right because now my breast is a terrible sight, I mean it is burned, it is completely shriveled up, so now it hurts and I don't think this has anything to do with cancer at all, but that it is a terrible shriveling up of the tissues, so I am . . . One of my sides is white, the other is purple and it has gotten worse. At first the burn was only a real burn, like a very bad and deep burn, and then the flesh grew back. For a while the breast stayed sort of pink . . . like a burned and badly healed skin it kept getting darker . . . One of my breasts is purplish red, which tells you that deep burns come up afterward and that the sclerosis comes up through every little vein.

In telling us about her long physical but also mental ordeal, a waitress who was treated in 1972 for cancer of the rectum, whose nature she did not acknowledge, made us understand that she no longer recognized herself. She could not stand seeing herself in a mirror; she was "no longer a woman":

They took off a little cyst in my left groin, telling me that there were some ramifications with the polyp I had in the rectum . . . And then I started in with the rays . . . After the rays I automatically felt better, but what happened is that I got too much, and I was burned . . . It burned my right side, and it dried out the sciatic nerve, and that automatically gave me edema; so since then I have edema. Right now you see me in good shape, I look quite all right, but if you had seen me then, *I wasn't even a woman, it was awful.* He had given me a strong radiation treatment because at the time I was big and strong, at such times a person's constitution comes through; after all I weighed 64 kilos, I was in good shape, I had a good heart and good lungs, my blood pressure was always impeccable, and then the edema, wow, when that took over, it got into the pelvis, and after the pelvis, it got up to the heart . . . I also had it in the stomach, in the stomach it also hurt, and then after that it got into the chest, and it got into my face, *I was . . . something horrible* . . . I am telling you, my body was . . . oh, I was really hideous . . . At the end of the hallway there was a mirror; well, I swear to you I didn't look at it, because I said to myself, "God Almighty!"

Surgical interventions and the removal of organs, while they do permit medicine to cure, cause a different kind of injury by compromising the patient's perception of corporal integrity. This problem is experienced in diverse fashions. After a hysterectomy, one 45-year-old woman, who referred to herself as a "happy surgical patient," did not feel any threat to her "entity as a woman":

Since the birth of my last child I knew that I had a fibroma on the uterus and cysts on the ovaries, and last year in May I had a total operation. So there. And all of this I have taken very well, without particular anxiety. I found it a little hard, of course, to get back on my feet after the operation, but ... I mean physically only, because this thing did not affect my entity as a woman at all, as certain people say; when it comes to that, I am not the least bit upset, no indeed ... I know that some women who only have the uterus taken out feel less of a woman because of it, but I, who had both the uterus and the ovaries removed, frankly, it didn't bother me at all, and in fact *I must even say that I am better off than before,* I have no other troubles, like hot flashes and that kind of thing, nothing in my life has been changed ... on the contrary, I find that not to be bothered with menstrual periods is a good thing ... You see, I am quite sure ... listen, I am 45 years old now, I don't want to have another child, do I? ... so whether menopause comes a little earlier or a little later ... no, it didn't bother me at all, I feel just like before.

By contrast, a 39-year-old woman suffering from chronic renal insufficiency who receives hemodialysis treatments is sorry that she agreed to the removal of her kidneys:

I had very high blood pressure. They did all kinds of tests on me, and then they told me, "Okay, your kidney problem comes from high blood pressure." Then I had the operation, and they took out both my kidneys, and now I come to dialysis twice a week. But if I had to do it over again, I wouldn't have the kidneys removed; it was the blood pressure, blood pressure, that's all, because I was not in pain, no pain in the kidneys, no headaches either ... nothing, nothing that hurt ... they told me, "Okay, we're going to remove your kidneys and then we'll do a transplant." So now I'm still waiting ... No, if I had to do it over again, I always say, and I always did say, if I had to do it over again, I wouldn't have my kidneys removed.

Brutal incidents such as a hemorrhage, medical mutilation, and the experience of overwhelming pain that takes over and dominates an individual's entire life: all these serve to remind us that despite the new image of illness, its other face still hovers in the background. Although we may wish to hide it from view, the horror of the sick body sometimes resurfaces. Yet it is no longer dominant, and it may well be that it disturbs us all the more precisely because today it constitutes a relatively rare experience.

Illness Internalized and the Body as Machine

Now that illness can no longer be read as easily on an outwardly intact body, our vision has turned toward its inside: it is within the body, and no longer on its surface, that we decode illness today. This being so, we have had to learn to familiarize ourselves with the accomplishments of a medical knowledge that has become increasingly precise and reliable in the course of time. In medicine, the last two centuries are marked in particular by the development of the anatomo-clinical method—which combines the use of a spatial approach that circumscribes illness within the body with a temporal approach that locates and classifies symptoms in chronological series—and by a newfound access to the inner recesses of the body and the understanding of its functioning thanks to increasingly powerful means of investigation. In the eighteenth century, autopsies began to be performed more frequently, and soon the exploration of the cadaver was supplemented by that of the living body: the ear was reinforced by the stethoscope, and by 1880 the eye was able to delve into the body's conduits and cavities by means of the endoscope. The microscope made it possible to penetrate the infinitely small. Finally, at the end of the nineteenth century, the use of x-rays completely revolutionized the approach to numerous ailments.

For the lay person this new approach to the inner body, first learned in school but gradually integrated through personal contact with the physician, resulted in a renewal of the schemata through which the body is perceived. To be sure, since the Renaissance the image of the body as machine had slowly begun to develop, replacing that of the body as microcosm. In the seventeenth century the term *machine* was often used to speak of one's body. "The machine was falling apart," said Madame de Sévigné.[53] In the eighteenth century Rousseau, who tells us that he had done some reading in physiology, explicitly envisaged his organism as a machine whose parts maintain complex relationships with one another and whose illnesses are analogous to breakdowns caused by worn-out or faulty parts: "After having read a little physiology, I began the study of anatomy, and took a survey of the number and working of the individual parts which composed my bodily machine. Twenty times a day I was prepared to feel the whole out of gear. Far from being astonished at finding myself in a dying condition, I only felt surprised that I was still able to live, and I believed that every complaint of which I read the description was my own."[54] Today this vision is absolutely dominant, although other, more archaic images have sometimes survived as well. A farmer suffering from lung cancer who was hospitalized at Blois in 1972, for example, linked the image of a pump with a metaphor of a different type, comparing the body with a natural element, the river: "I caught a cold there, and so they brought me here . . . I couldn't breathe at all, and since December they have been tapping me. I have water in my lungs, and when the lung is filled with water, the heart swims around in it . . . The longer this goes on, the more I gasp . . . I gasp . . . But once they have tapped me, I'm all right . . . One feels the heart starting up again . . . The other day I jokingly said to the intern, 'Are you sure you haven't hooked up a hose and a pump to these lungs of mine . . . it feels like the whole Loire is running through.' "

But for most people the vision is resolutely mechanistic. In 1960 a 33-year-old technician felt that the body "functions" as long as none of the organs is "out of order": "Illness is an abnormal state in which one organ is affected or no longer functions in the same way, yes . . . one could consider the individual like a very fine machine and whenever there is an organ that has something wrong with it so that it no longer functions normally, it must be repaired if it is badly out of order." In other words, today's sick speak of their sick body in terms of functioning or nonfunctioning organs. People with renal insufficiency undergoing hemodialysis, for example, have an image of the slow deterioration of their kidneys. A 53-year-old woman says:

> It started during my first pregnancy. I had a lot of albumin during this pregnancy and the others as well, and I had attacks of nephritis, very severe bouts, with each pregnancy. Of course, every time I had these bouts of nephritis my kidney deteriorated a little more . . . and with all that albumin also, and all of a sudden the urea started to go up: 0.80 g., and then 1 g. of urea, and I had it all the time. I was put on special diets, and the diets did improve me for a while, but at the end they did almost nothing for me. *It was obvious that my kidneys were completely deteriorated.* I had more than 10 percent of renal permeability. It was quite clear that sooner or later my kidneys would quit, and sure enough, one day the urea hit 2 g. and my kidneys stopped filtering.

Nonetheless, this perception has its problems: it is not always easy to make the perception of the symptoms coincide with the localization of the affected organ. In 1960 many of the persons interviewed expressed their distrust of an organic reality whose obscurity they stressed. One engineer said: "Often one discovers by chance that a pain in the head has to do with the teeth and that a bellyache has to do with something in the kidneys; the pain is not necessarily localized." There can be conflicts with the medical diagnosis. In 1972 an electrician hospitalized for a liver abscess refused to accept this diagnosis in favor of a syncretic vision of some devouring ill:

> This thing got hold of me all of a sudden, that's all . . . I started losing weight and then I completely fell apart, no strength left . . . Suddenly no appetite, nothing . . . I was all worn out. "Good grief," I said to myself, "what is going on here?" I took some quintonine, which I put into a liter of good wine. After that I picked up a bit . . . I ate better. The upshot was that I had to go back to the hospital. So there you are. It came from when I had shingles . . . I did notice it, but *I didn't think that my shingles would gobble up my red blood corpuscles,* but they did, and I was out flat. The doctors told

me that I had a liver abscess, but there is nothing wrong with my liver . . .
I never had a liver attack.

Yet medicine increasingly leads the sick to direct their sight toward the inside
of the body and to adopt their own vision of the ill. In the *Magic Mountain*, already, certain patients enjoyed carrying around the x-ray photographs of their
affected lungs, studying them and eagerly showing them to others. To be sure,
it was exceptional at the beginning of the century to have access to the inside
of one's body in this manner; today it is quite common. For some this perception remains upsetting. The authors of a recent study on hospitalization, the
patient, and the treating physician at a Bordeaux hospital report the following
brusque reaction: "They put a tube down my throat and they said, 'Would you
like to see your stomach?' I told them: 'No, I don't give a damn about my stomach.'"[55] This patient did not want to become involved with a system of knowledge that he could not assimilate. But in most cases—and in this respect a
definite evolution has taken place over the last twenty years—the perception of
the inner body made possible by medical technology is now accepted, even by
people who by their level of education are a priori out of touch with such
specialized knowledge. The sight of the inner body, especially through the
radiological examination, together with the outward symptom, which may be
nonexistent or unclear, provides material proof of illness or cure; here the individual can see the traces of the ill or their disappearance. Like the upper-
middle-class patients of the *Magic Mountain* in 1905, a road construction
worker hospitalized in 1972 for tuberculosis was given the x-ray photographs
of his lungs, the sign of his cure, when he was discharged from the hospital: "I
had a little cough, right, and then they made an x-ray in one of those vans
where they take pictures. They saw that I had something in the lungs . . . I've
been here two months, almost two months, and I'm leaving now. I am taking
my x-rays and everything with me, everything is fine, I'm all better, everything
is as it should be." In 1980 a retired railroad worker accepted the medical diagnosis of myocardial infarction because of the scars visible on the x-rays.

> I was yawning all the time, I sweated, I kept going to the window to get a lit-
> tle air and I felt funny, there was something in the windpipe that bothered
> me, but I didn't have any compression, nothing, nothing at all. And after the
> electrocardiogram the doctor said: "It's a heart attack." I was stunned. It
> turns out that my coronaries are 80 percent stopped up, and when the coro-
> nary arteries are stopped up by fat, the heart muscle is no longer irrigated,
> that's what it is . . . I can't believe it, and yet I have proof in hand, no prob-
> lem about that, *I have the proof of the electrocardiogram* of the first day and
> then the coronary arteriographs and the x-rays they took, no problem there
> either, you can see the scar, *the scar is still there.*

The space of illness, then, has been displaced into the body's interior. At the same time, however, the sick have gone along with, and indeed have adopted, the medical perception and the technical approach to the body. In fact, illness is not the only object of technological procedures today. Prenatal observation and childbirth now involve the deployment of a whole array of techniques for investigating the inner body: amniocentesis, sonograms, monitoring, and so forth. Today the pregnant woman has access not to the image of an ill but to a moving and until very recently inaccessible perception of the unfolding of life within her. In October 1981, a 40-year-old researcher talked about her first and recent pregnancy: "During that pregnancy I was rather impressed by two things. One was the sonogram, the first time when I saw the movement of that little thing jumping around like a flea. Now that impressed me! And then the most impressive thing was, at three months, when they made me hear the baby's heart, this small and very obstinate kind of life in there, which one hears because it is magnified by a device. It was quite moving." Illness today is increasingly often decoded in still another way, namely, through the results of more and more common and diverse biological examinations. In this case bodily sensations and organic and functional signals are relayed not by an image—in which a "reality" of the body becomes concrete—but by figures and formulas that testify to biochemical processes at the level of the cell. Here the space of illness to which medicine provides access is, for the sick person, infracorporal. Illness loses its reality, as it were, becomes detached and abstracted from the concrete body that we know. This is the case, in particular, when medicine discovers an ill in the absence and before the appearance of any symptoms. This is of course the role and the purpose of systematic biological screening, but it profoundly alters the relationship between the perception of the body and the decoding of illness: even before the body has spoken, the individual knows that the illness is or will be there. The psychoanalysts Ginette Raimbault and Radmilla Zygouris have analyzed the following case: alerted by her niece's illness, a mother asks a specialized clinical laboratory to perform a biological test of her 6-year-old child's urine. She does this, as she says later, "*without knowing why.*" The test is positive: the child has an as yet minimal biological abnormality, but there is no clinical sign, "he is not sick." The mother has the tests repeated several times, and eventually the disease does declare itself: it is Alport's syndrome, a severe hereditary kidney disorder. Thus, for several years the disease is there yet not there; although objectively proven by the formulas, it is not present in the concrete reality. As yet dissociated from the child's living experience, it is potentially present both in the test results and in the mother's anxiety.[56]

It is striking to see that today certain chronically ill persons, such as diabetics or sufferers from chronic renal insufficiency treated by the kidney machine, seem to have totally assimilated this approach to their body. Both of these groups closely follow the evolution of their condition and have come to perceive their body in terms of levels of glycemia, measurements of arterial pressure, phosphorus-calcium ratios, and so forth. A 51-year-old woman whom we interviewed in 1981, diabetic for the last 21 years and also suffering from several other diseases,[57] is the prototype of these "new sick":

> To begin with, I know the symptoms of each of my diseases. So as soon as I have an unusual asthenia, I quickly take my transaminases and alkaline phosphates. One can find out right away if it is a flare-up of the hepatitis; if it isn't that, it is something else. *I always have a lab that will do emergency analyses for me* . . . One day they found that I had a glycemia level of 7.4 g.; I'm telling you that this is something to go through, usually one is in an acido-ketotic coma with that . . . Myself, I tolerate hyperglycemia very well . . . first there are the immediate signs, often one is thirsty, one pees a lot, okay, and if the glycemia level is very high, one has acetone as well. In my case, though, the risk of decompensating my diabetes isn't too great, because I think that I have a diabetes that is not subject to decompensation, I'm lucky; I rarely get acetone. As soon as I take five units of ordinary insulin, the acetone goes away, so I'm not in danger I think—in any case, touch wood—I'll never be in danger of an acido-ketotic coma, but some people can fall into a coma with a glycemia level of 3 or 4 grams.

For this woman the objectified knowledge of levels and formulas, of the physiological processes, and of the effects of different therapeutic measures has become integrated into the perception of the concrete and suffering body and has become an extension and deepening of that perception. In her case the representation of the body is definitively marked by medicine, its concepts and its modes of investigation; but this knowledge has been appropriated by the sufferer, integrated into her own perception as a science with which she has become thoroughly conversant.

This involvement even goes a step further in the case of chronically ill persons whose very survival depends on continual therapeutic procedures, external objects, or prostheses that take over from the incapacitated body, such as the daily injections of the diabetic and the bi- or triweekly dialysis sessions for renal insufficiency: these add up to a biochemical body for the diabetic and a body-as-machine for the dialysis recipient. How do their users perceive these devices that permit them to live or to survive? What is vital to my life? What is part of my body? This is the fundamental question asked by these sufferers. For some dialysis recipients—one 48-year-old textile worker, for example, who performs the dialysis at home—the machine has in a sense become an extension of his body, a symbolic part of his self. The machine invades one's life, one maintains a narcissistic relationship with it, and it gives pleasure by making it possible to indulge in forbidden foods. It is a life-giving device:

For me the machine is the main thing, it's essential, after all, it's what keeps me alive. It's *kind of like food*, just about the same thing. If I need the machine I use it, if I need a piece of bread I use it; so there, it's as important as food. Sure, it has a big importance, one must give it that to begin with, and then it takes over the whole day, every day, all year, all one's life, really. That's all one thinks of, just as soon as one is finished with it, one has to start thinking about getting ready again, so one always has that machine on one's mind, I'll never be rid of it. I think of it before, I think of it after, I think of it while I'm using it, I mean, I always think of it. Worse than my wife! I think of the machine even when I don't see it, so *I think of the machine more seriously than of my wife*. It is a second wife. So you can see that it's important all right, very important.

A 36-year-old technical expert, on the other hand, who has been in dialysis for five years and has taken his treatments at home for the last year, has established a strict separation between the machine, a technical means that ensures his survival, and his life and body. There is no confusion in his mind between the technical level and all the others; every human being controls his own life, and it is up to the individual to stay in control of his body:

The machine means survival; if you will [*the kidney*] *is a pumping station*, three times a week I have the pumping station cleaned out, and that's all! So either it is nothing at all, or it takes on an enormous importance. If one finds that it is enormous, one had better envisage something else. If one finds that it is nothing at all, it is perfectly all right. If someone goes in for dialysis and spends all his time lamenting his condition, then it isn't worth it, he might as well go ahead and die, and be done with it. After all, there are so many things to do, and one wants to stay alive, one has reasons to stay alive, one has a family, one loves life. If you really want to stay alive and put up with the treatment, all your problems become very small, but if you make it the biggest thing in the world, it isn't worth it.

The machine is also a life-giving device for a young man of 18 who has been living for 14 years in a provincial intensive care unit, where he is kept alive by an artificial lung. Yet one can detect a certain anxiety in his attitude toward this body-as-machine that may "quit": "The artificial lung sends me air, and if the setting moves I can regulate the dial, I can regulate the respiration a bit. For me it's, it's a completely external life-giving device, but I must always have it right next to me, and it mustn't ever quit." For the other face of survival is the sick person's dependence; and from the body-as-machine to the artificial body and artificial life it is only a small step. One 40-year-old female employee spoke of hemodialysis in these terms: "One has the impression, at least I had the impression, that one is living artificially . . . because one is tied to a machine. One does realize, doesn't one . . . that without the machine . . ."

Illness has today become an individual phenomenon rather than a scourge that marks the social space; moreover, it usually cannot be read in our outward appearance. In a certain sense it has lost its reality; the "body of disease" and the "body of the sick," which, as Foucault has taught us, were not always the same thing in the past, once again tend to become two separate entities. In order to decode our illnesses, we no longer rely on the global vision of our bodies, or even on the perceptible reality of our symptoms, but turn to the infracorporeal messages furnished by medical science.

Our image of the sick, as well as their own self-image, has undergone a profound transformation. Moreover, this development has reinforced the individual character of illness, for the sick person is very often the only one to know of the existence of an illness that shows no sign to the outside observer. By the same token, the decoding of illness has assumed a double face: the sick person also, indeed above all, appears to the world as an inactive and unproductive member of society. Illness and the sick body have thus become the signs of a social status, that of incapacity. It is no longer the transformation of the individual's outward appearance, but rather the disruption of his or her capacity for activity and social integration, along with a close involvement with medicine, that has now become characteristic of bodily illness.

6·

From Causes to Meaning

While physical impairment and the transformation of the body are indeed the means by which the sick recognize their illness, they also wonder about the "causes" of what is happening to them and search for explanations. In the so-called "traditional" societies illness, a crucial though incomprehensible event both for the individual and for the group, always gave rise to questions and interpretations that went beyond the body itself. The problem of the causes of physical suffering is therefore at the core of every society's system of beliefs as well as of the data that anthropology has undertaken to observe and place in a theoretical framework. It is also at the core of the history of medicine. "If one wants to date the origins of true humanity from the moment of the conscious emergence of causal thinking," says Walther Riese, "then the hour of birth of such thinking is also that of a rational, that is scientific, medicine."[1]

The Notion of Cause and the Explanation of Illness

Yet this statement is fraught with many pitfalls, not least among them the very notion of "cause." Walther Riese's assertion testifies to the central importance of the notion of cause in a certain conception of science, but the fact is that for a very long time in the history of medicine, this notion was not at all clear. Foucault, for example, shows very well that at the end of the eighteenth century the classificatory medicine of species still "implied a representation of disease that had nothing to do with the link between effects and cause, with a chronological series of events, or with their visible passing through the human body."[2] The system that made illness intelligible was not founded on the distinction between cause and effect, for in certain cases the effect was given the same theoretical standing as the cause. Foucault also analyzes, in connection with madness, the distinction between "underlying" and "immediate" causes that was made for so long in medical thought, pointing out that the "immediate cause" of the ill was usually almost indistinguishable from the symptom it was supposed to explain; it was little more, Foucault says, than the "causal valorization of the attributes."[3] By contrast, the realm of the underlying causes was infinite, and in the course of the seventeenth and eighteenth centuries in the case of madness it became more and more encompassing and could include all the events of the soul, among them passions, sadness, intellectual work, and meditation, but also events of the outside world as well as climatic phenomena and various aspects of social life. In short, Foucault shows a "polyvalence and heterogeneity of causal linkage in the genesis of madness"[4] that can be found not only in the writings of physicians, but even in its effects on the operating procedures of the asylum.

Moreover, it is undoubtedly a mistake to associate, as Riese does, the notion of cause with the emergence of a scientific thought that is in conflict with all magic and religious conceptions. In this area the findings of medical history concur with those of anthropology. The historian Henry Sigerist, for example, shows not only that in the medicine of ancient Egypt empirical and magico-religious elements were closely associated, but indeed that this magico-religious therapy was founded upon the notion of cause, for the demon or the ancestor that had to be expulsed from the patient was considered to be the "cause" of the illness.[5] The empirico-rational therapy, on the other hand, dealt only with the symptoms, which it attempted to eliminate by material means, such as plant-based remedies. Many anthropological data also show that it is difficult to differentiate, as the anthropologist G. M. Foster,[6] for example, still did only recently, between "personalistic" theories – in which illness is attributed to the active and deliberate intervention of a human being, a spirit, or a god – and "naturalistic" ones, in which illness is due to the influence of natural forces or elements. It is even more difficult to find in these data an irreconcilable opposition between totally magic conceptions and others that reveal the beginnings of scientific thinking.

It is not our purpose to attempt here a synthesis of the contributions made by anthropology or to retrace the history of the etiological theories in medicine. But the problematic nature of the notion of cause must not make us underestimate the powerful need, a need we have found at every turn, to explain illness. It will therefore be useful to try to retrace the manner in which the sick, or at least nonphysicians, have asked questions about biological disorder and to identify the events and the phenomena to which they have related it, regardless of whether this relation fits into the model of causality. Perhaps this will be a way to seize the weight that yesterday's questions and interpretations still carry in our contemporary representations and to find in them the beginnings of today's explanations. Yet here we once again encounter the problem of the autonomy of nonmedical thinking – that of the sick and those who care for them – in relation to medical thinking. The question is whether nonmedical thinking has any independence at all, or whether it is entirely subordinated to that of the physicians. This is indeed one of the areas in which medicine, despite the meandering path it has followed, has had its most obvious impact, for today the "scientific" explanation provided by the physician has acquired total legitimacy. The lay perception of the causality of illness is thus always related to the state of the medical etiological models. Nonetheless, it would be erroneous to deduce from this the idea of a simple subordination of lay thinking to medical thinking. Many examples[7] show that as late as the early nineteenth century, learned medicine had not yet gained complete ascendancy over a whole variety of popular systems of medical knowledge. What we discern throughout the centuries is thus not a one-way dependence but rather circular movements and a constant back-and-forth between learned thought and other ways of thinking.

Even though, as we have seen, our vision of the body has gradually espoused a set of anatomo-physiological categories and become structured through a system of medical knowledge, one can nonetheless state the hypothesis that medicine has never provided a totally satisfactory answer to the question of the origin of illness. "Why me?" "Why now?" These questions still arise when illness strikes today. They demand an interpretation that goes beyond the individual body and the medical diagnosis. The answer that it is given transcends the search for causes and becomes a quest for meaning. We still want to fit illness into the order of the world and of society.

The explanation of illness thus extends beyond the answers given by medicine because it seeks a meaning that they cannot provide; but our explanation also shuns medicine because, at the other pole as it were, explaining one's ill is also a matter of day-to-day observation and perception, which are accessible to every one of us. We all feel that by merely using our senses, we can perceive palpable evidence for a certain number of our ailments. Here medical knowledge is in a sense superfluous. This is what Montaigne expressed when he wrote, speaking of the kidney stones that tormented him: "I observe also this special convenience in this disease—that it is one about which we have little to guess at; we are dispensed from the disturbance which other maladies cause us from uncertainty as to their origin and conditions and progress—an infinitely painful disturbance. We have no need of doctoral consultation and interpretration; our sensations tell us both what it is and where it is."[8] Even today, when we are imbued with scientific schemata, the reference to sensory perceptions still has its place in the explanation of illness. In 1972 for example, a young girl of 17, hospitalized for pleurisy, said: "I caught a chill. *I first felt it myself*, and then the doctors told me that it could have come from catching a chill. That evening, I felt it: I went outside, and I felt the chill." In the same manner we often refer to the sensory qualities of our environment, the air in particular, in order to predict through immediate perception that they will have a harmful

From Causes to Meaning · 101

effect on our organism. In the 1960s in particular, people often evoked the feeling of "intoxication" produced by the environment. "The noise of the streets, the bad smells, all of that attacks me," said a 55-year-old female translator; "whenever I go out in the morning, *I feel that there are a thousand things that attack my health*. The smells ... whenever I pass by a truck, I feel that I am breathing poison. But it is a defense, this sense of smell, because I can feel that I am being poisoned."

Biological Disorder, Upheavals in Nature, and Divine Punishment

One wonders whether this sensory awareness of the quality of the air, the ability to observe climatic phenomena and the immediate perception of changes in their condition are at the root of the importance attributed for so long to *air*, *climate*, and the *seasons* in the medical and lay explanations of disease. It is very likely. For in various guises all of these elements do indeed constitute one of the oldest explanatory configurations for biological disorder, and its traces can still be discerned today. Very early in the history of medicine, above all in the Hippocratic corpus, it marked the beginnings of a vision that, breaking with the conception of disease as sent exclusively by the gods, integrated it into the system of natural phenomena. Although the "aerist" theory, which considers air and climate the primary explanatory factors of disease, was propagated throughout the ages, this climatic determinism may have reached its climax by the end of the eighteenth century. Deeply concerned about the murderous epidemics and epizootics that threatened France's economy, the royal administration—in the person of Turgot—decided in 1776 to create the Royal Society of Medicine, appointing Vicq d'Azyr as its head. For sixteen years, more than a hundred physicians painstakingly noted the interrelations among epidemics, morbidity, climates, and seasons, eventually drawing up a hitherto unprecedented chart of France's health conditions.[9]

This set of ideas, in which air, climate, and the seasons were seen as the primary determining causes of illness, was widely accepted, and the writings of nonphysicians over several centuries show their deep hold in all segments of society. They also show us their complexity. Pierre de L'Estoile, for example, frequently referred to them; in his case humidity usually seemed to be the essential factor: "This season's constitution, which is changeable, gloomy, and humid, there being no day or night when it does not rain, has caused severe illnesses in France with strange and sudden deaths" (January 1606).[10] But it could also be the cold: "Several sudden deaths occurred in Paris this month. Many people toward its end found themselves suddenly seized and afflicted by catarrhs, diarrhea, and dysentery, owing to the outbreak of extraordinary and unseasonably cold weather" (October 1608).[11]

The air could also be "malignant" and "corrupted." "Many continuous, even spotted, fevers, indicating a great corruption," L'Estoile also wrote in August 1609.[12] The notion of "corrupted air," of "corruption," was central to the medical discourse for several centuries, especially when it came to epidemics. Ten years before L'Estoile, in 1599, it was invoked by a physician of Burgos, cited by B. Benassar.[13] "It is not the plague, properly speaking, because the plague demands a universal cause, such as corrupted and putrefied air," this physician wrote in connection with the epidemic that was devastating Spain. But this notion was also held by lay people. In 1717, when she traveled in Turkey, Lady Montagu spoke of "infected" air, also to account for the plague: "I was made to believe that our second cook, who fell ill here, had only a great cold . . . I am now let into the secret that he has had the *plague*. There are many that escape it; neither is the air ever infected."[14] At the end of the eighteenth century, Louis-Sébastien Mercier in his *Tableau de Paris* still adhered to this conception. He also felt that the air was one of the principal vectors of disease: "Whenever the air ceases to contribute to the preservation of health, it kills; yet health is the good for which human beings have the least concern. Narrow and half-closed streets, excessively high houses that inhibit the free circulation of air, butchers' shops, fishmongers' stalls, sewers, and cemeteries cause the air to become corrupted and charged with impure particles, so that this stagnant air becomes heavy and conveys malignant influences."[15] In *Jane Eyre*, published in 1847, Charlotte Brontë, unaware of the role played by lice, still attributed the origin of a typhus epidemic to the miasmas and fogs of an unhealthy climate: "That forest-dell, where Lowood lay, was the cradle of fog-bred pestilence; which, quickening with the quickening spring, crept into the Orphan Asylum, breathed typhus through its crowded school-room and dormitory and, ere May arrived, transformed the seminary into an hospital."[16]

As we can see, the corruption of the air itself could have different causes. It might be the "malignant" combination of heat and humidity, miasmas arising from the ground or from marshes in the countryside, putrid effluvia from human or animal cadavers, but also emanations from living bodies and soiled garments, stagnating air in very narrow city streets—in various combinations all of these notions contributed to the idea of corruption. It is unnecessary for this book's purposes to attempt to follow the evolution of the different formulations or try to unravel their complex articulation. In Mercier's text, for instance, the mention of "narrow and half-closed streets" seems to mark an early foreshadowing of the hygienist discourse that was to come into its own in the nineteenth century, yet his reference to "particles" and to the notion of "heavy" air shows the influence of Boyle's corpuscular theory, which was transferred to medicine at the end of the eighteenth century, by Philippe Hecquet in particular.[17] According to this theory, all bodies exhale minute particles to form their atmosphere, which becomes more and more rarefied from the center to the periphery. The earth itself is a large body, which under certain conditions of humidity exhales a vitiated atmosphere. This "thickness" or "heaviness" of the air, which carries morbid substances issued from bodies contained in it, breeds disease.

But side by side with these notions one finds, at least until the mid-eighteenth century, references of an entirely different order. Related to air and climate, biological disorder also had correspondences with other upheavals of nature: unusual meteorological phenomena such as eclipses, earthquakes, thunderstorms, and tempests, conjunctions of the stars, "heavenly bodies," and comets. Recall the comet whose appearance Defoe evoked in connection with the London plague. Biological disorder was also related to the disorder of human souls who do not conform to God's will. Boccaccio, in speaking of the plague of 1348, joined the explanation by "heavenly bodies" with the reference to God: "Either because of the influence of heavenly bodies or because of God's just wrath as a punishment of mortals for our wicked deeds, the pestilence ... killed an infinite number of people,"[18] he wrote. A passage in L'Estoile's journal also shows us how the phenomena of biological life, unusual and unsettling events in nature—thunderstorms and tempests—and phenomena of social and moral life could become amalgamated in a syncretic vision: "The disposition of the air was malignant, filled with thunder, thunderstorms, heavy rains, and tempests, which, symbolizing the humors of this world, took a great many persons of all ages, sexes, and qualities out of it. Diarrhea, apoplexy, and various kinds of sudden and inexplicable death also killed a great many, bewildering the people who nonetheless did not mend their ways" (August 1609).[19] In January 1606, L'Estoile had already established the same kind of correspondence and had also brought in God. Having evoked the "severe illnesses" brought about by the "constitution of the season," he continued: "A great many murders, assassinations, thievery, excesses, lewdness, and all kinds of vices and impieties have been extraordinarily prevalent in this season ... It is a poor beginning for the year and threatens us with a worse end by the constitution of the weather, which is so pitiful that it seems to weep over our sins in the absence of the fear of God, which in our day is no longer found among men."[20]

The disorders of the body thus have their correspondence in the corruption of both the air and morals. This breakdown of order encompasses the phenomena of nature, those of the organism, and the conduct of human beings. But over all of this hovers the will of God. In the last analysis, it is he who sends illness to us. For several centuries, this conception was the underlying assumption of both medical thought and of society as a whole in the Christian West. It was perfectly legitimate to search for various kinds of "causes" of illness, but God alone was the "primary cause."

Here, then, just as we expected, we come to the limits of the explanation of illness in terms of "cause" alone. For to place God at the root of illness is more than an etiological conception. The reference to God is sometimes stated in the discourse on the same level with all other "causes," but in the deepest sense its role is of an altogether different order. It states the truth about the order of the world and shows us that illness cannot be conceived of as a phenomenon apart from that truth. Thinking about biological misfortune always implies thinking about the world and society, and in ages when God was the great principle of everything, illness was bound to fall within its purview. But this inclusion of biological disorder under the heading of the divine law is much more than the attribution of a cause, even a first cause; it is a statement about the meaning of illness which assigns to the sick a place in the order of the world.

Contagion

Yet, as we have seen, different orders of reference can be brought to bear simultaneously. The ultimate recourse to God did not prevent the gradual emergence of a variety of etiological conceptions. Among them was the notion of *contagion,* which was frequently associated with the corruption of the air. We know that in this respect the observation and the thinking of ordinary people preceded those of the physicians and scientists. It is true that in the middle of the sixteenth century Fracastor had already formulated a theory of contagion and differentiated among three forms of this phenomenon: contagion from person to person, indirect contagion through objects capable of transmitting disease, and contagion at a distance without the intervention of human contact or the exchange of objects. Although the medical profession did not accept these ideas, they were widely held among the common people, who used them to justify a variety of hygienic and isolation measures. In popular language the term *contagion* was synonymous with plague; indeed it was used in this sense by Montaigne in a passage concerning the return from one of his voyages. But Montaigne also expressed the idea of a transmission without contact, related to the quality of the air. Very healthful air can "become poisoned" and carry "contagion"; and this contagion will be all the more virulent for having "mastered" a more healthful air: "But within and without my house I was assailed by a plague of unexampled severity, for as healthy bodies are subject to the most violent maladies inasmuch as they can be mastered only by them, so my very healthful climate, in which contagion, although in the neighborhood, has never in the memory of man gained a foothold, becoming poisoned, produced strange effects."[21]

In August 1603, Pierre de L'Estoile, for his part, mentioned a case of indirect contagion transmitted by imported merchandise: "Toward the end of this month, in the shop at the sign of the cock, rue des Prêcheurs in Paris, was found the plague, of which nothing had been heard in Paris for a long time. It was said that it had been brought in in some merchandise arriving from London, where they were counting 2,000 deaths per week."[22] As for contagion from person to person, it was clearly assumed in a report of 1740 concerning one of the miracles experienced by the convulsionaries of Saint-Médard.[23] Here we read about "a very simple-minded young man suffering from scrofula, because he had slept with one of his master's relatives who had the same disease." Yet in the eighteenth century the notion was not yet accepted by all physicians, and the dispute between contagionists and anticontagionists continued. The already mentioned corpuscular theory, reformulated by Philippe Hecquet in the form of a theory of miasmas, was one of the contagionist theses. Others spoke of a "pestilential leaven" or related the origin of epidemics to living creatures, worms or insects. But the anticontagionists—in agreement, incidentally, with the political powers, which always worried about the panic aroused by the idea of contagion—were not short of objections. They stressed the close relationship between plagues and famine, and one of their main arguments was the character of contagion as a "popular prejudice," which they found to be, not always without reason, redolent of "superstition."[24]

In medical circles the debate about the reality of contagion and the nature of its processes was to last until the time of Pasteur's discoveries and pass through many vicissitudes. Bretonneau's perspicacity in the early nineteenth century did not persuade the medical profession to accept the idea that diphtheria and typhoid fever are contagious. In the middle of the century, Semmelweis did not do much better with puerperal fever. Tuberculosis was not officially designated as a contagious disease in France until 1889, whereas in Spain and in Italy it had been so designated at the beginning of the century.

But then the discovery of the *microbe* and the elaboration of Pasteur's model of specific etiologies brought a complete transformation of all medical concepts, and the hygienist movement acquired a new content. Whereas the hygienists of the eighteenth and nineteenth century had envisaged the combined but imprecisely understood action of multiple environmental factors, ranging from material elements to social conditions, the nascent bacteriology fixed its attention upon the microbe as the last and decisive link in the chain of events by which disease was triggered. Since then, elementary education has so thoroughly disseminated the notion of a microbe-related "specific cause" of illness to generation after generation that it is now stated as an undisputed truth. In reading certain assertions made by today's or yesterday's sick, one might be led to believe that the microbian model is indeed unequivocally identified in our representations as the preponderant cause of illness. In 1961 a young engineer of 31 asserted: "Illnesses are for the most part caused by bacteria." At that time a 41-year-old woman also said: "I think that today illness is really *exclusively a matter of microbes* or viruses, which gain the upper hand and spread, because they have become more or less resistant to antibiotics, or to vaccines, or to other means of defense that have been invented."

Nonetheless, even in 1960 — and this attitude is even more prevalent twenty years later — "the microbe" did not fill the entire space of our interpretation of illness. There was still, for example with respect to the most frightening illness of all, cancer, a quasi-magic image of contagion that had nothing to do with any notion of a microbe. In 1960 a 53-year-old employee suffering from breast cancer told us about a cancer victim's struggle against phantasms of contagion: "I said to myself, 'I have become an object of horror.' I asked the doctor, 'Listen, is this contagious?' He told me, 'You are out of your mind, not at all. People don't know this, people are just too dumb . . . By all means, do eat from the same plate as your daughter, it's all right.'" In this case we also see what positive or negative effects this attitude can have for the sufferer: overcoming such groundless fears is the best way for family and friends to make the sick understand that their affective and social ties have not been broken and that they are not excluded. The woman continued: "I had friends who came and drank out of my glass when I was sick to show me that they still loved me. It was great; it doesn't look like anything, but it is one of those things that made me feel much better." Twenty years later, in 1980, even though information about cancer was much more widely disseminated, a 49-year-old peasant woman from the southwest still said: "I think that there are certain persons who go so far as to be afraid to touch something that has anything to do with someone who has cancer. I think it can go as far as that. There are people who are afraid of that, who say that it is contagious."

Then there are those who may acknowledge the existence of the microbe but nonetheless feel that illness "has no cause." Here is what one young woman of 24 thought in 1960: "That is what I find so awful about illness, I don't think there are any causes for it. You get it because there is a microbe, for example in contagious illnesses. With others, like tuberculosis, one doesn't know. Often they say, 'It's because he is overworked.' So then, did he get it from a microbe? With things like that, you can't tell." Sometimes the specific agent, be it microbe or parasite, is only the foreground to a social dimension, which may, exactly as it did in the past, assume the maleficent face of the "outsider." In the past, strangers poisoned the wells or brought the plague; in 1979, according to the 34-year-old wife of an accountant, living in the suburbs of Paris, they brought lice and scabies: "The parasites in the schools, believe me, it is catastrophic here . . . lice, scabies . . . at the beginning of the school year, all the children should be systematically and thoroughly checked over. All right, you'll say, no wonder with all the foreigners that are here. When I first moved here, there weren't too many people and there were no parasites. Then the foreigners came in, and there are lots of them . . . They are dirty, too, that's why they have brought lice, scabies, ringworm . . . we'll have the cholera before long."

The microbe, then, does not provide the entire explanation of illness. People feel the need to find, as in the old schemata, a "first cause" to explain its presence and its action. Without it, the sick person continues to face the unknown, as we heard from a 61-year-old woman interviewed in 1972, who was not sure how she had "caught" viral hepatitis a few years earlier: "Viral hepatitis is something you can catch without knowing how, it is a virus . . . one can catch it in the hospital, one doesn't realize it, perhaps one has come in contact with someone. And why? *After all, it doesn't just jump on you like that!* Well, one never knows, one may have touched something belonging to someone, or else it's the shots . . . I used to get shots once or twice a week . . . Maybe that's how I caught it? I have no idea. One can't know, it's difficult." Also in 1972, a young mason of 17, hospitalized for pulmonary infection, wondered, without coming up with a real answer, how he had "caught this thing":

> I don't know how I caught this thing. They don't know either: a microbe, it seems. They don't know how, whether it was a chill, or a microbe I caught at work, or maybe in the street somewhere. They thought that it was a tooth; they pulled one of my teeth, but that wasn't it . . . they searched some more and they asked me if I had birds at home. I told them, "No, but there are pigeons, which I sometimes catch on the window sill." So they told me that it might come from that, through a microbe. Or perhaps that I had swallowed a fly, but it may also have come from the motorbike, because I ride a motorbike. I have often heard that one can get tuberculosis from riding a motorbike. But that's not the case here. I don't think it comes from that.

Behind the too specific explanation by the microbe, one thus finds the clear outlines of a sense of frustration and need, the need for a conception that would permit the individual to integrate several causes. "There are several causes to a man's death," an Ivory Coast villager told an ethnologist.[25] "Several causes must come together to get cancer," a young postal employee asserted in the same manner in 1972. There is also a need to relate a given illness to one's environment and one's life as a whole, and thereby to give it a meaning. Only by taking all these factors into account in a multicausal model can we hope to arrive at a full explanation. In 1891, for example, Rimbaud reviewed all the conditions of his life at Harrar in writing to his mother about the cancer that was to kill him, although he mistook it for varicose veins.[26] The disease deposited and marked in his body the entire meaning of his personal history during these hard years: "Bad food, unhealthy housing, inadequate clothing, worries of all kinds, boredom, continual rage amidst the blacks, who are as stupid as they are raffish; it does not take very long for all of this to affect one's morale and one's health very profoundly. One year here is like five elsewhere."

Illnesses Generated by a Way of Life

Today, this integration of diverse factors involves the notion of "the modern way of life," in which the causality of illness takes on an understandable meaning. This notion is already present in connection with the microbe because—like contagion in the old "aerist" conceptions—the microbe is associated with the air. In that case the specific factor is integrated into a larger cause, which takes the environment into account and postulates a fundamental contrast between an urban way of life and life in the countryside. In 1960, an artisan's wife saw a connection between life in the country, air, and absence of pathogenic microbes on the one hand, and lack of air and space in the city, microbes, and illness on the other: "In the country there is air and the microbes don't have anything like the influence they have here . . . In Paris, small living quarters also play a role because if there are a lot of people in one room, there is no air, and as soon as somebody is sick there are microbes." In 1979 a farmer from Hérault thought that the air of the countryside drives the microbes toward the cities: "In the country we have pure air, and that's the main thing: we don't get contaminated as much. And if they say that the flies bring diseases, well, it just isn't so! After all, we have plenty of flies here with the sheep pens. And we also have a lot of air here, *the microbes don't have time to stop*, they keep going, and they stop in the city."

Nonetheless, today, and this was expressed in 1960 already, unhealthy air is not so much a matter of microbes as of pollution. In this manner the contamination of nature and of the human living space by "the modern way of life" and urban society becomes concrete. We now perceive a chain that binds together a specific agent, whether it be microbic or toxic, the quality of the environment, and society as a whole. Pollution, "toxic materials"—in 1960 they were also referred to as "chemicals"—are the fallout of urban concentration and activity, generated by our industrial societies; and they are the cause of illness. In 1960 a 35-year-old painter said: "The atmosphere in a city like Paris can be quite harmful. The doses of CO_2 that people breathe in Paris are bound to cause anemia, and moreover the acid fumes from the fuels that are burned are surely very bad for the mucuses, and that must make it easier for microbes to settle there, it must make for a lot of flu, bronchitis, and such." An engineer was thinking of more serious problems: "They have analyzed the air of Paris and they have found that the fumes from factories and the fumes from exhaust pipes are causing extreme air pollution, charging the air with certain molecules that give people disorders of the blood and of the nerves, and even a certain kind of cancer." In 1979 a young female postal employee sounded the same theme: "If one lives, for example, in an area or a neighborhood where there are lots of green spaces there will be, no doubt about it, fewer illnesses than if you live in a city next to a factory that spits out all these toxins, all that smoke that

may well be toxic." Air pollution is thus one of the essential symbols of city living, of the "modern way of life" that must be paid for with illness.

The "modern way of life," then, is today at the core of our representations
concerning the causality of biological disorder.[27] This conception does, of
course, have its antecedents in the Rousseauist visions of the relationship between nature and society. In the late eighteenth century, in particular, it was
expressed in medical topographies and also in the writings of such social observers as Louis-Sébastien Mercier or Rétif de la Bretonne. Indeed, the indictment of the city and its harmful effects was the original motivation for writing
the *Tableau de Paris*:

> If you ask me how one can stay in this filthy den of all vices and all ills, piled
> on top of one another, amidst an air poisoned by a thousand putrid vapors,
> amidst cemeteries, hospitals, butchers' shops, and sewers . . . amidst the
> smoke of this incredible quantity of wood, amidst the arsenic-filled, sul-
> furous, bituminous vapors perpetually exhaled by the workshops where cop-
> per and other metals are being tormented; if you ask me *how one can live in*
> *this pit*, whose heavy and fetid air is so thick that one can see and smell its
> atmosphere for three miles and more around . . . and how, finally, man can
> abide in such prisons, whereas, if he freed the animals he has fashioned to
> his yoke, he would see them, guided by instinct alone, flee in great haste.[28]

But today the concept of "the modern way of life as cause of illness" is no
longer confined to the medical perspective or to learned elites who study "the
people." It has become a collective representation, and one, moreover, that is
formulated in very complex ways: at the level of the individual, the "way of
life" is a cause of illness; at the level of society as a whole it shapes the pattern
and distribution of illness – and we have seen the encompassing significance of
the "illnesses of modern life" in the collective consciousness. In an even larger
sense, this "way of life" is so pervasive that it corrupts and shapes all the factors
that can affect health. It is precisely this common significance of the various
elements of an individual's spatial-temporal environment, of such factors as
pace of life and forms of personal behavior, that has caused "the modern way
of life" to become an integrative notion, the *foremost paradigm of the causality*
of illness. Yet behind the search for causes, behind the myriad ways in which
the protean content of the notion of the modern way of life permits us to combine and modulate the most varied factors, we once again encounter the search
for meaning. If this way of life begets illness, illness in turn assumes a meaning, for it incarnates and objectivates within the body our negative relations
with what we call our "social environment."

An important part of this paradigm is *food*. It would be tedious to try to retrace
for food, as we have done for the configuration air-climate-contagion-microbe,

the evolution of the ideas by which food has been related to health. The link between them is strong and very old. Throughout the centuries that were haunted by the fear of famine, good nutrition was quasi-equivalent in people's minds with good health. Indeed, for a long time, food was practically the only treatment given to the sick in hospitals. F. Lebrun, for example, lists the components of the diet prescribed for the "sick poor" of the Hôtel-Dieu of Angers in 1588: each one of them was to receive per day a pint of wine and "a loaf of bread made of bolted rye, weighing two pounds *poids de marc*."[29] Roast or boiled meat was served every day, except on Fridays and certain Lenten days. In the same spirit, medical textbooks of the seventeenth and eighteenth century[30] usually included many chapters dealing not only with diets for the sick, whether poor or rich, but also for the healthy, children poor or rich, and convalescents.

The reversal that has taken place in our time is radical. For centuries, everyone associated illness, especially epidemics, with lack of food, famine or shortages. The already cited physician of Burgos from Bartolomé Benassar's book wrote: "The present disease has one specific cause, namely the lack of food for the poor."[31] At the end of the eighteenth century, the same reason was held responsible for a particularly murderous dysentery epidemic in Anjou: "I cannot conceal from you the fact that shortage of food has been the germ of this disease," wrote the intendant of Tours, du Cluzel, in 1783.[32] A century later, malnutrition was still considered one of the principal causes of phthisis. The reader may recall the terrible utterance of a tubercular female textile worker in Lille, cited in the survey published by the Bonneff brothers: "Since I was married, I have never had enough to eat," she simply said.[33] As late as 1914, Maurice Boneff published a novel, *Didier, homme du peuple*, which retraced the life of a syndicalist and tubercular worker. Here again the role of malnutrition is stressed; the author writes about his protagonist: "He has reached the difficult age for the undernourished. When one is young one doesn't get enough to eat, but one doesn't worry about it. Around 25–30, one begins to pay the painful price. One has trouble in the bowels, or else in the chest. If one coughs, that is called having a frog in the throat or else a hell of a cold."[34]

Less than fifty years later, the excess of food has come to be seen by the public at large, and not only among the well-to-do, as responsible for all our ills. In 1960, a taxi driver asserted: "People are overfed with too rich things, and this is very bad for them, that's official." A postal employee, for his part, considered almost with envy the situation of people in other countries who do not have enough to eat: "They say that the French are digging their graves with their forks, one often hears that. You have nations, the Hindus for example, they don't get their fill, well, there are troubles from which we suffer that they probably don't get."

Above all, however, our food today is, like everything else, marked by the impact of "the modern way of life," which has transformed the production of food. In 1960 already, many persons stressed that we are eating products whose "natural" character has been altered by the use of "chemical" elements. Fertilizers, for example, were violently denounced. Among dozens of other persons, a 46-year-old postal employee said: "I have come to wonder even about a chicken egg; they want you to eat eggs when the hen has gobbled grains that were grown with chemical fertilizers; in the meadows where the cows are grazing, they also put chemical fertilizers. Is this natural? Is this the way to respect the ways of nature?" He contrasted the old techniques of food production, in which not only the composition of the product but also the "natural" time span needed for its maturation were respected: "When I spent my vacations with my grandparents in Auvergne, they had an old bread oven, they would make enough bread to last two weeks; they would let it rise for one whole day, and it would stay in the wood-fired oven for three hours. Today the bakeries bake the bread with fuel oil in fifteen minutes . . . Well, *they just fail to observe a natural condition* . . . the dough needs its natural time to rise and one must give it the necessary time to bake; I believe this is very important for people's health." This man, along with many others, believed that this bad or "chemical" food could be the cause of illness, especially cancer; he also said: "Recently I read in the paper about a margarine that seems to have poisoned people in Holland or Belgium, the nature of the poisoning was not stated very clearly in the press . . . but anyway, *this chemistry* that they are putting into food, so far as I am concerned, it is bound to contribute to the flare-up of cancerous conditions."

Twenty years later, these ideas—now supported, incidentally, by the findings of certain epidemiological studies—have acquired an even greater strength. The image of foodstuffs containing heterogeneous chemical elements that "alter" their nature has become more concrete through the notions of additives or preservatives. The image of "fake," "artificial," or "doctored" products, which arises when any intervention is equated with dubious manipulation, expresses the individual's alienation from a society that alters the very staff of life and thereby creates illness. In March 1979, a 46-year-old linotypist said, more or less as one would have said in 1960: "Look at how in these shopping centers, in these department stores, you are forced to eat this or that product, because they just put it before you, because that's all there is, and people have no choice but to eat it. They eat things that are really very bad for them: preservatives, products that are not made for human consumption, and one can really get messed up in a few meals with bad processed foods."

The Wear and Tear of Work

The realization that there is a connection between illness and *work* has taken a different path. Today work, like food, is included as an essential factor in the representation of the individual's way of life as a cause of illness. But in the past, and for many centuries, the sick had nothing to say about this. The medical profession, on the other hand, began very early to study occupational illnesses. In the thirteenth century already, Arnaud de Villeneuve was interested in the hygiene of the various crafts; he analyzed harmful factors such as heat, humidity, dust, poisons, and postures at work, realizing that they may affect workers' health.[35] In the sixteenth century, some physicians studied the lead poisoning syndrome, and in the eighteenth century Tenon described the mercury poisoning syndrome.[36] In 1701, Ramazzini published his *Traité des maladies des artisans,* in which he studied more than fifty occupations.[37] In the nineteenth century, Villermé and the other hygienists conducted their studies.[38] Nonmedical observers, at least those whose testimonies have come down to us — aristocrats, bourgeois, and writers who, although they themselves were not idle, did not feel the burden of excessive labor in their flesh — were unaware of or did not want to see and acknowledge it. Louis-Sébastien Mercier, for instance, did describe the harsh working conditions of the people of Paris: "The traveler, whose first observation yields a much better judgment than ours, corrupted as it is by force of habit, will tell us time and again that the people of Paris are the hardest working, the most undernourished, and seemingly the saddest people on earth."[39] He described these people: "Bent under the eternal weight of fatigue and work, engaged in lifting, building, and forging, plunged into quarries, perched on roofs, transporting enormous loads."[40] But, as we have seen, what he really incriminated as a disease factor was the air, and more generally "the city."

As for those whose bodies were directly harmed by work — peasants, artisans, workers of both sexes (for Madeleine Reberioux has taught us that there were many female workers even in the Middle Ages)[41] — it was not until the nineteenth century, industrialization, and the struggle for social justice that they began to speak and to write. During the campaigns of pamphlets and open letters spawned by the political upheavals of 1830 or 1848, the theme of work and fatigue as sources of impaired health and causes of illness was broached in *Parole ouvrière* in a manner that today would be called "militant." Thus in 1833, a garment worker, Grignon, responded to the manifesto of the master tailors, who claimed that their workers were the best paid and most fortunate of the capital: "Our kind of work may well be the most disastrous of all for health; we assert that our occupation furnishes the greatest number of patients to the hospitals."[42]

All the trades participated in this denunciation, usually on the grounds of the workers' premature death. In 1848, during the National Assembly's hearings on working conditions in France, the testimony of a mine worker of the Loire region was heard. He felt that if the living and working conditions of the miners were not improved "one would soon see the greater part of the workers invalided at the age of thirty-five or forty." He added: "It is an acknowledged fact that the average worker does not live beyond the age of thirty-eight or forty."[43] In 1870, the newspaper *La Marseillaise* reported a worker's speech during a general meeting of the strikers in a sugar refinery: "Piece work is killing and ruining us; that's what makes us sick: and then they accuse us of intemperance, and when we are sick and worn out they give us two days' notice. If we don't want to go under, we must absolutely work a little less and earn a little more."[44]

Henceforth, the main emphasis was placed on the workers' exploitation and the effects of work on the body. Recall also the controversy over tuberculosis which raged at the end of the century:[45] Was it caused by living in the slums, as the medical profession thought, or was it brought about by "the wear and tear of excessive work," as the labor unions claimed? Work does wear the body out, and certain occupations do kill, and so the Bonneff brothers gave the title *The Killing Occupations* to one of their studies of work-related illnesses. "The departments where heavy industry has been established," they asserted, "have the highest level of mortality from tuberculosis. *To remedy this state of affairs, more is needed than the promulgation of sanitary regulations. What needs to be resolved is the social question.*"[46]

Today this theme of wear and tear from overwork is still sometimes sounded by aged workers. Here, for example, is a 65-year-old man, hospitalized in 1972 for excessive respiratory insufficiency. He was worried about his retirement and wondered how he could live on a reduced income when he was no longer working. Like his fellow workers of earlier generations, he had "worn himself out" working:

> My asthma goes back to the war, for one thing I had to sleep in the water when I was a prisoner, and then it kept getting worse. I got emphysema and then it was the heart, what with working so hard. With a lot of extra work I got heart attacks, and now I can't take anything anymore. I have my mother who is 85 and my wife who has been very sick for the last seven years, and so I have worked a lot, thinking about retirement. I was afraid that I wouldn't be able to pay my rent in Paris, the telephone bills and all that, so I worked very hard to buy myself a little house, and that is above all what makes you get sick. *It's no wonder that I'm sick, I have worked a lot, I am worn out.* If you think that I started when I was 11, and that I am 65 now.

In 1972 as well, a worker in the printing trade blamed his working hours, especially the so-called "3 × 8" system, to explain his palpitations: "I never used to have palpitations. I wasn't doing the same kind of work; but today I'm doing it, and I can tell you one thing, it's a tough pace. Not the work itself, but the working hours. I am working the 3 × 8 [that is, three eight-hour shifts at the plant, implying that each worker's hours must rotate among morning, afternoon, and night shifts], so of course that's rough. No question about it, it's very hard, and the body doesn't take it very well."

In 1960, a 35-year-old house painter also spoke of today's working hours, which, owing to commuting time, become very long in the big cities: "They tell us that working hours are much better now than in 1900. In fact, there is nothing great about it, because in 1900, if somebody worked ten hours, he lived right next to his work, and when he had worked ten hours he could go to bed and get some rest. Now somebody may work eight hours, but then he has an hour on the Métro, plus an hour on the bus, plus a half-hour on the train . . . Now of course this is bound to produce lack of sleep, *nervous tension and anxiety*, which is very bad for people." The contrast between this "now" and (a quite probably mythical) "1900" brings out once again the idea of a "modern way of life" marked by work, subordinated to the demands of every individual's occupation, and conducive to illness.

In 1960 this conception was predominant, but for the members of the middle class it was not so much a matter of organic wear and tear as of disintegration of psychic capacities. Such people spoke of "lack of balance," of "fatigue" or nervous "tension," and of "anxiety." A good example was a taxi driver who went beyond his personal case and spoke about his occupational group as a whole: "Of course with the life in Paris, a nervous person is bound to get very worn out, because our job in itself makes for a lot of nervous tension. So it turns out that I am worn out, like many others, but that's not a personal thing, it's like this for all of us who are in this job: we all complain of nervous fatigue, it's because of the traffic, of living in Paris." Another taxi driver spoke for the entire collectivity: "In the cities, what with modern life, there are many people who certainly worry too much. Modern life, the way it is, leads to a lot of worry, which often has to do with the job, with responsibilities, and with stress, so that people live with a kind of anxiety. A kind of nervous tension that can probably indirectly cause trouble for the heart or the arteries."

Actually, this conception of the relation between work and illness, indeed the whole representation of a harmful way of life, is of a rather schematic nature. It is often used, not so much to speak about individual states of health and concrete working conditions, together with the social relations to which they have given rise, as to denounce, in rather abstract terms, the "agitation," "stress," and "anxiety" spawned by modern life, which has somehow become a global environmental phenomenon that affects every individual in the same way. In the same manner, this "indictment" of "social conditions" is a matter of expressing our relations with them; illness serves as a signifier, as grounds for condemning what we call "society." Nonetheless, we feel compelled to place the vision expressed in this condemnation into a natural context, and therefore tend to objectivate "society" in the form of material environmental conditions, such as polluted air, adulterated foodstuffs, and so forth. Illness literally embodies our unsatisfactory relations with society, but this relationship must assume a material character, must affect nature by perverting it, before we can feel it in our bodies; and in fact, we are all affected in the same manner.

In the 1960s the representation of what triggers illness thus posited a "modern way of life," amounting to the vision of a bad society—seen as a global entity that manifests itself most obviously in material ways—facing individuals who are both similar to and isolated from one another and more or less alienated from the network of social relations. It is a rather striking fact that at that time work-related illnesses were almost completely absent from the representations of the middle-class people whom we interviewed. As we shall see,[47] a more specific awareness of the relationship between working conditions and health was to assert itself in the 1970s.

But even in the 1960s, the feeling of being outside of society, of being under constraint, was forcefully expressed in the vision of the individual in society that underlies the conception of "way of life as cause of illness." A 50-year-old woman translator, for example, analyzed in the most concrete terms the constraints imposed by her way of life, which she was powerless to change:

> So I went to the doctor, and he told me: "If you change the relationships that surround you, with your daughter, your husband, your way of life, your work, your colleagues . . . you will get better." What am I to do with this kind of advice? It may be perfectly correct psychologically, but in practical terms it is worthless, because one cannot completely reorganize one's life. One is in a certain situation that is a given. One doctor said to me: "You should quit your job." Very nice, but what if I said to him: "You should quit *your* profession?" One would have to change one's entire way of life, and that just can't be done.

This woman's feeling of being unable to "cope" with life was also expressed by many other persons whom we interviewed. Their life, many said, "was not suitable for them," indeed, they thought that it was not suitable for human beings in general: "I think that the human machine can't really take this way of life," a young female teacher told us, for example; "big cities usually just make people sick." More than with the causes of biological misfortune, such a vision is concerned with the definition of society and human nature itself. Several persons expressed the idea that the very nature of human beings is changed by the modern way of life and modern society. Their statements hark back to the vision of the relation between nature and society that came into being in the eighteenth century: "I believe," said a postal employee in 1960, "that man, despite the achievements of progress, finally becomes corrupted." "Why is it," wrote Restif de la Bretonne on the eve of the French Revolution, "that man is so easily corrupted? I believe that perhaps he must, like the tree or the animal, always dwell in the soil where he was born."[48] In this manner the social evolution is seen as victimizing the individual, whose exemplary representative is the sick person. The conception of a "way of life as cause of illness" is thus far more encompassing than the identification of social causes within an organicist medical model of illness that tends to disregard social causes. In the 1960s illness was seen as the sign and counterpart within the individual's body of a failure of modern society and of the degradation of humankind. Twenty years later, these ideas are being formulated much more precisely and some of them are expressed by the collective consciousness.

Lay Representations and the Medical Debate

This set of conceptions closely corresponds to a whole trend in modern medicine. In the last decade in particular, the greater control over infectious diseases and, on the other hand, the increasing incidence of chronic illnesses have turned medicine's attention toward other etiological models than that of specific causes. Emphasizing the limits of modern medicine in the control of illness and stressing the need for prevention, there is a whole literature that insists on the urgent need to conceive of the causality of illness in terms of many factors. It calls for a systemic approach, which, by endeavoring to analyze the interrelations among different variables, is the only means to advance our understanding of illness. This larger conception of health and illness must include, first and foremost, the variables relating to the individual's social and physical environment. In a polemical article that gave rise to considerable debate in English-speaking countries, John Powles shows how certain improvements in the "way of life" (nutrition and hygiene in particular) have contributed to the reduction of illness as much as the advances of medicine.[49] But, he adds, "unfortunately this new way of life, because it is so far removed from everything to which humans have become adapted through evolution, has produced its own burden of illness. These illnesses caused by faulty adaptation are greatly on the rise."[50]

These ideas are not shared by everyone, however, and the debate has divided the medical community. For example, Dr. Lewis Thomas, the director of cancer research at the Sloane-Kettering Foundation in New York, believes that every disease has a causal mechanism that is unrelated to our "way of life." "Every disease has its own unique causal mechanism that dominates everything else. If you are looking for effective means of treatment or prevention, you must first find this mechanism and start from there . . . I believe that one day it will be discovered that cancer is the result of a single bad switch somewhere deep within the cell. I do agree that there are vast amounts of cancerogenic substances in the environment, each one of them capable of triggering cancer, but at the core of the problem there is this switch that cries out to be discovered."[51]

What are we to make of this correspondence between lay perceptions and the medical debate? Should we assume that we are dealing with a successful dissemination of scientific notions and theories that have reached and convinced the general public? There is no question that in certain areas—for example, the connection between tobacco and lung cancer or the effect of specific pollutants—information has been widely disseminated, particularly in the last few years. Yet the concept of a way of life as source of illness is much more than a matter of dissemination of scientific thought; the problem is infinitely more complex. It is a fact, to be sure, that in the 1960s information about these themes—in books or articles for the general public, or news in major newspapers and other media—was still rather dispersed. Moreover, certain "established facts"—among them the connection between tobacco and cancer—were precisely those that elicited a good bit of skepticism or outright incredulity.[52] Still, the collective representation of a harmful way of life appears to be a phenomenon endowed, at least in part, with its own dynamic. Linking fundamental anthropological schemata—illness as something "out there," disease entities attacking the intrinsically healthy individual—with the sensory perception of an environment and conditions of life shaped by industrial activities and urbanization, this consciousness goes back to the eighteenth century. This framework can serve to integrate bits and pieces of information gleaned from the corpus of scientific knowledge and the medical debate, but these can only be assimilated and assume a meaning because they match already existing sociosymbolic schemata.

As the example of contagion has already shown, we must therefore understand the connection between learned and lay conceptions as a reciprocal relationship. Actually, the present environmental and preventive orientation of the medical profession is nothing new. It harks back to the hygienist conceptions of the eighteenth and nineteenth centuries, and if the debate has assumed renewed vigor today, it has in fact been carried on for more than a century. This debate also testifies to the deep anthropological roots of medical thinking, which may well be fed by the same sources as lay thinking. Today's medical debates are based, to be sure, on sophisticated epidemiological models, yet they also make use of observations taken from the schemata of collective thinking. Moreover, medicine itself has not completely dismissed the problem of meaning. Medical science, as the nineteenth-century hygienists said, is by its very essence a social science, and many of today's physicians would agree with them. Medicine therefore cannot turn its back on the vision of society which is at the core of the concept of way of life as the cause of illness.

Facing One's Own Illness: The Hidden Meaning

All of these etiological concepts — air, contagion, microbes, or way of life — have one point in common: they all refer to *illness as attacking human beings from the outside*. Yet anthropology has taught us that in most human societies concepts of disease oscillate between two poles, the "exogenous" concept, in which illness is embodied in an external factor and seen as an aggression, and the "endogenous" concepts, which in various ways see *illness as residing "within the individual" and connected with that person*. This idea of illness coming out of the self is sometimes expressed in the lay discourse in the extreme form of a "being" of illness that all of us carry within ourselves and that at some point comes out into the open. In 1960, a 31-year-old businessman exposed his vision of the origin of illness to us in these terms: "In my opinion, everyone is sick, but most people don't know it; by this I mean that *we all carry illnesses within us* . . . and, depending on the stage of life where we find ourselves, circumstances, or nervous state, these illnesses do or do not come out."

In 1917 Franz Kafka invoked the idea of "two beings" doing battle within him, one of which — the good being — he identified with the trauma of his tuberculosis, although it was the other that had inflicted it and benefited from it. He wrote to his fiancée, Felice, a few weeks after his illness had been diagnosed:

> These two beings that are doing battle within me . . . are on the one side a good being and on the other a bad one, but sometimes they switch masks, which makes this confused battle even more confused . . . It is now clear that the loss of blood has been too great. The blood that the good being (for we must now see it as good) sheds in order to conquer you benefits the bad being. At the very point when the bad one by itself probably could no longer find anything decisive and bad to defend itself, the good one offered it this new element . . . The blood does not come from the lungs but from the — or a — decisive blow of one of the combatants. The latter now has the succor of this tuberculosis, a succor as immense perhaps as that which a child finds in its mother's skirts. What more does the other combatant want? Has the battle not ended brilliantly? I have tuberculosis and that is the end of it.[53]

In both of these cases, the great writer and the anonymous individual feel, although in very different ways, that the illness has an autonomous existence. Lodged within the individual, it nonetheless has its own being. To be sure, this "ontological" vision is not the most widespread. More often the endogenous conceptions of illness postulate an upheaval of the organism, a breakdown of its harmony that also involves its relations with outside factors. In the Hippocratic theory already, the "temperaments" were the product of an equilibrium among the natural elements (air, fire, earth, and water) and the "humors" that made up the individual (bile, blood, black bile, and phlegm). For centuries these notions, spilling out beyond the limits of learned medicine, structured the discourse of ordinary people and informed their self-perception. In the seventeenth century, for example, Pierre de L'Estoile described the medical care he received from his physician, M. de Hélin: "Very learned, very wise, and very expert, he treated me well and gently according to my humor and complexion."[54]

Then, in the middle of the nineteenth century, the notion of heredity, whose specter, as J.-P. Aron has put it, "had stealthily made its way in medical thinking for a century, suddenly broke into the everyday vocabulary."[55] Yet Aron also tells us that heredity was at first, and remained for a long time, a social and institutional notion, a means of codifying filiations and intergenerational ties, before it came to express a body of knowledge concerning a biological reality.[56] Mendel's laws of hybridization, formulated only in 1865, were forgotten for a long time until the science of genetics came into being. In the early nineteenth century, not even the most famous dictionaries of natural science included an entry on "heredity." To the lay person, the whole question of the nature of blood ties had always been a mystery. Here, for example, is Montaigne, wondering about the phenomenon of family resemblance, which seemed wholly incomprehensible to him: "What a wonderful thing it is that the drop of seed from which we are produced bears in it the impressions, not of the bodily form alone, but of the thoughts and inclinations of our fathers! That drop of water—how does it contain this endless number of forms? And how does it convey these resemblances, whose course is so headlong and irregular that the great-grandchild will resemble his great-grandfather, the nephew his uncle?"[57]

The idea of a hereditary taint, on the other hand, of the transmission of illness within a family, has existed—as even the Bible attests—long before there was a general understanding of the problem of heredity. What is involved here, ever since the Atrides, is the perennial nature of evil and its resurgence generation after generation. It is indeed the theme of evil, biological and social evil, that was sounded in the guise of "tainted blood" in the middle of the nineteenth century, and we find it not only in the medical theories of degeneracy but also in Zola's works and in the anxiety that came to pervade society as a whole in the face of alcoholism and syphilis. This moralistic attitude toward pathological heredity persisted for a long time. Alcohol, debility, and physical degeneracy of almost monstrous proportion are associated in the horrifying description of the children in Léon Frapié's *La Maternelle* (1905):

All these children carry a thousand stigmata of degeneracy. Here is little Doré, who is cross-eyed, along with twenty others who are victims of the same alcoholic heredity. If it is not the eyes, it is the hips that give out: we have here a whole collection of crippled hips, and we also have three kids that limp, not counting Vidal the hunchback; as for those with rickets, twisted limbs, or scrofula, we don't even mention them, we might as well take the whole lot, more or less. The resemblance with animals is not to be dismissed: many of the children, just like Richard here, have the faces of monkeys — old, deeply wrinkled faces that have a hard time puckering into gaiety. We have a whole lot of fish heads with droopy mouths, cat heads with flattened noses, he-goats with the flat pate of a cassowary, of greyhound jaws, and of chins that look as if they had fallen off or as if they were a long, morbid excrescence.[58]

As late as 1960, the discourse of two teachers — is this just a coincidence? — was of the same order. Here is one of them, a 50-year-old male, who had taught for more than 20 years in the same village of Normandy: "One sees an awful lot of children who are not normal . . . For example in my case, where I have been here for 23 years, I am teaching children of my former pupils; in certain families one can see that *alcoholic degeneracy* is being passed on, skipping one generation . . . I have in class, for example, several very clear cases of children whose father is sober, but the grandparents, whom I knew very well, were alcoholics, and well, now the grandchildren are suffering the consequences."[59]

Yet it is doubtful that the idea of an impairment exclusively linked to the lineage was ever dominant. If, as we believe, there is always a search for meaning behind the search for causes, how could anyone go along with the idea of illness as consubstantial with his or her family except in the most atrocious despair, the despair of Oswald in Ibsen's *Ghosts*, for example?[60] Indeed, people usually feel that a pathological heredity is present in *others*; the bourgeois sees crippling defects in the children of alcoholic proletarians, and the lower classes see "last of the line" degeneracy brought about by the debauchery of the aristocracy. For ourselves, on the other hand, all of us must uphold the idea of an outside aggression if we are to face the ruin of our bodies with anything but utter horror. The neutrality of the genetic concepts developed in the last few years has not made any difference in this respect: our "way of life," not our DNA, is at the core of our collective representations of illness.

Nonetheless, many persons perceive and accept the idea of the individual's participation in his or her illness. Frequently this is seen as a participation by default: in 1960, "weak points," and more or less persistent "reduced states" that diminish the individual's resistance were invoked, but outside aggression by the way of life remained essential. A judge said: "One may have something within oneself, one may be in a state of greater or lesser resistance . . . the illness strikes at the weak point." Today the notions of "heredity," "constitution," "terrain," and individual "predispositions" are associated and at times merged in the discourse; a related notion is that of "living conditions" that have left irreversible traces. A young postal employee interviewed in 1979 included all the conditions of her own life since childhood in this complex: "Some people are much more prone to illness than others, this is also a matter of *constitution . . .* there are *hereditary factors,* I mean what their life has been since birth, how their childhood was, how they have developed in adolescence, what they do as adults, all of this goes together." At that time also, a 78-year-old woman, the widow of an executive, accounted for her "gall bladder attacks" by evoking the living conditions of earlier generations, which she associated with the idea of "race": "Unfortunately this runs a bit in my family; my father had liver colics, my grandmother had the same thing, as does my son, and my grandson as well. I am Jewish, you see, and so we certainly belong to a very old race; and this has to do with the wearing out of the race. Besides, our ancestors lived in hot countries, a very special climate, so now we pay for that."

But the notions of heredity, favorable terrain, or predisposition are only one part of the tradition. Throughout the ages, the recognition of an intrinsic relationship between the individual and the illness he or she carries has been stated even more frequently in terms of the role played by the sufferer's soul, humors (gaiety or sadness), morale, and psychic state in the triggering of illness. One only has to look at a few examples to become convinced that this is indeed a fundamental intuition. In the age of the great epidemics, it was widely assumed that a happy person would not get the plague. In the sixteenth century, Montaigne linked the good health of the native peoples of Brazil to the serenity of their souls: "That which we are told of the people of Brazil, that they die of nothing but old age, is attributed to the serenity and tranquillity of their climate; I attribute it, rather, to the tranquillity and serenity of their souls, freed from all perturbation and care and laborious or unpleasant occupation."[61] Descartes shared this conviction when he wrote to the German princess Elisabeth, who was ill and about to leave for a water cure at Spa, that if she took care "to consider only objects that would bring her contentment and joy . . . I do not doubt that this alone would be capable of restoring her to health."[62] In 1960, an industrial salesman still expressed the same theme: "After I got married I have never been sick, and I have the feeling that I don't get sick anymore because I am happy."

Conversely, sadness and sorrow have been recognized at various times, by lay people and even by the medical profession, as the direct causes of illness. In 1608 Pierre de L'Estoile analyzed the death of the Queen of England in these terms: "The unanimous opinion of the Queen's physicians and of those who assisted and served her privately in her chamber is that her illness was caused by a sadness that she had always kept very secret."[63] In June 1848, Balzac wrote to Madame de Hanska: "Now I will tell you that the sorrow that devours me is causing dreadful ravages in my physical state . . . That is why I have gradually reached a point where my heart is in such a state that I am unable to make a violent movement; I cannot climb a staircase without getting palpitations that make me stop cold. Just from writing you this, I am bathed in perspiration. The trouble is not in the organ so much as in my morale."[64] In 1972, a 49-year-old unemployed pianist interpreted the incipient tuberculosis for which she was hospitalized in this manner: "I believe that this is a general state resulting from a long, long, long unhappiness, long, long, long suffering, a great many tribulations in every area of life. It is almost, one might say, the end point of twenty-five years of uninterrupted suffering."

Illness Spawned by the Self

Today, more frequently perhaps than ever before, "morale" and "psychic state" are taken into consideration in accounting for organic illness. At the slightest incident, we all think, and often say, that the trouble is "psychosomatic." The way we express this may vary according to social class: "Illness begins a little bit in the imagination, in the head," said a young house painter in 1960, whereas in the same year a 37-year-old female writer said: "My subconscious calls the illness and takes refuge in it." These two statements translate essentially the same intuition, that of a complex and somewhat mysterious interaction between the body and the psyche. This is the explanation that Rousseau already gave for the rather strange ailment—with buzzing in the ears, palpitations, weakness—that plagued him for several years while he was living at Charmettes with Madame de Warrens:

> Meanwhile, my health was not completely re-established; on the contrary, I was visibly wasting away. I was as pale as a ghost and thin as a skeleton. The beating of my veins was terrible; the palpitations of my heart were more frequent. I continually suffered from shortness of breath, and my weakness at length became so great that I could scarcely move . . . There is no doubt that my illness was, to a great extent, attributable to hysteria (*vapeurs*). This, which is the ailment of happy people, was mine. The tears which I often shed without any cause for weeping, my lively charm (*frayeur*) at the rustling of a leaf or the chirping of a bird, my changeable disposition amidst the calm of a most happy life—all these were indications of that weariness caused by happiness, which, so to speak, leads to an extravagant sensibility. *We are so little formed for happiness in this world, that of necessity the soul or body must suffer*, when they do not suffer together, and a happy condition of the one nearly always injures the other. When I might have enjoyed life

heartily, the decaying machinery of my body prevented me without anyone being able to localize the cause of the evil.[65]

Scholars have indeed often stressed the likelihood that Rousseau's ailments were of a "psychosomatic" nature, pointing out that at the time he was forced to live as the lover of a woman for whom he felt a great deal of affection but little desire. Although the writer himself was apparently unaware of this possible cause and did not feel, as we do today, that physical illness was the expression of a revolt of his entire being, he did voice the idea of a kind of price to be paid: the body, he said, pays for the happiness that the soul is unable to accept in all simplicity. In 1972, a 40-year-old man who worked as an official of the Algerian railroads also saw his illness—a violent attack of dysentery—as a kind of ransom; ransom for a professional success. Engaged in the investigation of a railroad derailment in which twenty-four people died, he had, as he said, "taken this business terribly to heart." He had to fight hard to have his views accepted, but in the end "with everybody watching, I won. Everyone was forced to accept my version. I was very fatigued from all the work, all the traveling, to the point that on the night of this victory I broke down with a horrendous case of dysentery, which started up that very night. It was overwork, and then also, I have always been just a little bit violent, and I have had inexplicable mishaps before, after I had been through violent emotions."

In the Romantic vision of tuberculosis, which is no doubt one of the most elaborate expressions of the "illness of the individual," the idea of a "ransom," a "price to pay," is also present, but here it is the ransom for being an exceptional person, the price to be paid for passion and genius. But, as we have seen,[66] consumptive individuals "welcomed" their illness, made room in their life for an ailment in which they recognized themselves. This theme of the "consent given to illness" is a kind of corollary to the ransom that must be paid. This is another notion that one encounters again and again in the most various kinds of discourse. Proust, for instance, wrote to Madame Strauss, who suffered from an ailment that the writer contrasted with "organic illnesses": "I remember that you told me that M. Hale had become better because he was so afraid of going to a spa. But he had an organic illness that may have left traces. You, fortunately, have nothing that can stay with you; in your case all that is needed is that your body refuse to consent to being ill."[67]

In the 1960s several persons expressed not only their acceptance of illness but even their desire for it. A young architect said: "It has always given me pleasure to evoke the possibility of being immobilized for a certain time, of being placed into a certain universe apart by an illness." Such statements translate the vision, shared by psychoanalytic theory, of a flight into illness on the part of a person who is caught in an unbearable situation. This was expressed very clearly in 1979 by a young woman of 33, a teacher by training: "My illness is very psychosomatic; I had a pinched vertebra, I couldn't move, at times I was almost paralyzed and, well, that happened whenever I couldn't stand it anymore, it was my way of calling for help because, when all is said and done, it has to do with loneliness. *Loneliness of the body when it is pinched*, when it cannot breathe properly and can't function . . . it's like life, which should go on without being blocked."

In this case the illness, even if the sick person surrenders to it in the face of an unbearably painful conflict or situation, is not the root of the evil; on the contrary, it is the individual's ally, the physical outburst, almost the outburst of vitality, that permits her to escape an even greater catastrophe. Moreover—as psychoanalytic theory claims, and as everyone firmly believes—illness provides us with "secondary benefits," for it makes it possible to escape from the sometimes unbearable constraints of everyday life. In 1942, Dr. René Allendy, a psychoanalyst, evoked in his diary the illnesses of his childhood: "I remember the deep pleasure of snuggling in my bed, knowing that for an undetermined length of time I would not have to make any effort or bear responsibility for anything."[68] In 1960 a young professor, in speaking of what childhood illnesses can mean, expressed an even more subtle vision: "I had the feeling that I was discovering a different universe . . . because [when I was sick] there was a certain gentleness to my life that was exceptional . . . I had five brothers and sisters, and therefore had never known what it was like to be coddled; now I had *a kind of universe apart*, just for me, something that deep down I needed . . . because I believed that I needed exceptional conditions to become myself . . . and in that situation, when I no longer had to stand up for myself and to stand up to the others, I was much freer to become simply myself."

In this perspective individuals identify biological illness with the most valued and the deepest part of their personality, contrasting it with the social personality that is shaped and demanded by an alienating society. In certain other cases, however, biological distress seen as "illness spawned by the self" becomes an unacceptable reality that can lead only to despair. This happens when a very severe and intensely life-threatening illness such as cancer comes to be seen as the sign of a failure of our entire being. It also happens when the sick, unable to read within themselves anything but the failure of their entire existence, come to consider the bodily reality of that existence particularly intolerable. Illness, more than any other manifestation, compels the recognition of definitive defeat by materializing it in the body. We have seen the distress of Fritz Zorn, who was convinced that his cancer was but the ultimate expression of his total inability to cope with life.[69] We also sense the distress of Kafka, writing in the previously cited letter to Felice: "Deep down, I do not consider this illness as tuberculosis, or at least not primarily tuberculosis, but rather as the expression of my complete bankruptcy." "And now," he continues, "I am going to tell you a secret which at the moment I don't even believe myself . . . I will never be well again."

No wonder, then, that in such cases all of us are loath to recognize our illness as "spawned by ourselves," as expressing a breakdown of a different kind: that of our entire person. We find it difficult to speak of death except when we deny it, said Freud; in the same manner we find it difficult to admit our own and irremediable failure. If the meaning of our illness is within ourselves, it remains almost always obscure to us. Just as we ourselves only perceive the defects of our neighbors, so it is usually *the others* who tell us that we ourselves have spawned the illness. And when that happens, despair turns into anger, into the refusal to accept this interpretation, which the sufferer experiences as an intolerable aggression: Susan Sontag wrote *Illness as Metaphor* as a reply to those who claimed that her cancer signified her defeat as a person.

III·

IDENTITIES OF THE SICK

7.

Fate or Disease without the Sick

*I*n studying the evolution of our vision of the body and its relation to illness, we have shown the growing impact of medical knowledge on our thinking and the progressive dominance of a mechanistic yet, paradoxically, abstracted vision of the sick body. By the same token, however, the limits of this vision have become palpable, for although medicine has provided us with the categories through which we perceive the body with greater or lesser precision and accuracy, it cannot provide the answer to our questions about the nature of illness. The fact is that we want to know not only about the causes and mechanisms of illness but also, and especially, about its meaning. Such questioning is grounded in the importance of several major notions, which serve as schemata of reference for different visions of the world. God and the order of the universe have long been considered the "first causes" of illness, and indeed have given a structure to its meaning, but we today seek to understand and interpret our illnesses in the light of our vision of society.

These orders of reference operate on more than a symbolic level. They are reflected in the institutions that take charge of illness and the sick. The charitable institutions of the past, for instance, were inspired by a religious vision, whereas the late nineteenth century progressively put into place the social laws that define the status of the sick to this day. These institutions, and the major references to which they are linked, are therefore the anchoring points to which the sick relate their state, as well as the "reality" that structures their identity. We shall see how this identity asserts itself in different ages, and we shall follow the development of the figure of the sick person as it emerges from the intertwining of a certain form of pathology, a set of values and dominant visions of the world, the state of medical knowledge and its impact on the existing pathology, as well as from the institutional system of health care.

Submitting to Fate

For many ages the sick and those who cared for them invoked the terms *destiny* or *fate*, inherited from the ancients, in order to give meaning to the changed relation with the world entailed by illness. These notions were used in an effort to explain the transformation that was visited upon the sick, a transformation that amounted to a loss of identity. For in the most remote past, illness was not considered to be part of human nature. Otherness and impotence were the outstanding characteristics of the sufferer and his or her personality. To be sick was to undergo an ordeal, to be no longer oneself, but rather the receptacle for an outside event, the completely alien illness that struck the sufferer. Fate, understood as humankind's relation to an order beyond it, was brutally and irremediably visited upon the sick person.

In this manner the sick were no longer in control of their lives; first of all because they were materially threatened with death, but also because they were alienated from their present life by the foreignness of their condition. The future became uncertain, but the continuity with the past and with their earlier personality was broken as well. This recognition of an irremediable transformation of one's own person, of being dead while still alive, is without question one of the essential ways of apprehending illness, and one that recurs throughout the ages. We see this feeling expressed in almost identical terms over a distance of several centuries. Here, for example, is the anguish mixed with resignation of Samuel Pepys, who was going blind and wrote in his diary in May 1669: "And thus ends all that I doubt I shall ever be able to do with my own eyes in the keeping of my Journal, I being not able to do it any longer, having done now so long as to undo my eyes almost every time that I take a pen in my hand; and, therefore, whatever comes of it, I must forebear; and, therefore, resolve, from this time forward, to have it kept by my people in long-hand, and must therefore be contented to set down no more than is fit for them and all the world to know . . . And so I betake myself to that course, *which is almost as much as to see myself go into my grave.*"[1] In 1960, a farmer immobilized for life by an accident also said that, although alive, he felt as if he were dead: "Here I am, forced to do nothing, and the worst of it is to watch the others work and to be unable to do the same thing . . . I am more than half dead, much more dead than alive."

Sometimes the horror inflicted by fate was such that to fight back was not only useless but insane. Death appeared to be the only solution; it could be voluntary, or else family and friends must inflict it on the person who was already condemned by the biological *fatum*. In the early seventeenth century, Pierre de L'Estoile repeatedly mentioned cases of rabies in his journal. This disease, perhaps more than any other, was perceived as a tragic and irreversible blow dealt by fate. The individual upon whom it was visited became entirely alienated, separated from himself and his companions, and cut off from any future, for it was believed that rabies transformed human beings into animals.[2] In the face of this threat, rabies victims were usually strangled. The inevitability of such an end was understood by everyone, including the sufferer's next of kin, regardless of their feelings. In one case a young woman was poisoned by her own husband: "At that time it happened in Paris that a very beautiful young woman, about twenty-seven years old and the daughter of a saddler, living in the rue de la Harpe and newly married to a saddler by the name of Cordon, was bitten on the hand by a little dog that she had and became rabid. And because she was above all afraid that she would be strangled, as is usually done in such cases, a means was found to make her die a more gentle death by giving her a poisonous medicine, which she took very happily (even though she knew what it was) from the hand of her very husband and died three hours after she had taken this medicine" (April 1604).[3] In another case, also cited by L'Estoile, the sufferer himself acknowledged the dehumanizing transformation he was about to undergo and asked for his death even before the symptoms of the ill had appeared: "On that day a page, having been bitten by a rabid dog in Paris, had taken to the road in order to go to the ocean (which is considered the supreme remedy in such cases). As he passed through a forest, he was scratched by brambles and thorns, which drew blood. As soon as this poor page saw it, having been warned that the sight of his blood would make him utterly rabid (which is held to be absolutely true and inevitable), *he asked his companions to strangle him as gently as they could.* This the others did in tears and with the greatest regret" (July 1603).[4] During a rabies epidemic in eighteenth-century Anjou, the sufferers were still bound in chains like dangerous animals and left to die. "One could see them," says an eyewitness, "tear themselves to pieces amidst pitiful cries and finally expire."[5]

Yet this fatalism was never complete; human beings tried to fight back even in antiquity. Forcefully struck by their impotence throughout the ages, they nonetheless continued their struggle against their inevitable destiny. As we have seen in connection with the great epidemics—which, more than any other ill, were the very incarnation of the idea of destiny—this resistance could take a great variety of forms, ranging from sanitary measures to prayers, medical remedies, recourse to healing saints, and witchcraft. Today, and for more than a century now, our attitudes toward illness decidedly favor action, struggle, and victory over biological misfortune. It is therefore all the more paradoxical that the notion of *fate* is still present in today's sick. This very term was used in an interview of April 1981 by a 52-year-old diabetic. The behavior of this woman, who participated in a patients' self-help group, struggling and "negotiating" with her illness as well as with the medical profession—and we shall come back to this[6]—was the very opposite of fatalistic resignation. Yet the idea of fate still had meaning for her: "I have always considered illness a fate . . . For me, illness was something that was written in my stars and what is more, it was bound to happen to me, because I have never had any luck anywhere."

More generally, of course, some people feel that death is always foreordained: "I do believe, in any case, that death is foreordained . . . it's fate, in any case," said a 41-year-old female worker in 1979.

The Order of Things

Even if we would like to forget it, the struggle against illness and death always encounters its limit in the end. That is why some people feel that death is the "normal" issue of illness, that it is part of a natural order, "the order of things," which we must accept. This attitude was expressed in 1960 in the meandering musings of an elderly lady of 76, Madame K., who suffered from a heart condition. "To pass away, that's inevitable; suffering perhaps is not, but death is . . . listen, so far I have never met anyone who lived beyond a normal life span . . . let's say it is 100 years or so . . . I don't know any centenarian and, my goodness, I wouldn't particularly like to become one . . . but *there is a normal limit to life*. No, I don't mean to say that I find this normal because I would find it useless to go on living . . . I find it normal because that's how it is."

In 1960, more than today, this idea of a natural order including death was an integral part of the discourse about illness. It could be stated in many different ways. To a 33-year-old technical agent, for example, who reported his perception of the death of old people in the common room of a hospital, death was "normal" and even "to be looked forward to": "I have seen people die when I was at the Caen hospital; this was in a general medicine ward when I was doing my military service. There were a lot of old people, and during that time I saw many of them die, I mean perhaps ten; well, if it's an old person, it doesn't strike you in the same way; it seems more natural somehow . . . when you see people who have already been bedridden for some time, you feel that their strength is gone, and it didn't upset me very much . . . you know it's going to happen, and you almost look forward to it."

The same idea appeared in response to one of the questions asked in our survey, the one concerning "the possibility of a world without illness."[7] The majority of the persons interviewed believed that this was impossible and held that illness and its corollary, death, are not only "natural" but also "necessary." "It is necessary for people to die," said a 46-year-old technician. "As soon as we are born we are destined to die . . . it is necessary for people to die, that's the law of nature, we must die and make room for others . . . look at the plants, the flowers and everything, *that's how it is, one appears and one dies, it's a law of evolution*, it makes a circle . . . and if that natural selection were done away with, how could we go on? Life would become impossible because there would be too much of it, that's it."

By 1980 the ineluctable and "natural" character of death was not forgotten, but this recognition was decidedly less present in the collective consciousness with respect to illness; and in any case it was stated much less readily and frequently. Yet today, no less than yesterday, the image of illness is still that of a sudden, unforeseeable, often inexplicable and inevitable calamity, which has not lost its age-old character as a blow of fate. When it strikes, human beings are faced with their impotence. In the 1960s, a 54-year-old woman shopkeeper evoked the death of her husband 15 years earlier, as well as the more recent death of a relative: "My husband started with what we would call today an infectious flu, an abscess in the throat and so forth, and within ten days, despite the greatest specialists in Paris, he was dead; it was a galloping form, even though he was a man in excellent health. I have an aunt, she lost her son eleven months ago, a boy who was absolutely in the best of health. This again was a sudden and absolutely unexpected illness." For her, the situation had not changed between 1945 and 1960. But in 1979, a skilled female worker still asserted: "When one gets a disease, you know, sometimes one doesn't expect it; there are diseases that come on all of a sudden." Sudden illness is still wrapped in mystery, the shopkeeper continued: "Illness can strike, but where it comes from, one can't know . . . it's quite sure that if people lead a regular life, in principle their health is stronger, only there are cases that absolutely . . . this fellow of 48 who led an absolutely regular life and suddenly he gets a brain tumor, where did that come from? And how did he get it? Was he hit on the head when he was a child? So much out there we don't know . . . Myself, I am very fatalistic: the illness is there because it's there . . . but how? It's very hard to know."

Above all, most people felt, nothing can be done. Many ills are impossible to prevent, asserted Madame K. in 1960. "Illness, I don't believe that it can be avoided, because everyone without exception gets sick, I don't know anybody who hasn't been sick, if only because of accidents, and one can't escape those in life . . . there is always the same number of sick; the hospitals, I believe, are more crowded than ever. Nowadays people take better care of themselves than they used to, but I don't think it has done any good." Madame K. unhesitatingly applied this general observation to her personal experience—to herself, who suffered from a heart condition, and to her youngest daughter, who had died from leukemia two years earlier. "Take the disease that my youngest daughter died of . . . Now there, really, I don't see what precautions one could have taken to avoid it, I don't see at all what could have been done to avoid such a death . . . cancer, leukemia, in my opinion, there is nothing that can be done about it . . . and in my case, for example, I don't see what I could have done to avoid it, if my heart was like that."

On this basis, certain persons interviewed in 1960 claimed that ignorance was a positive thing. One must not tell the sick the truth; they are better off if they do not know. The shopkeeper asserted: "Myself, when dealing with sick people—and I have seen a lot—*I think they shouldn't be told* ... really, if they are very sick, they shouldn't be told ... I think the severely ill don't realize how bad it is ... I would even say that this is a mercy from God. When my brother-in-law died he weighed thirty-eight kilos, but he never saw himself. The day before he died he talked to his doctor about taking a trip to Russia ... no, they mustn't be made aware, because it seems to me that to know that one is finished, on the way out, that it's just a matter of days ... it's too horrible." Another woman, 44 years old, put it more starkly: "What difference does it make whether a disease is deadly or not? ... what difference does it make whether or not one knows it; if one has it, one has it ... *it's better not to know*, both ahead of time and when it happens; and, in any case, one can't do anything about it."

In the last twenty years the idea that action is always possible and that in order to prevent illness one must know "ahead of time" has made considerable strides, and such clear-cut statements to the effect that nothing can be done and that it is best to remain ignorant have become rare. The disillusioned resignation or stoic acceptance of these women no longer strikes a responsive chord in us. For many of us, impotence in the face of illness has become an unbearable, indeed almost scandalous, failure. And yet it still exists, but it is now expressed by the seriously ill, and by them alone, with a clairvoyance that shows their despair. A 60-year-old milliner, hospitalized for lung cancer, did not know the exact nature of her ailment, which she believed to be caused by "a microbe." Yet she described the evolution of the illness that brought her to the hospital without much illusion: "In the long run I couldn't help but see that I wasn't getting any better, and then I also had to realize that I was losing my strength, and so I had to do something ... I just had to try. One can't always get things fixed, but one can at least try ... Of course there are illnesses that can't be fixed ... that sort of thing has absolutely nothing to do with human will, it can't be helped, it's fate ... well, that's just how it is."

The same attitude was expressed by a 65-year-old farmer who also had lung cancer but thought that it was a heart condition. In our conversation with him, we sensed his distress in the face of this sudden assault that foiled his plans for retirement:

> The heart, all of the sudden it doesn't work any more, it just gives out, I couldn't breathe at all, oh my ... That's how life is, just when you're real happy, and then bingo! ... just then I was saying, "I'm going to be 65 years old, I'm going to retire." My wife is already retired, she is 72, so it's just the two of us in the house, the children are grown up, they are married; well, I said, "I have a few little pieces of land that I own, and so I am going to work a bit in the summer when the weather is nice, and in the winter I'll just putter around the house nice and quiet .." Well, and now ...

We can also sense his incomprehension and his resigned impotence:

> Where it comes from ... I sure have no idea ... All I can do is ask the doctor, but he won't say. The other day I said to Dr. P., "It still hurts in here." He said to me, "I know it, Monsieur X.," but he didn't say what it was. "I know it"; sure he does, better than I, but ... well, I just have to wait ... I have to, and I may die tomorrow ... what else can I do if I have to ... can't do anything about it.

Since 1960, however, the context in which the conception of illness as foreordained is expressed has evolved. In 1960, it was linked to a system of values centered not so much on resignation as on physical endurance and especially on will power and self-control—in short, on a certain stoicism. It is no coincidence that the attitude to adopt in the face of pain was one of the key points of this conception. The shopkeeper whom we previously cited told us: "My sister and I had babies within two weeks of each other. We had a doctor—although at the time births took place at home, with an attendant—and he had told us: 'The ones who scream the most are the lower-class women, the better a woman is brought up the less she screams,' so my sister and I we had made it a point of honor to give birth properly; you didn't hear a sound ... so one can hold back ... and yet I had a terribly hard delivery, but no carrying on, not one scream, I mean ... this pain went on inside, if you will."

We know, and indeed this woman expressed it very clearly, that such values are typical of middle-class people, for whom nothing is more important than to set themselves apart from the lower classes. It should probably also be noted that these notions were held by persons over 40 who had little use for "new" ideas. Thus, when the so-called "childbirth without pain" became a rather widespread practice, several women, all of petty-bourgeois background and all over 40 years old, told us in identical terms: "I could never have done childbirth without pain." A vision of the world founded on stoicism continued to shape their attitudes.

All of this was perfectly expressed by old Madame K. She felt that illness, which cannot be prevented and which, like death, must be accepted because "that's how it is," is nonetheless a defeat. "It is a calamity, *but one has to put up with it*. For me, illness is something a bit shameful, and that is why I don't like to talk about my physical miseries, why I don't want to see a doctor ... For me, to be ill is always a sign of inferiority." Madame K.'s stoicism, in short, had nothing to do with a submission that would include, for example, attaching a positive value to biological misfortune. She was not afraid, she said, of inevitable illness, but she was determined not to let her life be dominated by it until there was no other possibility. She accepted death, but it was out of the question for her to become "a sick person," and even less "an invalid"; and she had fought what she considered the stigmata of illness every step of the way. "I got my first eyeglasses," she said, "at 75. Before that I considered my eyesight sufficient, and now I am sorry that I have to wear glasses ... *I feel diminished* ... Deafness, blindness, all these things that come with old age are awful; many people make you repeat everything ten times; I would rather not understand, not hear it, and I don't say anything ... I wouldn't wear a hearing aid for anything in the world, no indeed."

The dependence on others that comes with illness was also unbearable to Madame K. During an acute phase of her heart condition she felt humiliated by being taken in charge or, as she put in, "treated like a charity case." "I was out of it, by this I mean that I was not involved in any way, they followed a course of treatment without asking my opinion, put me in a room by myself, treated me sort of like a charity case; I find that rather humiliating." She refused as much as she could: "They gave me morphine, things like that that made me feel inferior, and I struggled not to let them do it to me." When she was taken in charge by medicine "without being involved in any way," Madame K. sought neither to negotiate nor to know. "Something to do with the heart," she said about her illness, "I can't understand it very well, and I have never asked my doctor, haven't tried to get to the bottom of it." No doubt she felt that to find out the exact nature of her illness and to take an interest in it would be tantamount to letting herself be defined by it. Much better to refuse this consent as long as possible. "Sometimes I go along, but most of the time I don't, that's all there is to it," Madame K. said very simply, in speaking of her doctor's instructions.

Illness without the Sick

In serious illness, however, refusal gave way to a total passivity, which constitutes an ultimate form of denial. Rather than accepting themselves as "sick persons," ratifying this definition of themselves, the victims of illness preferred to become objects, objects of medicine. "When one is sick, either one doesn't pay attention and thinks that it will pass, if it isn't serious; or else one goes along with everything, *one becomes the object of medicine*, if you will." In that case, Madame K. also said: "My illness cannot be a worry for me, it is a worry for others." With this statement, Madame K. expressed an ultimate denial: "It is not I who is ill."

Twenty years ago, then, the response to biological *fatum* was often an uncomplaining acceptance of illness and death, coupled with a refusal to admit the loss of identity, the living death that is associated with it. Today by contrast, as we shall see later, many people accept being "a sick person." They go along, often in the most minute detail, with everything that is involved in this well-defined role, adopting, sometimes even enjoying, all the behaviors associated with this identity, which they have made their own. But it is as if, much more than in the past, they refused to die of their condition. Human impotence, which not long ago was seen as an evident fact, has now become intolerable. Death is not so much the "natural" outcome of illness as the result of incorrect behavior on the part of the sick person and the physician. But, of course, it always wins out in the end.

Among those who feel that their end is near, the seriously ill, the notion of fate reemerges, as we have shown earlier. But it is no longer embedded in a system of values; it has become necessary as the ultimate explanation of this experience that is about to engulf them. In the face of death—as they know, even if society as a whole wants to forget it—human impotence is complete. The milliner cited above said simply: "When one is seriously ill, it is fate. One is destined either to die or to recover ... At least that's how I see it, I really don't know. If one recovers, it's better, of course. If one doesn't, well, that's too bad."

The sick who feel that they have reached the end sometimes envisage their fate with great lucidity. Witness this 79-year-old architect who was hospitalized for cancer of the prostate and who, although he avoided pronouncing the name of his illness, had no illusions about its outcome: "This is the beginning of the end," he said of his state at the time; "I know perfectly well that this illness will go on to its conclusion ... It is an illness that can't get better, its name is marked on the chart over there; no, it can't get better." Such people "accept it," they say. Some of them, like the milliner, are simply resigned: "I accept it ... uh, sort of, *I have to, I guess*; I'm not saying that I like it, but I do accept it." Some of them are serene, like the old architect, who refused to undergo a mutilating surgical intervention: "I did not want the operation, because at my age I prefer to stay as I am and go off quietly ... I am all prepared to get on my little raft and to let myself drift off with the current." He also said: "One must see things as they are. We are on earth to live as long as possible and as agreeably as possible; and then *one day one has to go.* And without regret. One should go without regret." But this acceptance, this concept of illness as an ineluctable fate, is usually no longer part of a view of the world. It only comes after the sufferer has been brought up short against reality. Yet perhaps these notions do constitute a refuge from the potential feelings of guilt for the failure that death has come to represent in our day. In this sense today's sick, like those of 1960, assert that they are not responsible for their illness and for their death.

The reason is, no doubt, that the illness has already destroyed them. "Nothing is left of Tchekhov, the illness has swallowed him up," said Katherine Mansfield when reading the Russian writer's last letters. In the same manner, we are struck by the bleakness of the picture that these sick persons, even though their resignation protects them from the most absolute despair, draw of an existence from which social networks, relations with others, and frames of reference, especially with respect to them, have been progressively eliminated. They are lonely; as the milliner said: "There are times when it would be nice to be with someone, but I said to myself that with all this coughing it is better to be alone. Because if someone were right there it wouldn't do; it must be disagreeable to hear somebody coughing and not be able to help at all; for others that is quite a stress too." The dying face the bleakness of an existence from which they no longer expect anything. "I have come here to get treatments; well, I knew it would have to be like this, that's all there is to it . . . no use looking for more." Time, the future, or plans no longer exist. "Life is over now; I have no plans for the future," said the architect at the end of his interview.

Today, then, just like twenty years ago, though in a different sense, one might say that illness as fate has become *illness without the sick*. In 1960, this was because the sufferer refused to be "a sick person"; today it is because, even though the sufferer is still alive, nothing is left of a being invaded by biological fate.

8·

The Burden of Sin: Sinners and Penitents

*I*n the Christian West, the ancient notion of *fatum*, of illness as fate, was an integral part of the religious notion of evil, in which human destiny was controlled by the will of God. Here illness had a precise meaning, for God sent it to humankind as punishment for its sins, its sinful nature. The two conceptions, that of fate and that of divine will, thus did not contradict each other. The Apostle Paul said: "Wherefore, as by one man sin entered into the world, and death by sin; and so death passed upon all men, for all that have sinned."[1] In the most ancient Christian vision, illness was indeed linked to sin, but it was not, as in certain antique conceptions, the direct and unequivocal result of individual wrongdoing. A specific illness could not be strictly related to a personal transgression; rather, both had their origin in the imperfection of human nature.

In fact, some of the early Christians—and this is sometimes seen as one of the reasons for the spread of Christianity in times of calamity, such as the great plagues—looked upon illness more as an opportunity for redemption and salvation than as a punishment. In 251 Cyprian, the bishop of Carthage, wrote in connection with the plague that was raging in the region: "Many of us are dying in this mortality; that is, many of us are being freed from the world. This mortality is a bane to the Jews and pagans and enemies of Christ; to the servants of God, it is a salutary departure. As to the fact that without any discrimination in the human race the just are dying with the unjust, it is not for you to think that the destruction is a common one for both the evil and the good. The just are called to refreshment, the unjust are carried off to torture."[2]

Punishment and Salvation through Illness

In later centuries, particularly since the sixteenth, following the Council of Trent, this version gave way to other and more directly punitive concepts, which again rose to the surface in the nineteenth century. In the face of cholera, certain writers, among them Joseph de Maistre, still asserted that God was punishing vice and sin.[3] Pascal also spoke of punishment in his famous *Prayer for Making Good Use of Illness*, which he composed in 1654 when he was ill himself: "Thou gavest me health to serve Thee, and I have used it only for wordly ends. Now Thou hast sent me illness in order to correct me. Do not permit me to use it to irritate Thee by my impatience. I have made bad use of my health, and Thou hast justly punished me for it; do not let me make bad use of Thy punishment."[4]

But Pascal went beyond accepting punishment; he demanded it because it was also the remedy for the real illness, that of the soul. Here *the sinner becomes a penitent*, and the suffering of the body becomes the means of redemption. "Make me understand that the sickness of the body is but the punishment and at the same time the outward sign of the sickness of the soul. Oh Lord, cause it to become the remedy by making me aware, through the pain that I feel, of the pain that I did not feel in my soul, sick though it was and all covered with sores . . . Make me feel this pain strongly, and help me make the rest of my life a continual penance that will wipe away the offenses I have committed."[5]

Pascal felt that the only possibility of salvation was in total submission to God's will. In such an attitude, the difference between health and illness, indeed between life and death, is abolished. "I confess that I have considered health a blessing,"[6] he said at first, but then he continued: "I do not know what is best for me, whether it is health or illness, wealth or poverty, or any of the things of this world. This is a knowledge that is beyond the understanding of men and angels, it is hidden in the secrets of Thy providence, which I adore without seeking to fathom them."[7] The prayer also says: "I ask neither for health nor for illness, neither for life nor for death; I ask that Thou mayest use my health and my illness, my life and my death, to serve Thy glory, my salvation, Thy Church, and all Thy Saints, whom I hope to join through Thy grace."[8]

Here suffering has a meaning and a mediating function; it embodies the sufferer's hopes of joining the community of saints. But it even has a function in this world, for it enacts the image of Christ on the cross. In the Middle Ages already, the revulsion and horror usually spawned by biological misfortune gave way to the veneration inspired by some of the penitent-sick, the "poor sick," who also came to be called "Our Lords the Sick."

Throughout the ages, we can discern the influence of the Christian conception of suffering in diaries, letters, memoirs, and even novels. The sick considered and defined themselves as sinners from the outset; they had no doubt that they were being punished for their sins. Thus Pierre de L'Estoile stated in 1610: "This illness . . . kept me tied to my room and my bed, which I was unable to leave for two whole months. During this time my weak nature, which is keen to feel pain yet has no feeling for sin, and is slow to mend its ways yet quick to complain, caused me great suffering in body and mind. *For this I blame my sins alone,* for I have received great blessings from Thee, oh Lord, but I have thanked Thee for them only as a matter of form."[9] The sick asked for God's help in tolerating their ordeal. "For . . . all the discomforts that will accompany my being blind, the good God prepare me!" wrote Samuel Pepys on 31 May 1669. In 1822 Abbé Delille reported the words of the dowager Duchess of Orléans, who suffered from breast cancer: "She said that God alone could offer comfort for the greatest suffering; that one could find it by resigning oneself to His holy will and by pouring out all one's feelings into His fatherly bosom."[10]

At the threshold of death, the sick affirmed their confidence in the divine promise of life eternal. "As for me, I am certain that I am going to God and to the dwelling place of the blessed," the dying La Boétie assured his friend Montaigne.[11]

In Charlotte Brontë's novel of 1847, Helen Burns, the little consumptive who is dying, speaks similar words to young Jane Eyre. Jane, frightened by the idea of death, asks her: "But where are you going, Helen? Can you see? do you hear?—I believe, I have faith; I am going to God!—Where is God? What is God?—My Maker and yours; who will never destroy what he created. I rely implicitly on his power, and confide wholly in his goodness: I count the hours till that eventful one arrives which shall restore me to him, reveal him to me.—You are sure, then, Helen, that there is such a place as heaven; and that our soul can get into it when we die?—I am sure there is a future state; I believe God is good: I can resign my immortal part to him without any misgiving."[12]

Edifying accounts of the death of men and women, bourgeois and great aristocrats, and less stylized testimonies as well, show that the words and phrases that the dying have used to express their suffering and respond to it have not changed throughout the ages. This very permanence, this quasi-ritualized form of expression, makes it difficult for today's reader to appreciate their full meaning. Our modern sensibility does not always clearly perceive the fears, hopes, and expectations that are expressed or hidden by these words, which strike us as stereotyped. Yet historians have taught us that emotions and feelings also have a history, and that words which have become a mere formula for us may at one time have constituted the collective expression of the most intimate sensibility. At the same time we also know that in the early-modern period, and certainly in the preceding ages, the religious faith of the poor, especially in the countryside, was sometimes casual and routine. There is evidence to show that many of them had an intense fear of death and that they did not want to think about it. The hold of the Christian conception of death no doubt varied considerably depending on circumstances and social milieu.

God Alone Can Heal

Nonetheless, this conception furnished the predominant pattern that structured people's representations and shaped their individual experiences. Its motivation operated on two levels. On the one hand, a religious conception responded to the need for meaning. At a time when "dying well" was the most important concern,[13] the Christian vision assigned to illness a positive function as a warning and as a means of salvation. However, recourse to the Church also mitigated the feeling of impotence in the face of illness when all human action had failed, for God could help the body as well. The physician's first duty was to call the priest to his patient's bedside to minister to his soul; but sometimes the intervention of the priest contributed to the healing of the body. The last sacraments, it was thought, often restored the sufferer to health. Perhaps it is in the spontaneous notations of Pierre de L'Estoile's journal, rather than in purposely edifying deathbed accounts, that we can perceive this twofold motivation for the constant recourse to God. In 1609 and 1610, L'Estoile repeatedly complained about the illness that tormented him, describing it as a "melancholic ailment" compounded, moreover, by bouts of "tertian fever." As we have seen, L'Estoile stated that his illness was a deserved punishment: "I attribute all of this to my sins and to the offenses I committed in my youth, which God has seen fit to chastise by sending me a sickly old age."[14] Yet this ordeal was also the sign of divine mercy. L'Estoile accepted it as such and hoped that it would bring his salvation: "But in all of these accidents I have always found, and still find, comfort in the thought that affliction in the house of those whom God recognizes as His own is a sign of His secret mercy, and that the prosperity of others is a sign of His secret indignation. God preserve me from ever wishing to be at ease in this latter fashion; may He on the contrary do me the grace of not refusing me any pain in this miserable life, so that I may win Christ and a blessed eternity."[15]

Yet, and Pierre de L'Estoile frequently made this point, "the worst in all of this is that I can do nothing about it."[16] The efforts of medicine and the physicians were also useless, indeed harmful; in December 1610 he wrote: "For myself I can truly say that, being very ill at that time, I would have died if I had not stopped taking the physicians' bleedings and remedies."[17] "On Wednesday the 8th, my ailment not having been improved by the bleeding, I was forced to take a purgative prescribed by M. Hélin, even though I did not expect it to give me relief any more than all the rest, for in this wretched illness I learned that most remedies do more harm than good. Only those of the Great Physician can help."[18] God alone can cure the ill he has sent. "Only the one on high, He who has inflicted the wound can heal it,"[19] Pierre de L'Estoile also wrote at that time. More than any other medicine, recourse to God's mercy and prayer are thus the best means to seek relief.

On Wednesday the 24th, Saint John's feast day, after precisely one month, I left the house to go to the Augustins' Church, having kept to my bed, my room, and my house, unable to leave them, from the 24th of last month until today, having suffered eleven bouts of tertian fever attended by great agitation of body and mind. For the relief of these troubles I availed myself of the advice of M. Hélin, a very learned, wise, and expert physician who treated me well and gently according to my humor and complexion. And yet, to tell the whole truth and to give all the glory for it to God, as is fit, I will say that in all my illnesses I have never yet found, and still do not find, anything that serves and sustains me more and gives me more relief and comfort than the reading of God's word, meditation about it, and prayer.[20]

"Making good use of illness" could open the gates of heaven for human beings. But in the face of overwhelming suffering, which remained a profound mystery even when it was recognized as the fruit of sin, recourse to God was also the best hope for relief, even in this world.

For us it is strange to observe that for centuries religious sentiment, prayer, and appeals to divine mercy were no obstacle to the most superstitious practices and even magic. Remedies provided by physicians and empirics, penitences and pilgrimages to healing saints, and formulas of magic incantation formed a set of expedients of which people availed themselves indiscriminately. Some of these expedients were extremely equivocal; according to the strict orthodoxy, healing saints, for instance, were only supposed to intercede with the divine will on behalf of the faithful. Yet it is obvious that they were often considered as magic healers in their own right, as miracle workers whose effectiveness was linked to the observance of material rites.[21] In fact, we must always be mindful of the fundamental ambiguity of religious sentiment, especially in the countryside, and of the fact that it was "imbued with magic, which in turn imbued religion."[22]

But what else was there to do? Robert Muchembled has shown very well that in the French countryside, especially in the Middle Ages, but even until the eighteenth century, "recourse to secret practices, formulas, and rites that could hardly be called Christian was the only means of survival available to populations that were always in danger, living as they did in villages where there was neither a doctor nor a trained midwife."[23] Muchembled makes a good case for the importance of the soothsayer-healer, who combined the functions of the physician, the priest, and the man of learning.

But the positive image could easily become negative, and the healer could turn into a sorcerer endowed with maleficent powers. By the same token, the conception of illness as willed by God could easily give way to the idea that it was triggered by the maleficence of a sorcerer in the service of the Devil.

The Spectacle of Christian Death

The Christian conception of illness undoubtedly had its apotheosis in the "Grand Ceremonial"[24] of death in the early-modern period. This collective ritual, which starkly expressed a vision of this world as the equivalent of evil, served to transcend human impotence. The dying, who were fully aware of their state, were the main actors in the spectacle of their death; dominating their suffering and their weakness, they knew the strict etiquette and the precise steps they must follow in proceeding from the adieus to the survivors to the spiritual exercises that would prepare them for the encounter with God. In the process, the sense of their suffering was also revealed, for all the bystanders felt that the wrenching separation from this world was transmuted into a blissful return to God. The carefully staged ritual of the grand ceremonial thus acted out and embodied the Christian conception of suffering.

Michel Vovelle has masterfully analyzed these scenes of the exemplary Christian death, especially among the great of this world.[25] He makes us follow, step by step, the death of Anne d'Autriche, who died of cancer. Her demise was described by two witnesses, Madame de Motteville and Madame de Montpensier;[26] the latter reports the manner in which the Queen Mother was informed of the impending fatal outcome. Once the physicians have retired, God enters the stage. The grand ceremonial is directed by the Archbishop of Auch. He says to the Queen: " 'Madame, your condition is worsening; you are believed to be in danger.' She hears these words and receives them with most Christian sentiments."[27] "She asked for her confessor," adds Madame de Montpensier, "and told us, 'Please leave me; I no longer need anything, all I have to do now is think of God.' " Madame de Motteville in turn describes the precise moment when the sufferer perceives the double face of death: "She had a clear view of the terrible moment that would soon separate her from this earth forever. She wished, to be sure, to go to the place where she would enjoy that everlasting rest; but before she could possess it, that part of her which was corruptible would have to end; and this transition, which is dreadful for all of us, and which she considered to be such despite her constancy, was momentous enough to absorb all of her thoughts."[28]

Then, after the confession, comes the farewell to the world, first of all to her family: "Presently the Queen Mother wished to speak to the King and dismissed everyone else. She also wished to speak to the Queen, and then to both together. It can be assumed that in doing so she wished them happiness and peace in their marriage, fear of God, and His abundant blessings. The words of this worthy mother were no doubt received by the King with a truly filial heart, filled with respect and gratitude."[29] Very quickly, however, God again takes center stage:

The Archbishop of Auch brought the Body of Our Lord, followed by the Bishop of Mende, the parish priest of Saint-Germain, the Abbot of Gue-madeuc, and several other Almoners. The Archbishop, holding the holy host, exhorted the Queen in the most Christian terms. *He showed her the need to humble herself before God*, explained the uselessness of all the things that we esteem most in this world, and told her that, although she was the offspring of so many kings and emperors, the mother, aunt, and sister of the most powerful princes on earth, she should consider that she was about to become the equal of the most humble of creatures, and that all of her grandeur would henceforth be of no use to her; that only repentance of her sins, penitence, and humility would be useful and salutary to her in that terrible moment when, appearing before God to be judged by her works, God's mercy would be her only wealth.[30]

Next comes the agony. Madame de Motteville depicts it as an edifying image from beginning to end:

The Queen Mother entered into her agony, which was long and filled with suffering, though without doubt profitable to her who endured it, for she continually offered it up to God. She constantly expressed her contrition, faith, and love, with wonderful concern for her salvation. The Archbishop of Auch frequently spoke to her of beautiful things, quoting verses from the psalms and places in the Scripture appropriate to her state. Since this pious princess was fully conscious, she responded to this with such submission to God's will, so many marks of humility and faith, that she moved the spectators of so Christian a death to devotion.[31]

Madame de Montpensier, a less conventional witness, makes us hear the last moans of the dying woman. But it is clear that even this last outburst of human feelings soon conformed to the perfectly wrought "mold" of the grand ceremonial:

A moment later, she opened her dying eyes and, looking at her confessor, said to him: "*Padre mio, yo me muero*" [Father, I am dying]. After she had said these words, her agony became so overwhelming and so painful that, feeling her suffering increase and her strength diminish, an impulse of nature, which hates suffering, made her say, albeit reluctantly, to the Archbishop Auch: "I am in great pain; will I not die soon?" Whereupon, the Archbishop having told her that one must not be too impatient to die, and that one must suffer as much as God has ordained, she acquiesced at once and repeatedly expressed her submission to God's will.[32]

Today, of course, we tend to think that such rituals, such collective staging of individual emotions, were best performed by kings and princes whose entire life was a spectacle. Yet Michel Vovelle takes us to the other end of the social scale when he makes us witness the death of Catherine, a poor prostitute of Nivelle, who had contracted the plague in 1633. Catherine realizes that she is very ill, the narrator tells us. "She did not distress herself; although she knew she was condemned to death, she accepted this news."[33] She therefore decides to go to the cemetery, there to die and be buried. In doing so, she reinvents, spontaneously it seems, a ritual identical to that of a princely death. She orchestrates her death, takes her leave, prays, and confesses in the presence of an admiring audience:

> Having confessed, she received the Holy Viaticum and Extreme Unction kneeling on the ground; and then, having performed her recollection, at about four o'clock she readied her little cart to make her way to Gontal (that is the name of the cemetery) in the company of her sister, who charitably helped her until she died. When she left, she enjoined one of her companions to have a mass in honor of Saint Gertrude said in the big church for the state of both her body and her soul. Thereupon she took in one hand a blessed candle, and a vessel of holy water in the other, like a Wise Virgin setting out to receive her Bridegroom, asking her sister to bring along fire with which to light the candle when the time came, as well as to bring a cushion and a pillow for her head. Passing through the street, she bid farewell to some neighbor women, asking their forgiveness for the bad example she had given. Asked where she was going, she said, I am going off to Paradise, if it please God. I trust in his mercy. Some answered her that she might escape death . . . No indeed! (she replied, showing them her body bearing the marks of the plague), see this, I wear my judgment written upon me, I needs must die, adieu my dear friends. She continued on her way and walked with such courage that one of those who were watching her could not help but exclaim in admiration: *Look at her! She goes to her death as if to a wedding.* And he spoke true, for she was preparing to attend the wedding of the immaculate Lamb.[34]

Having reached the cemetery, Catherine asks to have her grave dug, lies down in it herself, and dies what one is tempted to call a controlled death. "She turned her face toward the earth and rendered her soul to God so suddenly that her sister, who was holding her by the arm, could not lift her up again before she was already dead. You might say that she had picked the time and arranged to die when she wanted to die."[35]

After the eighteenth century, as the Church's hold over society slowly began to relax, the notions of sin and redemption lost their power. The meaning of death also changed, and the dread to which it gave rise could no longer be contained by religious rituals. In the nineteenth century finally, as the belief in science developed, and as medical activism—which might or might not prove effective—was on the rise, both the physician and the sufferer ceased to feel dominated by the divine will. They believed that they were dealing with organic processes that could be known and mastered. Resignation thus gave way to the desire to live at any price. The sense of sin, acceptance of the divine will, and hope for salvation no longer informed their attitudes toward illness.

As the physician replaced the priest and the nun in taking care of the sick, the Christian conception of illness and death gradually lost ground. It did not, of course, disappear altogether. At the end of the nineteenth century, Marie Bashkirtseff, for example, still saw her tuberculosis as caused by God's will, but this belief was intertwined with a vision of illness as linked to the deepest truth of the sufferer, to her individual personality, which was tantamount to her fate. In this case several notions merged together; illness and death were Marie Bashkirtseff's fate because her passion for life was such that nothing could satisfy it. Therefore she must die. Nonetheless, it was God who decreed that it should be thus: "Ah, I told you that I had to die. Because God cannot give me what would make it possible for me to live, he solves the problem by killing me. Having heaped misery on me, he now kills me to put an end to it. I told you that I would have to die, this could not go on; this hunger for everything, these colossal aspirations, they could not go on. I told you this long ago, years ago at Nice, when I still only vaguely sensed all the things that I needed to live."[36]

By contrast, in December 1920, about two years before her death, Katherine Mansfield wrote in her diary a text entitled "Suffering," which she hoped, she said, would be accepted as *"her confession."* It expressed a wholly religious conception of pain as a redemption. Yet the name of God is not pronounced, and there is no allusion to Christian faith:

> I do not wish to die without leaving a record of my belief that suffering can be overcome. For I do believe it. What must one do? There is no question of what Jack calls "passing beyond it." This is false. One must *submit*.[37] Do not resist. Take it. Be overwhelmed. Accept it. Make it *part of life*.[38] Everything in life we really accept undergoes a change. So suffering must become love. This is the mystery. This is what I must do . . . perhaps bodily ill-health is necessary, is a repairing process . . . If "suffering" is not a repairing process I will make it so. I will learn the lessons it teaches. These are not idle words. These are not the consolations of the sick.[39]

Today notions of sin and punishment through illness are often expressed in the same, albeit less elaborate, manner, detached from all religious connotations.[40] But the very fact that the context in which these notions have their origin is forgotten is also a sign of their deep roots in our culture. For those who use them, the terms of sin and punishment function as direct expressions of reality. "My legs are my only punishment," said a cleaning woman in 1972, speaking of her phlebitis. For her the term *punishment* was the very equivalent of *illness*. At the other end of the social scale, Fritz Zorn, the young bourgeois of Zürich, also spoke of his cancer as a punishment: "I was a good boy all my life, and that's why I got cancer. I think that anybody who has been a good boy all his life does not deserve anything else but to get cancer. It is no more than his just punishment."[41] Zorn, however, is able to connect this idea with a psychoanalytic representation of illness. "Cancer is a disease of the soul which causes a person who swallows all his sorrow to be swallowed in turn, after a certain time, by this sorrow that is within him."[42]

By contrast, direct references to God on the part of the sick or their loved ones have become very rare today. Moreover, the language used to express the importance of religious feelings as a way to accept illness is usually quite stereotyped. This, for example, is what a 60-year-old agricultural engineer said in the 1960s: "I have in my family an aunt who has been sick for many years and who bears her condition with a great deal of courage and strength . . . of course she accepts being ill because of her religious sentiments; it is a cross she has to bear . . . I do believe it is much easier for a religious person to deal with illness and the 'big step' than for someone who is not religious."

The Ordeal of Suffering Today

In fact—and this is surely no coincidence—the infrequent references to God, to faith, and to prayer which one does encounter today are almost always made in one context only, namely that of suffering and impotence in the face of suffering. In 1960, a young Catholic professor, in speaking of her experiences when one of her friends died of cancer, developed in a very emotional manner the traditional Christian vision of suffering and edification through suffering:

> Last year I had an experience that touched me very deeply. It was a woman with whom I worked, and who got cancer, and for nine months I regularly went to see her; really, I was with her until she died, and this is perhaps the fullest experience I have had of someone who was sick and suffered so much . . . some days it was horrible; she was in terrible pain, real martyrdom, and yet she was able not to talk to me about this business of hospitals and illness . . . She was joyful, she actually told me so, and besides I could sense it myself, it was extraordinary . . . there is a way of accepting suffering, and she had it, it was edifying for all those around her . . . In the hospital, she would walk around in the ward, she would go to see the other patients, they were

delighted, they needed her, needed to speak to her . . . I think that if a sick person accepts suffering in a certain way . . . it is an amazing experience to come in contact with people like that.

In this case, suffering also gave rise to a very special kind of communication. "There was a whole kind of friendship between us founded in part on this, a whole rather unusual relationship occasioned by her illness, the impression of something perfect, a sharing, an impression that one has very rarely in life."

In 1972, an old lady of 82 whom we interviewed in the hospital, where she was immobilized by a very painful case of arthrosis, expressed herself in a more matter-of-fact manner. But for her, too, God was the only recourse in the face of an ill against which there is little possibility of action, and she too felt that suffering can be an enriching experience. "I am a religious person, and I said to myself, 'I'll somehow get through this, because the Good Lord will help me! I can take it.'" In the last analysis, she considered suffering a good thing because one can offer it up for oneself or for others. "I was brought up in a very Christian milieu. Well, I sometimes said to myself, 'If Mother had seen me as I am now when she was alive, she would have been unhappy.' But now I am sure that she rejoices to see me suffering, to see me handicapped, because she used to say to me, 'These are merits that you can accumulate for yourself or for others.' Such is the strength of those who have faith."

In the face of suffering, the ideas of God, faith, and prayer are thus still part of a set of possible and legitimate references. This can even be the case for persons without religious faith. This is what we saw in interviews with a 45-year-old waitress, who was hospitalized in 1972 for an excruciatingly painful cancer of the rectum which failed to respond to treatment. She was pleased to tell us that people were praying for her. Although she herself was not a Christian and remained skeptical as to the effectiveness of prayer, she valued it because of the love it represented. "I have an aunt who is very pious, poor thing . . . she is all for me, and she prays . . . *I know that she prays for me and, really, that is good for me,* but I am not a Catholic, and as far as the illness is concerned, I don't know if it does anything. On the other hand, to know that my little old aunt prays for me, that makes me feel good." It would be a mistake to think that the only reason for this grateful acceptance is the emotional support conveyed by this prayer. Prayer still has its own legitimacy, perhaps because it lies outside the sphere of medicine, unlike the healer who is in direct competition with it. Significantly, this cancer patient categorically refused the parallel treatment suggested by two of her relatives, although this suggestion could also be interpreted as inspired by the love of her family. "I have a sister-in-law who works with one of my cousins, and when the two of them were cutting my hair, they had the idea that they would get someone to give me treatments, all this kind of business . . . to make me take something. Well, I said, 'Not on your life!' . . . I said, 'Don't even think of it. It's me who is sick, not you. Just forget it'—and that was the end of that."

The impact of religious conceptions on our contemporary representations is thus very complex indeed. The Christian conception, which for centuries has modeled our entire relationship with biological misfortune, often still implicitly informs our attitudes. Explicit reference to God, however, has become very rare. Nonetheless, even for non-Christians, it can constitute a "last recourse" when all other resources—medicine and the physician—have failed.

Yet even for Christians, God is no longer at the center of humanity's relationship with illness. Now that he competes with other references and other recourses, he is usually shunted into the background. One last case will show this very clearly. In the course of our interviews with sick people, we encountered only one person who asserted that she intensely experienced her illness according to the model of a "test sent by God." In this case too, the impotence of medicine was absolutely flagrant. Forty-four years old, the mother of four children and the wife of an executive, Madame A., whom we interviewed in 1960, at first spoke rather mysteriously about what had happened to her. "Twenty-one and a half years ago a miserable thing happened to me when I was having a baby, and for the last 21½ years I have personally had certain troubles because of it." She was rather reticent about explaining the nature of her troubles more clearly. It turned out, in fact, that these were not definable in medical terms.

> It was during the delivery of my second child, that I had . . . it seems that I was out of it so much that I don't know exactly what happened. But Professor R. was my obstetrician, and he certainly is no fool, and I had . . . I don't know what it was. He said it was not eclampsia, or epilepsy, or a heart attack. In any case, I had some kind of a seizure . . . I don't know of what. My little girl was born, and on the first day when I got up, the same thing happened again, I fell down . . . and after that it happened so often that I can't even keep count any more. So, because my whole family is full of doctors, they looked and looked and looked to find the cause . . . where this came from, what it was, but they never found out.

Because medicine was unable to diagnose her problem, Madame A. ceased to have recourse to it. "Even though my family is chock-full of doctors, I don't bother with their advice and I do as I see fit," she said. The explanation of her illness, she felt, was of a different order. "I take it as a test, if you will, a test sent by God and visited on me for some reason. I do not seek to find the reason. Whatever the reason, *I accept it, and that's all* . . . And I assure you that this is why I have been able to take it ever so much better than if I had gone in for all the treatments I should have had." Once Madame A. had redefined her problem in this manner, her life, which had been deeply upset by her illness, returned to normal. "I had been in very good health until then, and it was very hard for me to see that I would topple over like a fly, that I could easily fall, and how many times I have burned myself . . . I am all covered with scars, but that's all. So then, as soon as I made up my mind that there was nothing wrong with me, at that moment my life changed, it returned exactly to what it was before."

Furthermore, God, who has sent the test, can also be the help that limits its scope. Confidence in him reinforces the all-encompassing, albeit somewhat strained, "will power" that sustained the sufferer. "I have prayed, seeing how I sometimes fell and realizing that this could hurt the children or the babies I was carrying; I really prayed, given my trust in God, that I should always be the one who got the bruises, and for $21\frac{1}{2}$ years now, it was always I who got them . . . *It's God, absolutely, who wants it that way*, never was one of the children hurt." All in all, Madame A. asserts, the "test" has been a good thing: "Every time I have been in trouble, I have gained something good from it, and I have come to love suffering . . . I do think, because I believe in God above all, that it is a grace . . . It becomes a strength, if you will."

The religious reference made it possible, in fact, for Madame A. to experience her illness in a double manner. It enabled her to "accept herself" and to consider herself "tested," but by the same token it also freed her from the need to question the nature of her affliction, so that she could refuse to attach any importance to it in her day-to-day life. Madame A. insisted on this point again and again. "I do exactly as if there were nothing wrong with me, and there is nothing wrong with me." Or, again, "It is by sheer will power that I live as if nothing were wrong." Life thus can go on as usual, at least she says it can.

Such a denial of illness, however, is a very different matter from the traditional acceptance of the Christian. It is based on different values, namely life and relationships in this world, rather than redemption and salvation. "I said to myself, 'Either I take care of myself, or I take care of the home, I have to choose between the two.' For me there was no question, I chose the home. So, ever since, I have stopped worrying about myself . . . I absolutely make no concessions to it in my life, and I act exactly as if this illness did not exist at all. By now, you see, it has been $21\frac{1}{2}$ years that it happened, and at least 19 that I act as I do now." Madame A.'s life and her conduct are governed by her relationship with the world, by her duty to her husband and her children, rather than by her relationship to God.

9·

The Damaged Individual: The Flawed Body

*W*e have seen how, as illness ceased to be perceived as a punishment or test willed by God, the physician gradually took the place of the priest and the therapeutic attitude superseded the punitive attitude. Crime today is often, madness and alcoholism almost always, considered to be a part of the realm of illness and treatment, rather than of sin and punishment. Yet when the notion of illness supplanted sin, it took on its moral connotations and the body became the locus of norms *par excellence*.

No longer the result of sin, illness has come to constitute, in itself, a flaw whose nature transcends mere organic disorder, for it is fraught with moral values. It is no doubt in connection with syphilis that one can best observe the emergence of this new space of transgression. We must therefore once again turn to the analysis of a specific illness in order to understand the shift that has taken place and the change that this illness has wrought in the identity of the sick. The inexhaustible medical discourse about syphilis deployed in the late nineteenth century played a crucial role in this shift, for it is here that the notions of transgression, indeed crime, against the body, the lineage, and the race came into being. But its repercussions went far beyond the medical profession and became an integral part of the collective consciousness.

To be sure, syphilis was not the only illness to be surrounded by moral reprobation at the end of the last century. Any ailment could become caught up in it. This is attested, for instance, in a letter written in 1905 by Proust to Robert de Montesquiou, in which the writer clearly states the difference between the traditional Christian vision of punishment by illness and the notion of illness as, in itself, a fault. "You are, Monsieur, more cruel than the most cruel Catholic theologians, who wanted us to take our illnesses for punishments of our sins. You want us to consider them as faults in themselves; you want us not

[In this context, the word *avarié* (damaged) has the connotation of *syphilitic* in French.]

only to suffer physically from our ills but also think that we should feel remorse for them, and that our illnesses, inevitable and painful enough though they are, should make us feel guilty as well."[1] As early as 1872, Samuel Butler had already masterfully shown in *Erewhon* how illness and crime might undergo semantic shifts and exchanges, for in the imaginary society depicted in his book the sick are punished and imprisoned, while thieves and murderers receive compassionate medical treatment.[2] Moreover, at the end of the nineteenth century there was a reaction against the Romantic glorification of illness—tuberculosis linked to beauty and genius—and a shift to "health" as a value. This value was applied to social problems by the hygienists, and to biological and racial concerns by the eugenicists, who in numerous writings published at that time extolled health as the means of "hygienic generation" and "safeguarding the purity of the blood."[3] Indeed, the hygienist and the eugenicist discourses merged in the notion of the "social scourge," which encompassed alcoholism, tuberculosis, and syphilis. The result was the image of biological evil bound up with social conditions, issued from the harmful behaviors bred by these conditions, and fraught with dire consequences for both society and biology, because it was bound to affect the well-being of the community and the betterment of the lineage and the race.

In this triptych of social scourges, tuberculosis symbolized the new figure of death. The ultimate illness, it had become the modern form of the ancient calamities. As for alcoholism, it was almost exclusively tied to the image of the wretched and, more important, the "dangerous" people. By contrast, syphilis, the "venereal peril," perhaps because it most clearly united social and biological concerns, now became the privileged arena of interaction between moral and medical considerations, resulting in a veritable reversal, for the body was once again seen to bear the burden of sin, even though illness had ceased to be the testimony of God's wrath. An outspokenly health-centered ethic was developed, and the physician was to be its expert and its guardian.

As for the sufferers, though they were no longer sinners, they had failed; not, as in the past, in their souls, but in their bodies. They were now "damaged."

Pleasure and Decay

For a very long time, syphilis was linked to sin in its most traditional meaning, that of failure to obey God's commands. Debauchery, along with the prostitute who was its purveyor, delighted and putrefied the body. In the kiss and the embrace, pleasure and poison became mingled. The fear of becoming contaminated was part of every sexual encounter. Oscar Panizza's play *Le Concile d'amour*,[4] which was published in 1895—and, incidentally, earned its author a year in prison—was precisely about the birth of this scourge out of guilty pleasure. It was set in the spring of 1495, "the first one in which the appearance of syphilis is attested by history," as the author tells us. God and the Virgin, scandalized by the debauchery that reigns in the city of Naples, encircled by the French ("the siege," says a messenger, "has carried the sexual frenzy to a paroxism of debauchery"), at first want to exterminate the human race. After some reflection, they decide that instead it should be chastised by the most dreadful punishment. To find the right kind, they call on the help of the Devil. "This poison, this thorn," the latter says, "will have to be put—hm, into the thing itself, into the—hm—into the connection."[5] "It will have to be extremely enticing," comments the Virgin Mary.[6] The Devil heartily agrees: "What is needed is a new and particularly subtle poison, which does not immediately kill either the one who infuses it or the one who receives it. What I need is a discreet, insinuating venom that acts slowly, is transmitted by heredity, and can always be found fresh in a few living individuals. In addition, it must be associated with moments of supreme ecstasy, with the elation of the most naïve love, the most delightful happiness they ever experience—in this manner no one will be spared."[7]

Satan decides to extract some of his own substance ("what could be more venomous, more penetrating"), a strange poison that will first be infused into the most seductive of creatures, his elective daughter, Salome. She will transmit it to men "by the usual channel." The Devil savors in advance his victory over a humanity that will rush toward its putrefaction and its death, and describes to the Virgin what syphilis will be like:

> The power of the poison in her veins is such that, two weeks later, he who has touched her will have eyes like glass beads! His very thoughts will coagulate. He will pant for hope like a carp out of water. After another two weeks, *looking at his body, he will wonder: Can this be I?* His hair and his eyelashes will fall out, and so will his teeth; his jaws and his joints will become loose. After three months his skin will be as full of holes as a sieve, and he will press his nose against shop windows to see if he can't buy himself a new skin! Not only will despair penetrate his heart, it will also flow out of his nose in the form of a stinking snot. His friends will look at each other, and those who are in the first phase will laugh at those who are in the second or third. By the end of the first year his nose will fall into his soup; he'll go and buy himself a rubber one. Then he'll change apartments, and jobs; he'll become compassionate and sentimental, he won't harm a fly; he will moralize and play with the insects in the sunshine, envying the fate of the young trees in the spring. If he is Protestant, he will become Catholic, and vice versa. By the end of the second or third year, his liver and his other glands will be like cobblestones in his body; he will switch to light foods. Then he will get a tingling in one of his eyes. Three months later that eye will shut. At the end of five or six years, his body will shake and sputter like fireworks; he will still

be able to walk, but he will worry whether his feet are still under his body. Not long after that, he will prefer to stay in bed, for the heat will do him good. At the end of eight years, he will one day pick a bone off his own skeleton, smell it, and toss it into a corner in horror. Now he will become pious, very pious, more pious all the time, and he will love leather-bound volumes with gilt edges and a cross on the cover. Ten years later, he will be a rotten skeleton, nailed to his bed, gasping, his mouth opened wide toward the ceiling, wondering how all this had come about, and finally he will die . . . *Then his soul will be yours!* [8]

Sexual pleasure, poison, woman, race, decay, and repentance—all the themes that came to haunt the minds of nineteenth-century writers in connection with syphilis are present in this myth of origins. For at the time all writers were fascinated by what Huysmans called the "unusable inheritance," the "eternal disease"[9] which, according to him, had ruled the world from the beginning. "All is syphilis," says his hero des Esseints, whose horrible dream Huysmans enjoys describing for us: "This ambiguous, sexless figure was green, and it opened, under violet lids, eyes of a light and cold blue, terrible eyes. Extraordinarily thin arms, the arms of a skeleton, naked to the elbows, emerged from ragged sleeves, shivering with fever; and emaciated thighs rattled in worn-out, much too large boots. The dreadful gaze fastened itself on des Esseints, penetrated him, and chilled him to the marrow of his bones . . . He immediately understood the sense of this frightful vision. He had before his eyes the image of the Great Pox."[10] Venereal disease played an enormous role in the collective mythology of many nineteenth-century writers. Patrick Wald Lasowski has analyzed this phenomenon and has found that the artist, the "damned"—and the difference between "damned" and "rotten" is not very great—lived under the sign of syphilis, in defiance and horror of contagion by it.[11] Yet in this contagion lust and sin, along with their consequences, putrefaction and the corpse, were felt to become one with creativeness and genius. Lasowski shows how deeply nineteenth-century literature was marked by the disease. Baudelaire, Barbey d'Aureville, the Goncourt brothers, Maupassant, Huysmans, and many others described it unendingly and with morbid pleasure, reveling in gnawed-away flesh, emaciated bodies, disfigured faces, empty eye sockets, purulent wounds. This meant more than giving in to the spell of a myth; for these writers it was the way to reach the deepest essence of their art. Profoundly marked by syphilis, by decay and death, their style of writing became the sign of their "modernity."

The Collective Fantasy

This was the period when all of society was ill with syphilis, in its fantasies as much as in the flesh. Its increase was undeniable; "more or less everybody had it," said Flaubert in the *Dictionnaire des idées reçues*. A number of controversies concerning the precise number of victims were fought out,[12] but most of the figures cited are frightful indeed; and although one can doubt their accuracy, they give us at least a measure of the terror inspired by this ill.

In the early twentieth century, several studies attributed from 15 to 17 percent of all deaths to syphilis.[13] Professor Alfred Fournier, the most eminent specialist of his day, estimated that from 13 to 15 percent of all adult males in Paris had it.[14] Emile Duclaux, the first director of the newly created Institut Pasteur, estimated that there were fourteen million syphilitics in French society.[15] Syphilis was held responsible for an enormous share of infant mortality and, following the discovery of the gonococcus by Neisser in 1879, there was growing concern about gonorrhea, "the other damage,"[16] which had until then been considered benign, but which now turned out to cause sterility in many women. The medical profession also pointed out that the venereal scourge was continually spreading; originally an urban phenomenon, it had now reached the countryside.

Moreover, half of the victims contracted syphilis in adolescence. Their entire life could thus be marked by the disease. Alphonse Daudet suggested this in his diary, *La Doulou*, when he evoked the case of a syphilitic of his acquaintance, a "dissolute old fellow, Baron X." "When he was fifteen, his uncle, Marquis de Z., took him to his first supper at the Café des Anglais. That night, he took his marching orders for Lamalou."[17] At the time Lamalou was the watering spa where many people went to be treated for a variety of nervous ailments of syphilitic origin; Daudet himself often went there.

Daudet experienced the first symptoms in 1884; he died thirteen years later, almost completely paralyzed. In his diary he remembers the beginning of his illness: "Memory of a first visit to Dr. Guyon, rue de la Ville l'Evèque. He probes, contraction of the bladder, the prostate a bit agitated – in short, nothing. And with this nothing, everything started: it was an invasion."[18] One day Daudet learned that he would not get better: "Long talk with Charcot. It is what I think; it will go on for the rest of my life."[19] Daudet had a case of tabes (or motor ataxia), which had just been found to be, like the general paralysis of which Jules de Goncourt, Baudelaire, and Maupassant died, one of the long-term effects of syphilis, which attacks the central nervous system. Daudet's day-to-day descriptions of his state give a different image of the disease than the decomposition of the body. In addition, the diary depicts a long torture and the progress of irremediable deterioration. The torture is the pain which, as the diary's title – *La Doulou* – indicates, has come to dominate the writer's life,[20] and against which he unsuccessfully tries all the painkillers known at the time, from chloral to bromide, and even morphine.

The deterioration was caused by the impairment of the motor function, which gradually made every outing, indeed every movement, extremely difficult. In his diary Daudet kept a record of all the things he could no longer do as the years passed: "Thinking about crossing the road; scared to death! No eyesight left, totally incapable of running, often even of walking faster. The terrors of an octogenarian."[21] A few years later, when the illness had progressed, he noted: "Impossible to go down a flight of steps without a rail, to walk on a polished parquet. Sometimes I lose the feeling for part of myself—the whole lower part; my legs get mixed up."[22] "To get to this armchair and to cross this polished hallway," he also said, "takes as much effort and ingenuity as Stanley needed in an African forest."[23] For years, Daudet was afraid of total immobility, but over the years his pain became so severe that this fear diminished. "For a long time I was horrified of the wheelchair; I used to see it coming, rolling along. Now I don't think of it much any more, and without the dread of the early days. I understand that there is rarely much pain when one has gotten to that point . . . to be without pain . . ."[24]

Even more distressing than Daudet's experience is Edmond de Goncourt's description of the case of his brother, who was dying of general paralysis at the age of 40. The dominant factor here was intellectual deterioration. It began with language difficulties, slight at first: "Some time ago, and this is becoming more pronounced every day, he began to mispronounce certain letters, slurring over the *r*s, and saying *t* instead of *c*."[25] Then came awkward and uncontrolled movements: "We were finishing dinner at the restaurant. The waiter brought him a finger bowl. He used it awkwardly. His awkwardness was nothing very serious, but people were looking at us, and I told him, a little impatiently: 'Listen, friend, watch what you are doing, or we will no longer be able to go anywhere.' At that he broke into tears, crying: 'I can't help it, I can't help it!' and his trembling and contracted hand sought mine on the tablecloth."[26] Next were aphasia and mental confusion.

This Monday he was reading a page from the *Mémoires d'Outre Tombe*, when he became a bit angry because of a word he had mispronounced. Suddenly he stops. As I draw near *I come upon a creature made of stone that does not answer me* and silently looks at the opened page. I ask him to continue, he remains silent. I look at him, I see that his expression is strange, that his eyes are filled with tears and dread. I take him in my arms, I lift him up, I kiss him, and then his lips utter with great effort sounds that are not words but a murmur, a mournful hum that means nothing. There is in him a horrible new anxiety that cannot find its way from under his shivering blond mustache. Can this be, oh Lord, a speech paralysis? . . . It calms down, somewhat, after an hour, although he is unable to say anything but yes and no, with troubled eyes that no longer seem to understand me. Suddenly he picks up the volume again, places it before him, and wants to read, absolutely wants to read. He reads "the cardinal Pa(cca)" and then stops, incapable of finishing the word. He shifts in his chair, takes off his straw hat, again and again passing his scratching fingers over his brow as if he wanted to dig into his brain; then he crumples the page as he brings it closer to his eyes.[27]

What is left of Jules de Goncourt in the eyes of his brother, who watches in horror this irresistible dehumanizing process? "Over his animated face, so full of intelligence, irony, and that attractive maliciousness of the wit, there crept, minute by minute, the haggard mask of imbecility."[28]

The Medical Discourse — Fighting the Venereal Peril

The progress of scientific knowledge — the discovery of the gonococcus, the demonstration of long-range syphilitic impairment of the central nervous system, such as tabes or general paralysis, the gathering of statistics — was the basis of the physicians' inexhaustible and terrifying discourse against what they considered to be the most dangerous scourge ever to threaten the human race. This discourse was also instrumental in the elaboration of structures designed to combat the disease. In 1899 and in 1902, two major international congresses were devoted to the subject of venereal diseases. They resulted in the founding of the International Society for Sanitary and Social Prophylaxis (the French branch was established in 1901), a veritable antisyphilis league that spearheaded the obsessive propaganda campaign. The same discourse also informed a reconstruction of reality, which brought forth the social construct of an omnipresent "venereal peril" whose principal conveyor is the prostitute, and the medical construct of syphilis as the causative factor of all diseases. Once the notion of *parasyphilis* had been elaborated, the disease came to be held responsible for practically all morbid processes. Here the medical discourse and the literary text reflect each other in a vision that expresses the full measure of the obsession with the venereal peril, an ultimate metaphor of illness itself, its condensation as well as its first cause, for a syphilitic origin can lurk behind any illness. Huysmans wrote in *A rebours*: "It (syphilis) was rampant, taking refuge in undefined ailments, hiding behind the symptoms of migraine and bronchitis, vapors and gout; from time to time it would make its way to the surface."[29] This statement was echoed by the highly respected Professor Burlureaux, who declared in Brussels in 1902 that physicians "should be so familiar with the study of syphilis that in dealing with any patient the idea of syphilis should come to his mind."[30]

Worse still was the matter of inherited syphilis, which attacked children, innocent victims. It was held responsible for all tragedies of infancy, all deformities, all degeneracy. For example, Professor Pinard, a great name in pediatrics, told Alfred Fournier: "In my entire practice, I have never seen a case of rickets unrelated to hereditary syphilis."[31] In 1902 the playwright Brieux wrote a play, *Les Avariés*, which was first banned and subsequently became an enormous success. Brieux has the physician—one of the main characters—paint the portrait of the child afflicted with hereditary syphilis:

> Syphilis is above all the great killer of children—Herod rules France and the whole world, perpetrating his massacre of the innocents year after year. And although this might sound like blasphemy against the sanctity of Life, I will say that the most fortunate are those who have died. Go to the children's hospitals. We know the type of child born to syphilitics. It is a classic type and the physician can tell them apart from all the others, these little old people who look as if they had already lived and kept the stigmata of all our infirmities, all our debility. Many of those with rickets, of those whose little bodies cannot carry the weight of huge heads, of the hunchbacks, the misshapen, the monsters, of those who have clubfeet, harelips, or limps from congenital dislocation of the hip joint, are the victims of fathers who married without knowing what you now know.[32]

In the idea of the individual "rotten from birth," the notion of sin—that of the parents—merges with the notion of the indelible mark of destiny. Even if, as in the case of Oswald, the unhappy hero of Ibsen's *Ghosts*, the evil does not immediately manifest itself, it is there and will lead to its inevitable conclusion, namely, madness and death. Hereditary syphilis thus contributed to intensifying the terror of contamination even further. It firmly implanted the necessity of prophylaxis in people's minds. Brieux's or Ibsen's plays made the public tremble, as did the many popular novels depicting the multiple tragedies caused by syphilis.[33] The public devoured the different "manuals of the hygiene and physiology of marriage," which were published "for the use of the upper classes." In this manner a vast field of activity opened before the eyes of the physician, who became the expert and the guardian of a new morality, that of the body and the lineage.

Yet the medical discourse and medical activity started out as sanitary rather than moral endeavors. The physicians, foremost among them A. Fournier, set out to take the guilt out of venereal disease. In 1880 Fournier, holder of the first chair of venereal medicine, a field he had founded, broke with the practice of the Lourcin hospitals, where venereal patients were locked into basement cells by way of punishment. He opened a dispensary in an ordinary hospital and guaranteed the patients confidentiality. Later the League for Sanitary and Moral Prophylaxis also favored "humanizing" the manner in which venereal patients were treated. In *Les Avariés*, Brieux, who speaks for Fournier, asserts that there are no "shameful diseases." The play's physician harshly upbraids the "damaged" man's father-in-law, who is indignant about his son-in-law's illness: "This is one of the things that irritate me most, this term of 'shameful disease,' which you have just used. Like all other diseases, this is one of our miseries, and there is no shame in being unhappy—even if one deserves it."[34] The syphilitic is not so much guilty as the victim of bad luck: "Among the most severe moral critics, among those . . . who treat the syphilitics as if they were guilty, I would like to know how many have never taken a similar chance . . . Among a thousand of these men, would I find four? I say! Except in the case of those four, the only difference between these men and the syphilitics is luck."[35]

Emile Duclaux also thought that syphilis had to be freed from its religious connotations and that hygiene should be separated from morality. In 1902, during the intense debate about the regulation of prostitution—it was thought that about two-thirds of the syphilitics had been contaminated by prostitutes —he wrote: "The trouble is that any regulation of this matter remains caught up in religious preoccupations and notions of sin."[36] He was opposed to the intervention of the State, feeling that it should not play the traditional role of the Church and impose a morality on the citizen. "The State, living mainly on our shortcomings, and diligently involved in peddling tobacco and alcohol, would also give itself the task of watching over our morality, as defined by itself, and would enforce it by the power at its command! That would be exactly like the Church! Worse and more of it, it would be the Church in possession of power!"[37] Duclaux therefore wanted no part of an official code of morality, of vice squads ("missionaries of the official code of morality"); instead he called for a public-health policy, which in his opinion would solve all problems. "Everything could become perfectly simple if we consented to leaving morality, religion, and all the prejudices that have sprung up from centuries of mixing these two with public-health matters in their proper place; if we ceased, in a word, policing morality and began policing public health."[38] Prostitutes should thus no longer be sent to prison, but to the hospital for treatment. It would also be necessary for the physician to intervene in families and to act as their "medical director,"[39] playing a role in the sexual education of the young, especially with respect to marriage. Duclaux formulated the hope that one day "the physician will be involved in every marriage contract in the same official capacity as the notary" for the purpose of assessing and guaranteeing "the health capital brought into the marriage by the future spouses."[40]

Hygienic Action and Public-health Morality

A missionary for this new policy, the physician, after conquering a public opinion that would finally understand the value of hygienic action, would be called upon to bring proper public-health measures into society. The physician would become the expert who administers a capital of health whose importance was beginning to be understood by society. In this view, illness ceased to be tied to a transcendent morality issued from God the Creator and linked to our duty toward him, but in its place another area of obligations began to take shape; this was the individual's responsibility for his or her own body. Henceforth one could sin against oneself, against one's own biological life, which became charged with rules and values. Such sin was also a sin against others, against their bodies, which one could contaminate, and especially against the family and one's own offspring: "If you marry before three or four years, you will be a criminal," says the physician to the "damaged" man.[41] Individual health was seen as part of a collective capital owned by the lineage, the race, or the nation. In this view, society as a whole was at stake in the hygienists' efforts to establish a public-health policy. Such a policy not only attempted to combat the "social scourge" represented by syphilis, along with tuberculosis and alcoholism, but also became intensely preoccupied with the problem of the low birth rate.

Now that illness had become a "social scourge," a new face, a new identity of the sick, began to take shape. We saw its first outlines emerge in our discussion of tuberculosis, where we demonstrated that henceforth the sick were no longer defined by their own imminent death but, rather, by a special form of life, a precise place within society. The obsession with syphilis, which came to join the obsession with tuberculosis, clearly shows another—albeit complementary—aspect of this new status, namely, that the values that had hitherto governed humanity's relations to God and to the sacred were now vested in the body itself. Paramount in these values were the life processes, the body, and the lineage; but in the last analysis the principal value was the well-being of a society that had understood the importance of its biological capital.

The obsession with the "social scourge" was also contemporaneous with the consolidation of the physician's social status and the definition of the modern form of the medical "profession." The law passed in 1892 at last gave the physicians the professional status to which they had aspired; and the Public Health Law of 1902 acknowledged the importance of their role for society as a whole. In this manner the physician definitively ceased to be the figure who introduces us to death and became the authority to whom society delegates the right to rule over the values pertaining to health and to the body.

Caught up in this configuration, the sick person was, knew, and felt himself to be rotten, tainted, and damaged. In their diary the Goncourt brothers confess: "Yes indeed, we are rotten! The ragbag that we must force to obey does not cooperate. The skin is going. We are scabby, scrofulous, and who knows what else? We must get fixed up."[42] The new sin, the sin against the body, as set forth by the physician, takes over from the old sin or merges with it. The Goncourt brothers' evocation of the death of Murger, the author of *La Vie de Bohème*, suggests an unspoken disapproval of Murger's unhealthy way of life marked by complete disregard of the rules of hygiene, the expression of a moral decay that mirrored the rotting of his body:

> A death, come to think of it, that resembles a death in the Scripture. It looks to me like the death of the *Bohème*, this death by decomposition, a jumble of everything that marked Murger's life and the world he painted: the debauchery of nocturnal work, periods of misery and periods of high living, neglected pox, the heat and the cold of an existence without a home, with late suppers but no dinner, little glasses of absinthe as a consolation for the pawnshop, everything that consumes, burns, and kills, a life of revolt against the hygiene of body and soul, which causes a man to leave life at forty-two in tatters because he does not have enough vitality left to suffer and only complains about one thing, the stench of rotten flesh in his room; and that flesh is his own.[43]

Obviously, the hygienist discourse had hit its mark. The public, even if it transgressed against them, knew the rules it had set up. In order to forestall the danger of impairment, some people were willing to live a life of precaution and abstinence from pleasure. Brieux has his "damaged" man say: "No one, no one in the world has been as afraid as I was of what happened to me; no one, in order to avoid it, has arranged his life with as much care and reflection, or been as meticulous about his precautions . . . I have deprived myself of all pleasure. I have resisted being led astray, I have resisted temptation . . . I would have loved adventures, orgies, champagne, lace lingerie, and sculpted beds! I have sacrificed all that to my health."[44]

In *Bubu de Montparnasse*, young Pierre Hardy, who has been contaminated by Berthe the prostitute, accepts his exclusion, the separation implied by the doctor's diagnosis. He will not return to his small provincial town and will not see his family again. All he will have is the love of Berthe, for she is the only woman whom he cannot befoul. "You have done me a lot of harm," he tells her, "but now the harm you have done me is the thing that must unite us. You are the only possible woman for me, *because my touch gives the plague*."[45] The damaged individual carries a taboo. Daudet expressed a similar feeling when he noted that the "true name" of his illness was kept silent: "Not once, not at the doctor's, nor in the showers, nor at the watering spas where the ailment is treated, was its name, its true name, pronounced; 'affection of the marrow,' indeed! Even the scientific textbooks are entitled 'The Nervous System.'"[46]

Syphilis was thus suffered in terror, hedged in with precautions and taboos. It could also be experienced as a conscious transgression. But if defiance and provocation show that the normative discourse was never totally victorious, they also testify to the powerful hold of the norm against which they were directed. There is defiance of the traditional morality and the bourgeois values in the statement of Flaubert, who wrote to a friend: "So you laughed, you old scoundrel, you perfidious host, about my unfortunate cock. Well, you should know that he is cured for the moment. All that is left is a slight hard spot, but this is the battle scar of the brave. It bestows upon him a certain poetic quality. One can see that he has lived, that he has been through hard times. It gives him a fateful and accursed air that is quite thought-provoking."[47] There is also defiance, expressed with joyful exuberance, in this passage from Maupassant: "I have the Pox, I mean the real thing, not some measly clap, not the crystalline ecclesiastical kind, or the bourgeois cockscomb, or some leguminous cauliflower, no indeed, but the Great Pox, the kind of which François I died. And I am proud of it, dammit, and what I despise most of all are the bourgeois. Halleluja, I have the Pox, and so I no longer have to be afraid of them."[48]

In *Bubu de Montparnasse*, however, which was written when the antivenereal discourse was at its height, we see the outlines of yet another attitude. The novel's hero, Bubu, just like Maupassant, comes to feel that he is stronger than the pox, but also stronger than medicine. He refuses to accept the verdict brought in by the medical discourse. Upon learning that he is probably contaminated, Bubu the pimp is at first afraid of the pox and frightened at the prospect of becoming "totally rotten"[49] by them. But he is also afraid of words and of the science that gets hold of sick bodies and marks them, just as the executioner marks the bodies of criminals with a fleur-de-lys. "He remembered its scientific name: syphilis. He was scared of science with its implacable and cut-and-dried ways because it throws us into hospitals, because it looks at us and sees us, because it thrusts its words and its instruments into our lives as if we were nothing but flesh, disease, and death."[50] Comforted by another pimp, le Grand Jules – who tells him, "We all have them" – Bubu gets used to the idea of the pox, no longer fears them, and laughs at them. He feels stronger than the disease, and also stronger than medicine: "To be totally rotten . . . These words now amused him when he thought about Jules and all the others who were not totally rotten. Syphilis and science rummage through us, looking for disease, but ah! syphilis and science are up against our will power, just like the doctors that one can catch and fleece at street corners."[51] This early form of a counter-discourse shows us *a contrario* the impact of the new health morality, which henceforth became the target of rebellion.

Venereal Disease Today

Today syphilis, and venereal disease in general, has not disappeared. In 1972, nine cases of syphilis per one hundred thousand inhabitants were annually diagnosed in France.[52] After a spectacular decline, the incidence of venereal diseases is, in fact, rising.[53] Nonetheless, to be afflicted with syphilis or another "sexually transmissible" disease today no longer has much in common with the terrifying experience of the early years of the century. Here one can measure the full impact of the possibility of a cure; a curable illness simply does not offer as much room for anxiety and commonly accepted myths.

In 1980, a journalist in his forties had contracted syphilis twice within fifteen months; it was, he said, "something with which I was able to deal pretty well . . . I had decided that it was no tragedy; *I felt that it was no more serious than any other illness*, I mean it could be treated, no problem."

A young woman of 25, also interviewed in 1980, who had had a case of gonorrhea two years earlier, was even relieved to learn that she had a physical illness, after various physicians had for several months attributed her symptoms to psychological causes. "I was reassured because *it was a microbe* . . . I thought that if I took antibiotics it would be finished, in short it was like a bad case of flu. And also to know that I had something tangible and concrete, something that I could fight without questioning my whole life . . . yes, I was terrifically relieved." Worrying about her psychic state, her way of life, and her relationships had caused her extreme anguish; but the diagnosis of gonorrhea seemed to her not only reassuring but even somewhat comical: "I even thought it was kind of funny, you just don't expect this kind of thing, and then it hits you like that; in fact, one always thinks one will never get anything of the kind, venereal diseases are only for other people. It's like, for example, being pregnant and having quintuplets."

Frightening images are still circulating, of course, especially with respect to syphilis. But for the journalist the reality of the affection and of the treatment turned out to be much less painful than the stories told by his friends.

> When I had my first case of syphilis, I imagined complicated treatments. I had been told all kinds of things: They'll give you shots for ten days, then they'll leave you alone for two weeks, and then again ten days [of shots]. I have to travel in connection with my work, I am not always in Paris, and so I saw myself going from one dispensary to another, arriving in a town, looking for a dispensary, you can see how it would be an awful bother . . . and then I found out *that the treatment was simple*, that it was administered orally . . . Also, I had been told: the treatment can take a very, very long time, you must abstain from sexual relations for several months, but that isn't true at all. In the end the treatment of the disease seemed less painful and less drastic than I had feared it would be.

Although he was cured at the time of the interview, syphilis is an ever-present danger for this man, for he is homosexual and knows that syphilis is particularly prevalent in the homosexual community. Therefore, he says, "I have had to realize that I may get it again." Consequently, he has integrated this risk, and its prevention, into his way of life. "I now have a blood test every three or four months; I used to have it once a year at most . . . now I think about it a little more."

However, he says, "it's like the gas and electric bill that comes every four months; when it comes due, it is integrated into my everyday life; I know it's a chance I am taking." A chance that sometimes makes him worry: "There is this fear that one does have, of meeting people who can contaminate. It's just . . . something that exists; sometimes when you first meet someone, your heart might miss a beat, just like that, and there is a bit of hesitation." For her part, the young woman quoted above also says: "Now I sure watch out with whom I make love . . . I'm really scared shitless when I make love with a guy whom I don't know real well."

Does this mean that, along with its risk to the organism, syphilis has lost the aura of dread and guilt with which it was surrounded for so long? The answer is not simple. Certain physicians, the journalist asserts, still like to make their syphilis patients feel guilty. "I have been lucky that I happened to deal with people who do not go in for the guilt trip, but this is not always the case. I know people who went to the X Medical Center, and there they make people feel guilty as hell. I know people who have stopped their treatments because of that." The main point, as we have seen, is that venereal disease never concerns us alone, because it is transmitted and transmissible. As soon as the diagnosis is made, the physician directs the patient's attention to the chain of contamination, asking by whom he or she has been contaminated, and to whom he or she might have transmitted the disease. The sufferer *must* let them know. This obligation is, at the very least, embarrassing. For the journalist, it constitutes the most unpleasant aspect of the disease. "That's the part, really . . . to let people know about it, that's certainly no fun . . . to try to remember . . . of course in some cases it's simple, when one is with one person only it's simple, but there are cases when it's not simple. One must get out the address book, make phone calls, explain . . . People usually take it all right. They say, 'Well, okay, I'll go for a blood test' . . . but it's pretty embarrassing just the same, that's almost what worries me most."

Moreover, this objectivation of an individual's network of sexual relations is rarely a neutral matter. It can profoundly influence his or her affective relationships. To be sure, the young woman suffering from gonorrhea gave an amused account of it, in which the vaudeville aspect predominated. "I had passed on my clap to Bill, and Bill passed it on to his girlfriend; I think he was not supposed to have relations for two weeks, and so he didn't want to make love to her, but she thought he was mad at her . . . this kind of stuff is pretty funny. Or, for example, when Catherine went to the Center to have tests, because C. had passed it on to her, and when she realized, seeing me there, that he had caught it from me, but she didn't know it; she didn't know that he had had relations with me, but she found out at the Center when we met there." We are far from the anxiety of Pierre Hardy in *Bubu de Montparnasse*, who is unhappily aware that his love "gives the plague."[54] But for all her detached humor, this young woman knew perfectly well that important stakes were hidden behind this apparently comic imbroglio. "There is a funny side to having the clap, but at the same time it is also a bit shameful, because it involves sex, and with it one's affective relations, and so it upsets one's life."

The word *shameful* has been uttered; it was also used when she reported, still in a humorous manner, how she told her family about her trouble. To let others know that one has a venereal disease is not easy, even today. And, as the two reported conversations show, it is hardest when it comes to one's parents, one's mother, whatever her reaction. Discomfort and shame indicate that in this situation the feeling of sin is not far away. "*I was a bit ashamed to tell my mother*, not really ashamed, but a bit embarrassed just the same. But I made a joke of it, and I told her: 'Here it is, I finally caught the clap.' Well, she really took it terrifically well. My parents took it all right, they were neither shocked nor did they feel their honor was sullied." She continued: "There certainly was some feeling of shame. Because it also meant I was telling them about my sex life. I'm not used to telling that kind of thing to my parents." The words of the journalist showed the same embarrassment at having to reveal his sexual life to his family, to his mother. In his case, he would have had to confess to a deviant sexuality—which he refused to do: "It would upset me if my family knew . . . I am a homosexual, and my family does not know this. Everyone knows it where I work, my heterosexual friends and everybody, no problem about it, but *the family is the last stop that hasn't been let out* and I don't want it to be let out . . . there are some, especially one of my brothers and my mother, who would have a hard time with that."

For this man, the experience of the disease is one with the homosexuality that has brought it about. Indeed, his homosexuality constitutes the deepest meaning of the disease. When he discovered that he had contracted syphilis, this homosexual was really concerned only about his homosexuality. "It is more difficult to live with homosexuality than with syphilis, and someone who is homosexual and has caught syphilis will worry only secondarily about his syphilis, and if anything must worry him, it will surely be his homosexuality, not his syphilis."

By incarnating it in the organic reality, syphilis reveals a person's homosexuality, not only to others, but above all to the subject, who can no longer escape the image it has brought to light. "One experiences it a bit like the tangible proof of a homosexuality that comes out of the closet; they (homosexuals) *now have a painful proof that it exists*, it's no longer just in their heads. I think that for some people who are very, very uncomfortable with their homosexuality, this keeps reminding them of it, even though they might not always like to remember."

In a world in which norms have become blurred, where it is possible to live "on the margins" in a twilight zone without asking too many questions, a homosexual's syphilis reminds him that there is still a limit that separates normality from deviance.

> One can no longer escape a homosexuality that one usually accepts, with which one lives, although one does not want to be constantly reminded of it . . . after all, everyone does what he wants to do, traditional morality is gone, times are changing. Where does the homo stop, and where does the hetero begin? I mean, there is a kind of blurred zone where one floats around more or less comfortably, so long as one doesn't run every hundred yards into a marker with a pointing finger to remind a person, "You are a fag." Syphilis can precisely become one of those nails that you constantly pound into someone to remind him that he has broken the law.

Yet—and this must be seen as a new shift in the meaning attached to illness—for individuals who accept their sexuality, biological misfortune as such is little more than a minor incident. "Homos must accept something that is seen by the majority of public opinion as a flaw. I think if one has worked this out, if one has accepted this, venereal disease doesn't amount to anything, becomes secondary." The therapeutic effectiveness that has reduced the intrinsic seriousness of the disease has, by the same token, also voided it of its meaning. The "damaged individual" no longer carries a load of biological guilt. "If society knows that one is homo," the same journalist said, "it couldn't care less that one also has some disease or other. There is a connection, but it will not aggravate the social condemnation." At this point we suddenly rediscover the original phenomenon, laid bare and stripped of the sediments of the hygienist discourse, namely sin in its modern guise—deviance. According to our informant, this is particularly true for homosexuals, but it is experienced by heterosexuals as well. "For homosexuals who live as a couple, who are married, unless they believe that you can catch this from toilet seats, just like babies come out of a cabbage patch, syphilis is a proof of infidelity. So this can be very upsetting . . . Syphilis in a way is proof that the person who has it has broken the law; that is, the norms of the relationship that traditionally binds the couple."

The young woman afflicted with gonorrhea had also associated venereal disease with categories connoting stigma and deviance—"whores and Arabs"—before she herself experienced it. "I knew that there were venereal diseases, but I didn't realize that you could catch them so easily, I mean to say that I too had internalized the idea that it was something that only whores had . . . I couldn't imagine that I might have one, somehow I was thinking that *this kind of thing is for Arabs and whores* . . . and by that I meant: this is not for me, because I am a very classy girl, and I fuck with top-notch people, so they're not going to do this to me, pass on some dirty business to me."

One last shift has thus occurred with respect to venereal disease. Because it is no longer as serious a biological threat as it was, it no longer embodies a crime against health—the syphilitic is no longer physically or morally "rotten"—but instead it pits the individual's sexual behavior against the social norm. Venereal disease now occupies a space that no longer has anything to do with religion, health, or morality; it is a matter of deviance and social interaction.

10·

From Inactivity to the Right to Illness

*A*s long as it was seen as fate or as sin, illness was always conceived of in terms of its relationship to the divine or to nature. These notions were sufficient to assign a place to the sick person and, at the same time, to give meaning to the universe as a whole. With the damaged individual the new value of the biological capital made its appearance; and although it was a social value, the individual was held responsible for its preservation. A different type of relationship emerged with this notion of responsibility, which pitted the sick person against society. Society's taking charge of illness, finally, marks the emergence and the recognition of a specific type, the sick person, toward whom society has duties and obligations. Illness can henceforth be interpreted through its relations with a social order which has become only that, without reference to a transcendent principle.

Welfare and Political Power

Various authors have claimed that public welfare was the first attempt on the part of the political authorities to defend themselves against the insecurity that certain categories of outsiders represent for society, citing such examples as the repression of vagrancy in England in 1388 or the creation of the Grand Bureau des Pauvres in France in 1544. "The appearance of public welfare was related to the rise and the consolidation of political groups that represented society as a whole";[1] it thus "originally had more political than social significance, being linked to the defense and the consolidation of emerging political collectivities."[2] The costs of welfare and assistance were thus borne by particular groups, such as religious communities, confraternities, and trade guilds, whereas "the public authorities assumed a progressively stronger role in the preservation of order and the consecration of the values common to society as a whole."[3]

In the years after 1789, a doctrine of social welfare which broke with this conception was elaborated.[4] This shift in perspective had its origin both in the destruction of *Ancien Régime* society, which established a direct relation between the individual and the State, and in the rationalist and universalist philosophy of the Enlightenment, which associated equality among all people with the State's obligation to come to their aid. Society now owed all individuals the help to which they were entitled. "The religious foundation of this right was replaced by a social foundation, namely the duty of the collectivity to assist needy citizens, as opposed to the individual's duty toward a society ruled by administrative fiat." And finally, "the right to assistance" became a kind of substitute for the right to employment, for which society is also responsible."[5]

A half-century before the Declaration of the Rights of Man of 1793, Montesquieu had already elaborated the importance of work in relation to property ownership: "A man is not poor because he has nothing, but because he does not work. The man who without any degree of wealth has an employment, is as much at his ease as he who without labour has an income of an hundred crowns a year. He who has no substance, and yet has a trade, is not poorer than he who possessing ten acres of land is obliged to cultivate it for his subsistence." Montesquieu also insisted on the State's obligation to provide for the needs of certain social categories: "In trading countries, where many men have no other subsistence but from the arts, the state is frequently obliged to supply the needs of the aged, the sick, and the orphan. A regular policed government draws this support from the arts themselves. It gives to some such employment as they are capable of performing; others are taught to work, and this teaching of itself becomes an employment." But this is not a matter of charity, for "those alms given to a naked man in the street do not fulfill the obligation of the state, which owes to every citizen a certain subsistence, a proper nourishment, convenient cloathing, and a kind of life not incompatible with health."[6] In the *Tableau de Paris*, Louis-Sébastien Mercier also asserted that civil society is responsible for the citizens' health: "What could be more important than the health of the citizens? Does not the strength of future generations, indeed that of the State itself, depend on such municipal aid?"[7] The Declaration of the Rights of Man of 24 June 1793, which states society's duty toward its needy citizens, makes a clear connection among subsistence, work, and welfare. "Public assistance is a sacred debt. Society owes subsistence to needy citizens, either by finding work for them, or by ensuring that those who are unable to work have the means of existence."[8] Recognized since the eighteenth century, this link between right to employment and right to assistance called for the establishment of a social organization that would act upon this new conception of the relationship between society and its members, for "a theory of State-controlled assistance and welfare seems to complement the most radical individualism in matters of social relations."[9] This liberal conception, which Nietzsche developed with particular clarity, linked the appearance of a contractual relationship with the existence of "legal rights [*Rechtssubjekte*]." Examining "this sphere of legal rights," Nietzsche retraced "the long history of the origin of responsibility and the origins of the whole moral world of 'guilt,' 'conscience,' 'duty,' and 'the sacredness of obligation.' "[10] Thus it appears that illness and suffering had become part of the social order, inseparable from notions of "right," "duty," "obligation," and "responsibility."

The early stages of industrialization brought an acute preoccupation with social issues, especially with the relation between right to employment and right to assistance, which was raised by the problem of the insecurity facing the "new poor"; that is, the workers. To put it more precisely, the development of a wage labor force now posed the problem of the individual's relation to his or her work differently, namely in terms of such notions as work-related accidents and insurance against illness and even unemployment. "The uncertainty of existence," a term that H. Hatzfeld borrowed from Marx and Engels, was the reason behind the social measures adopted in the second half of the nineteenth century. As Hatzfeld reminds us, however, this "uncertainty of existence" was twofold. On the one hand, it was uncertainty with respect to employment and the haunting fear of unemployment, and on the other "this uncertainty became a kind of certainty concerning some of the contingencies of existence, for it was clear that the worker would be financially unable to face illness, disability, and old age."[11] Whereas the right to employment was indeed the essential demand of the workers' movement, the response of the powers that be was often the right to assistance, as Karl Marx has shown in connection with the Revolution of 1848 and the passing of the Public Welfare Law of 1849.[12] In a sense, this right to employment is the counterpart to the right of property but, unlike in the case of property rights, which can be acknowledged in the preamble of a constitution, it is impossible to guarantee it institutionally. The very risk that the workers had denounced all along as their most serious vulnerability was also the last one against which they could insure themselves; unemployment insurance dates from 1958.[13] Unemployment insurance can never guarantee job security; at best, it can afford a certain protection against job insecurity. H. Hatzfeld's analysis has shown that systems of social protection are part and parcel of the development and the organization of wage labor in industrial societies. The main issue in the relation between workers and employers, they are the response to the workers' needs and aspirations, but they were not born from their demands alone. They were also born because industrial enterprises needed them in order to solve a major problem, that of recruiting a stable labor force. Hatzfeld concludes: "After a society based on property, we now have a society based on institutions. After the citizen–property owner, we now have comprehensive labor laws. This mutation has not come about by itself; it was the outcome of a struggle between two complex forces – on the one hand the exigencies of the economic process, and on the other the aspirations of ordinary people and a set of economic ideas. But it is not clear that in this struggle the parties were diametrically opposed."[14]

Recognition of the interdependence between health and work is more than a principle stated in the preamble to the constitution. It is a reality that the public power has accepted in the institution of Social Security. Pierre Laroque has made it clear that "one of the foundations of Social Security is the notion that the collectivity is responsible for the well-being of its members, that it has the obligation to ensure their security . . . there can be no doubt that a society based on such principles is totally different from the traditional liberal society."[15] By the same token illness itself has changed its character and has become inserted into a new network of social relations. Now that illness means inability to work and is recognized as such by medicine – for the physicians participate in conferring a social character upon illness by identifying and labeling it – it has become a right. To be sick means to stop working and to receive treatments, and the sick person is entitled to both.

In the course of this development the sick person began to appear as a new figure on the social scene. New forms of pathology, as we have seen in connection with tuberculosis, contributed to the emergence of an individualized figure of the sick. The sick person was granted inactive status, freed from the duties of production and accepted as such. Different rights and duties and a new relation to society as a whole eventually came to define the sick.

From Charity to Solidarity

At the time when illness left workers stripped of all resources, only charity and sometimes mutual aid could prevent utter misery. Yet, early in our own century, *Didier, homme du peuple,* the central character of Maurice Bonneff's novel, found it difficult to accept the aid of his fellow union members when, like his father before him, he developed lung trouble. "When he came home from work, there were two men sent by the union who told him, 'The guys want you to get a rest, and so the organization will pay you two weeks off!' This attention made him weep." The weeks pass, and Didier goes back to work, because tuberculosis, the author says, "goes along with social conditions; it adapts to one's way of life; no disease is more accommodating than tuberculosis, for it does not make it necessary to stop working right away but grants long delays. In the beginning one does not suffer, for tuberculosis knows *that the poor don't have time to rest.*" When Didier succumbs, he has to stop working and takes to his bed. An irritable patient, "he gets upset with the assistant secretary of the union, who comes to bring him some money; he does not want to accept a penny from the organization 'because he is not a shirker.' Francine must receive the compensation in secret and invents a story of having taken the money out of the savings account."[16]

For a long time illness in a family meant ruin, as a 45-year-old female farmer from Périgord still remembered in 1980. In order to afford treatments for a sister suffering from a brain tumor, her parents were obliged to sell property. "My father sold his animals and his nut trees, and by the time my sister died we had hit rock bottom." In 1979 a retired 66-year-old woman also told us, "*It used to be, when one was sick, charity was the only hope,* and all one could do was weep and beg from the shopkeepers, so that they would let you buy on credit; well, I can tell you, this just tied one's guts in knots, so I feel that Social Security is a matter of human dignity."

Since 1945, thanks to the institution of Social Security, inactivity no longer means financial catastrophe or charity; now that it has become legitimate, it entitles the sick person to daily compensation payments. By guaranteeing the financial means to deal with illness, Social Security restores personal dignity to the sick, for, as the retired woman said, "it is paid by the workers; I know that the employer contributes, but it is still paid by the workers." Certain people, like the woman with breast cancer cited earlier, very forcefully expressed their consciousness of being part of a "chain of solidarity":

> I feel very strongly about it, for it is so important for people with expensive illnesses, because they have 100 percent coverage, and very special illnesses, like high blood pressure, heart condition, cancer, things like that, they are covered 100 percent. So, of course, if I had had to pay for my cancer treatments myself, I might well have died, because I could never have afforded all the treatments I had. That's for sure. It is also sure that others have paid for me, but that is where solidarity comes in. *Social Security is the most beautiful solidarity that exists.* I used to pay for others, and now they are paying for me; I think this is something that must be preserved at all cost.

Today this acquired right is being questioned in many quarters, given the difficulties and the deficits experienced by Social Security. Nonetheless, illness can no longer be conceived of without reference to sick leave, the cost of providing treatment, reimbursements, and limited payment insurances. It is a fact that although Social Security is indeed one of the mainstays of our society's health policy, it is usually envisaged by the individual as a means of meeting the financial burden of illness and gaining access to treatment. Its global role is seldom recognized. We tend to forget that Social Security is a tool for categorizing illness, for it distinguishes among such categories as "long-term illness," "disability," "occupational disease," and "work-related accident," which have a specific legal meaning and entitle an individual to services and compensation payments. At the same time, however, these are also social categories, and their definition constitutes a major stake in the interplay of economic, political, and social power relations.[17] Moreover, Social Security is a protection against nonwork in case of loss of employment and provides for an income during retirement; it is also the core of our society's family policy. In a larger sense, Social Security is one of the most important institutions of modern times. It has transformed the relationship between the individual and society in a quasi-irreversible manner and has become the centerpiece of a new model of society, the Welfare State.

Work and Social Security

To what extent has this evolution, which is irreversible as a principle, modeled individual behaviors and attitudes? Despite the recognition of the right to illness and the guarantee of being taken in charge that Social Security offers today, members of certain social categories still find it difficult to stop working in case of illness. This was expressed in 1971 by a young woman of 27 who ran a café in the suburbs of Paris. "I caught bronchitis and pharyngitis, and I stayed in bed for a week; this was quite bad for the business, because I had no one to take care of it." Work has its own laws, as a 47-year-old sheep farmer of Hérault told us in 1980: "Work calls the shots. There are times when one would like to stay in bed because one is sick, even with a fever, but one must get up to take care of the animals. So long as one isn't sick, everything is all right, but it is the same thing for everyone who is alone and has animals. You say to yourself: If you had a government job, you would take care of yourself for every little thing, and it wouldn't matter to your work. But for our work, I mean our pocketbook, it does matter."

In both these situations health seems to be clearly identified with ability to work, as the necessary condition for production. Even when income is not as closely tied to this ability to work, illness can be the source of financial difficulty, even though the cost is borne by Social Security. A 60-year-old house painter, hospitalized in Paris in 1970 for gall bladder stones, refused to stay in the hospital for an extra forty-eight hours "because it does cost money, despite Social Security; after all, one has to pay the 20 percent supplement, and 30,000 francs a day is a lot of money to wait for the results of my x-rays. What is going to happen next? And then the ambulance at 82 francs, 8,200 old francs, and it took three minutes to come here from my place. What's the point of social insurance, with prices like that?"

In order to cover the cost of the deductible, some people join mutuals, as did a young printer who was hospitalized in Blois in 1972. "Because hospitals or clinics are expensive for workers like myself, one has to have money. Myself, I am well insured, I have Social Security like everyone else, and I also joined a mutual, which pays for my deductible, so I don't have to pay a cent. I am not sorry that I did that, because an operation is expensive, it costs 3,000 or 4,000 francs, and if one is not insured like that one has to pay the 20 percent." The fact that one has to advance the money for treatment or medications can also make recourse to medical facilities difficult or even impossible, as a young mother, working as a concierge in Paris, told us in 1979: "I was very, very short of money. One day my child had convulsions, and I took him to the hospital because I couldn't pay 20 francs for a doctor. He had to have encephalograms, and they asked me to pay 20,000 francs. It was hard for me, and sometimes I couldn't do it. Sure, you are reimbursed, but first you have to advance the money, and if you don't have it, you don't get the care."

Even today, some persons feel that they are "a burden" to society because of their illness. This persistence can be explained by a very strong self-identification with productivity; such persons believe that only their work can guarantee their income and their social integration; they are unable to conceive of themselves as "entitled" and remain welfare cases in their own eyes. A 65-year-old mechanic, hospitalized for severe respiratory insufficiency in an intensive-care unit in Tours in 1972, felt that "he was bound to get sick because he had worked very hard." His entire life had been organized around "work well done," which had afforded him independence and even pleasure. "I have always loved my work, and in fact in my day one didn't work for money only as they do today. I used to work for pleasure, sometimes for free on Saturdays and Sundays." Now that illness had made him physically dependent, the idea that he could become financially dependent was most upsetting to him. "And now I can no longer do anything, I have trouble cleaning myself up, the least gesture and I am out of breath, choking. And instead of being able to help someone out, now I might have to be a burden to someone else. Why, I have always done for myself, I have always managed by myself, and I wouldn't want to become a burden to society."

The recognition that one has acquired rights by one's productive activity and that one can make use of them when the need arises did not come easily to a 69-year-old sound engineer hospitalized with a serious illness in Paris in 1972. "From the time when I started paying dues to Social Security I have contributed a lot of money and I have cost them a lot of money, and now I am starting again to cost them money. In the beginning I was a bit ashamed to take advantage of Social Security, but then I said to myself, 'No, I have been paying in for at least 30 years,' and since I have a fairly big salary, I am paying the maximum amount of dues, so what the heck, I am getting some of it back."

Some persons, like a young woman employee of 33, even go so far as to feel somewhat responsible for the difficulties facing Social Security. On sick leave for the last two months in 1979 because of acute sciatica and arthrosis of the neck, she could not help but think: "If I were in better health, would Social Security perhaps not have as many problems? My employer contributes, but that's no reason. The sums I spend on medications are incredible, and besides the treatments I get will go on for the rest of my life, unless there is a miracle cure, some advance in science. If there are many people like me, with no end of prescriptions, it's no wonder that Social Security is going broke."

Social Security also guarantees, in case of work-related accident or occupational disease, the right to a pension or to disability payments. But in that case too, the feeling of being a welfare recipient is not entirely overcome. And even if the illness is a direct consequence of their work, workers do not necessarily feel that they are entitled to compensation. This was the case in 1979 of a 36-year-old worker suffering from cirrhosis caused by benzene, who was classified as totally disabled. Having worked for 13 years in the same small rural factory, he said: "It was like a family, I knew everybody, I met my wife there, I got married, I bought a house 800 meters from the plant." The factory was his whole life, and besides he loved his work because "it was an interesting job, very varied, we never had to do the same thing all the time, it was not assembly-line work, I could work as I wanted to." He acknowledged that neither he nor his employer worried about work safety. "To install exhaust fans is an investment that would be extremely expensive for the employer, and if it is only used for a week now and then, it isn't worth it, *so one takes a chance with one's health, that's for sure."* Moreover, he said, "I never asked for a mask because the smells never bothered me, so I just breathed them without realizing it; a new guy who came to work next to me said, 'I don't know how you can take it, this thing here really smells bad.'" In 1973 he started having trouble. "The doctor told me that I was having liver colics, and I said, 'I guess my gall bladder is a bit sluggish, just prescribe a little diet for me, it'll pass' . . . and I would hold on until Friday afternoon, and I would rest Saturday and Sunday, and on Monday I would go back to work in good shape." In 1977, on the occasion of the medical checkup at work, "I had my blood test, as I did every year, but the doctor told me to come back, because it was not normal." After many tests and stays in the hospital,

> They have put me on disability. They came to check out the products with which I was working. The clauses of article something-or-other in the regulations for work-related diseases were applicable, considering the products with which I was working. So now I am entitled to a disability pension, it isn't much, and at that it isn't really worked out, because it really has to be benzene poisoning if you're to be certified. If you have been poisoned by trichloroethylene or something else, it is no longer a work-related illness. If you are in a little workshop like this, and if you mix twenty-five different products, eyeballing it just like that to come up with a glue for plastics which is not yet commercially available, and if all you have is the formula furnished by the manufacturer of the plastic . . . *then the illness is not certifiable.*

He concluded by saying: "Some people told me *I should have gone after the employer,* but I didn't feel like it." During a two-year remission of his illness, this man refused the retraining course offered by Social Security because he did not want to leave his home, and he finally obtained an office job in the area.

This example reveals another meaning that illness can assume; for here it is seen as the price one pays for employment, a price that is accepted as normal. The idea that work will inevitably wear out the body definitely persists in the minds of certain workers. Yet today also, but in a different social milieu, a young academic felt entitled to press claims for damages. Having suffered a detached retina, she considered that her illness was brought about by a conflicted work situation for which her body paid the price. Unwilling to accept this, she enlisted several physicians and a lawyer in her effort to have this illness certified as a work-related accident, an effort that failed. "This is a legal problem, but as far as I am concerned *I have the impression that this is linked to my work, but for society it does not count,* for there is supposed to be a shock, a well-circumscribed and obvious cause. If, for instance, I had broken a leg on the steps, it would have been a work-related accident, but if I kill one of my eyes working, it is not an accident." This is an extreme case of determination to carry the fight for one's rights all the way, even if these rights are not evident. One wonders whether this attitude foreshadows a radically different relationship between the wage earner and his or her work.

Many workers, however, feel that they cannot give in to their illness and its consequences, even when they know that their work has something to do with it. In 1970 a 61-year-old cleaning woman suffering from phlebitis acknowledged: "I was in bad shape, completely worn out, I would come home at night and go right to bed, I couldn't even eat any more, and that's why I got this. I probably pushed myself too hard, I pushed myself." But despite this realization, she missed her work: "I don't think I will go back to work, because I can't walk any more . . . I would have liked to go back to work, you know; yes indeed, it was my whole life." Similarly a 51-year-old farmer whom we interviewed in 1960, when he was paralyzed by a work accident, found it particularly difficult to "watch the others work" because his life had always revolved around work: "Here I am, forced to do nothing, and the worst of it is to watch the others work and to be unable to do the same thing—not to be able to put my hand to the job, and just sit in the car, because I have worked all my life since I was very young, and now it's pretty hard to take that I can't do anything."

Here illness has the character of a forced disruption of day-to-day life, which puts an end to the individual's professional, familial, or political activities. To be sick means above all to be unable to cope with the various demands of life, to be condemned to immobility or inactivity. Yet activity is precisely what defines the individual's relation to society, and the recognition of the right to illness has not fundamentally changed this relation. More precisely, the development of wage labor has had two kinds of consequences. On the one hand, the link between the right to employment and the right to security has become institutionalized; on the other hand, an essential connection between the individual's occupational activity and his or her identity has become established. As a result, the enforced inactivity of illness has become unbearable, for by destroying the ties that make it possible to be integrated into society and thereby to exist, illness has become tantamount to social exclusion. It isolates the sick from the world and from other people and encloses them within a solitude that cannot be shared. This breakdown of social ties is perceived all the more negatively if the subject is deeply committed to, and totally identified with, a social role. This is particularly prevalent in those professions where individuals have responsibilities that make them feel indispensable. But this kind of identification exists everywhere. We have seen it in the disabled farmer in 1960, and we also see it in a young mother who, also in 1960, expressed her fear of being excluded and marginalized by illness: "What is really so awful is that illness, I believe, really makes you very lonely . . . One is really out of the world. *When there is illness one is, and one stays, alone.* It's very hard to get help . . . It destroys what one would like to do, it isolates you." Solitude and isolation are compounded by the inability to cope: "If I got into very poor health, I could no longer do what I do with the children, I could no longer take care of them as I do." And if she could not fulfill her obligations as a mother, she would be "out of it," passive, and therefore useless. "I would be cut off from my family, life would have to be organized without me, I would not play the role that I play now. I believe that one who is sick is outside of normal life." In speaking about an illness she had had some months earlier, this woman acknowledged that "during that month life was organized without me, I didn't feel that I was involved, I felt that I was out of it," and she added, "one feels that one is on the fringe when one is sick."

In 1942 Dr. Allendy, sick and bedridden, considered his situation "infinitely pitiful," for he too found work indispensable to his social integration and his identity. "I can see that my career will end in destitution, oblivion, and suffocation, in sorrow at being unable to continue being what I was and of being rejected, like a faulty part, by a world that might become as ferocious as it is incomprehensible to me."[18]

By enforcing inactivity, illness thus prevents individuals from "playing their role," marginalizes them, and can even provoke a feeling of loss of identity. "Who am I?" the sick person wonders. These questions sometimes reveal a feeling of total annihilation of the personality, even the desire to end it all, as we heard from a furniture worker who had suffered a work accident in 1972. "A few days after the operation, ideas came into my head, ideas, shall we say, of just blowing myself away. I am not ashamed to say it, and after a while one does realize that one is not so disabled that one has to do away with oneself and that one can go back to work after all. In fact, that's exactly what happened, because I was rehired by the factory and given a different job."

Generally, however, severe illness does signify social death. The young woman cited above talked about a woman and her 35-year-old husband, who had contracted multiple sclerosis: "This has completely destroyed their life. I feel that there is no way to have an active life when a severe illness has struck. I feel that a severe illness that really makes it impossible to live a normal life is a turning point, it's the end, I really feel it's death."

In 1960 a young man of 35, who had had asthma since childhood, also expressed the feeling that his life had been destroyed. "My illness interfered with my schoolwork when I was a kid, and later when I wanted to go to medical school I finally had to give it up. It also kept me from doing what I wanted to do; I tried business, that didn't work out, I tried teaching, but I quit after a while." Unable to complete any project, he found himself "without a profession, in no position to think about marriage or founding a family." This unfulfilled life, which was destroyed by illness, also led this man to examine his own personality: "I am not very energetic by nature, and the virtual energy that was in me was snuffed out by the illness because I was spoiled as a sick child and this reinforced my effeminate traits."

Many sick people reject inactivity and its destructive consequences by developing an ethic of endurance. Not paying attention to oneself, acting as if nothing were wrong, are aspects of this ethic, which amounts to a kind of denial of the organic reality or at least to stripping it of any importance. The young mother whom we interviewed in 1960 refused to give in to illness and therefore always minimized her troubles: "I have practically never stayed in bed since I was married and had children, and I have always been in good health. A flu can be treated quickly, and when I have a sore throat I try to stop it right away, and in any case, I can take it, I don't go to bed." When she did have to stay in bed for three weeks, her only aim was "to recover as soon as possible, in order to get back to normal," for, she continued, "I do not accept the fact that I am sick to begin with, and so I have to get it over with very quickly."

Twenty years later a 48-year-old cleaning woman, the mother of six children, also developed an ethic dominated by the concept of endurance. For her the obligation to cope and to face the trials of life was much stronger than the signals sent by her body. "In any case," she said, "I don't pay attention to myself, I am too busy, and even if I don't feel well, I say that I'm all right and that's the best way to stay healthy, because if you pay attention to yourself, if you say, 'I don't feel so good today, I am going to go to bed,' well, that's when you get sick." In 1960 a young assistant film producer, suffering from asthma and tuberculosis, asserted that he "did not really feel sick," even though, he said, "I am 26 years old, and I have had an illness for about 19 years, but it has never really bothered me. I don't know whether I am used to illness or used to overcoming it, but I rarely ever feel it as such." In 1942 Dr. Allendy remarked: "In the inter-war period, I never changed my work load for an ongoing illness. Under no cir-cumstances did I want to fall into the category of the sick."[19]

Another way to refuse to "be a sick person" and to "become part of the world of the sick" is to make the active struggle against the illness one's occupation. In that case the "job of being sick" takes the place of the healthy person's work. "Being sick is a job, now I know that it is a job," said the woman with breast cancer, in 1960. "But I'll tell you that for me it will become more of a job when I can really fight my illness; now I don't fight because I am working, I don't have the time. I don't have the time to give my illness all the attention it deserves, I have too many things to do." This substitution does not entail total emptiness, it does not lead to the loss of one's social role, for the fight against the illness to some extent ensures a continued integration into society. In replacing one job with another in this manner, the sick establish a continuity between health and illness and thereby preserve their identity.

Illness has always, of course, entailed inactivity and the sick person's forced retreat from active participation in collective life. There have probably always been people who for this reason did not want to give in to illness. Nonetheless, the link between illness as inactivity and the feeling of loss of identity, which has become central today, seems to us to be a relatively new phenomenon. It must no doubt be seen in relation with the development of wage labor, which assigns to each of us a specific place in society, defined by our activity. But the feeling of loss of identity as a result of illness also affects other areas of social involvement, and this too, it seems to us, is a characteristic trait of modern sen-sibility. This change in attitude is strikingly illustrated if we recall the case of Chateaubriand, wounded at the siege of Thionville in September 1792, and fleeing with the "army of the princes" to Jersey. Immobilized there by a severe case of smallpox, cut off "from all serious things, especially politics," and strug-gling against death, he only learned at the end of January 1793 of the death of Louis XVI when he saw his uncle dressed in deep mourning.[20]

Yet for all his intense commitment, the forced interruption of his political ac-tivity did not elicit any comment from Chateaubriand. It was nothing more than a sequence of facts, brought about by a bodily ailment to be sure, but it did not in any way threaten the author's self-image or his identity. By contrast, it was immediately at this level that a young deputy in the National Assembly experienced his removal from active political life in 1960, when he became im-mobilized by rheumatoid arthritis. "I received letters from a friend who was founding a youth exchange center. He was very active, and I really felt useless. This was also the time of the Front Républicain, I read about it in *l'Express*, very exciting articles by Mauriac, and I felt totally useless."

The inactivity entailed by illness thus means desocialization and loss of iden-tity, despite the institutionalization of illness. In fact, this identification with our social role and our work may have been reinforced by the recognition of the right to illness and the legitimation of the status of a sick person. As a result, the representation of "the sick person," that is, someone who stands apart in the social system (a representation that is shared by all of us), informs the subject's attitude as soon as illness strikes. We must decide whether or not we will accept seeing ourselves or being seen as "a sick person." Will being sick make us willing to be part of the world of the sick, or will we reject that world, in the manner of the American sociologist I. K. Zola, who prefers "having a handicap" to "being handicapped"? More and more sick people insist that there is more to them than their illness, that their illness does not define them. Does this mean that access to social rights is not sufficient to bring about a positive identity of the sick and that the right to illness should be understood as the right to be sick rather than to be "a sick person"?

Being Changed by Illness

If illness destroys the normal ties between individuals and the social order, it also serves to reveal the nature of these ties. As their social relations dissolve in the wake of illness, individuals learn to examine and even modify the ties by which they are integrated into society and bound to others. A severe and life-threatening case of acute uremia caused a 48-year-old architect in Lille to become conscious of his vulnerability; he realized that sometimes the law of the body is stronger than anything and that one has to conform to it. "It has been a lesson in humility; I used to be very proud, I mean, if one were to push it to extreme, I thought I was the greatest, the handsomest, the strongest, I thought that nothing could hurt me. I used to say as a joke that I would die at 85 under the revolver shots of a jealous husband. And then I realized that I am not even 50 and that I almost went off, not under the bullets of a jealous husband but under the assault of urea. *So that made me think*." But he learned his lesson — he had to change his life. "I think there comes a time in life when, even if one has an exceptional nature, one must know how to stop, *one must know how to change one's life*, one must know how to slow down in all areas, work, eating, drinking. I think that time has come for me. What happens in one's life is not fortuitous, I think it always means something, it is a warning signal."

Illness can also become the occasion for questioning the direction of one's life. An enforced although authorized and legitimate pause, illness provided the occasion to take stock for a 49-year-old unemployed female pianist: "I have to start all over again. I have had a reeducation in every area, with respect to my nervous and digestive systems, and with respect to seeing life differently. A new chance, a new life, is opening before me. If you will, this has forced me, because otherwise I think I would have let myself die, looking all the while as if I were fighting back. For me, this illness is beneficial, I am going to make a new start."

Completely identified with his social role, a 50-year-old executive recognized, following an operation for peritonitis in 1972, that he had been so absorbed by his different obligations that he no longer had any time for himself, his family, and his friends. "What am I doing to myself? How can I go on living like this?" he wondered while he was in the hospital.

> I am 50 years old, and for me this operation will have been a kind of break, *a kind of turning point in my life*, because I have had time to think, far from the commotion of my professional life. I have had time to reflect, to put my problems into perspective a bit, both with respect to my work and to my family. And I even have the hope that in the coming weeks I will mature further in this kind of forced retreat, as it were, that has been imposed on me. As the director of a firm, I had a great deal of stress and worry, and then, from one day to the next, *there was a sudden and complete break. I am free, I am truly in a virgin state*, without constraints of any kind. This break will have been beneficial for me, it will be a pivot in my life. First of all, one proves to oneself that one is not indispensable; after all, the business goes on anyway. So one can stop, one can trust others. Somehow it is a period of great meditation, which I would never have had otherwise, it had to come about through illness.

One wonders whether illness, in addition to being the occasion for meditation and self-examination, can also lead to the emergence of another identity, a new social personality. At one level, it happens quite frequently that individuals who are condemned to inactivity realize in the course of this brush with illness that they can, with perfect legitimacy, give in, abandon their responsibilities, and forget the social constraints by which they are bound. In that case illness means freedom from the weight and the demands of society, it means the chance to take advantage of this respite in order to think about this illness and about one's life in general. Having become a defense against the established order and a rejection of a social role, illness then assumes the character of an escape and an opening: "I believe that illnesses are keys that can unlock certain doors for us," wrote André Gide on 24 July 1930; indeed he also wrote, "I believe that there are certain doors that only illness can unlock." By facilitating the access to a different world, illness thus becomes the equivalent of an initiatory voyage. "I have never met one of those people who brag that they have never been sick who was not, in some way, a little stupid; like those who have never traveled; and I remember that Charles-Louis Philippe used to call illnesses, very prettily, the poor man's travels."[21] It is a turning inward toward oneself and one's relations with others.

This voyage can also assume a moral sense by transforming the sufferer and revealing a new person. "I believe that in some way illness can be a benefit for people who accept suffering, it can almost give them more of a life," said a young 26-year-old painter in 1960, when he saw how his father-in-law had changed during years of suffering from cancer. "I realize that this man, after a while, began to accept his illness, and this, in a sense, made him a much deeper person. He had a more solid grasp of things, one could almost say that at the end he was a better man than before."

Illness as a refuge and an escape, which can mean access to oneself and to others, can also become a self-realization, a total liberation of the personality. An intense experience, illness liberates us from the false personality society forces us to be, said a young female journalist in 1960:

> One has the impression that one is infinitely more alive . . . , and suddenly one sees everything in a passionate light, which has nothing to do with daily life . . . One is delivered from all the things that stupidly take up one's time in life, and only those that matter are left, among them just living, that is really all there is. I firmly believe in the influence of illness on people; *it permits them to be what they were originally and what they could not be because of social circumstances*. So illness is a life outside of life, a parenthesis where one has the right to develop all the things that one has within oneself, knowing perfectly well that afterward one has to go back, that it cannot go on.

A parenthesis in ordinary affairs, illness makes it possible to exist and to live fully. It is also a moment of pleasure that one must seize, provided that "one experiences it for oneself, and not for others, it is a kind of solitary pleasure," the young woman continued, considering that "in comparison with a severe illness, there are very few experiences of such lasting importance in life; a truly severe illness rates as highly as a first love."

This young woman also advanced the outlines of a more assertive conception, depicting illness as the right to laziness. By this she did not mean simply that one should take advantage of a forced retreat from one's social role, but rather that it may be necessary to seek a break from it. Illness can thus turn from an interruption to a kind of strike against one's social role. "I do not think that it is very honest to say, 'I am in a hurry to get out of here to do this or that.' I mean, I personally think that I would be more honest if I said, 'It would be terrific if I had a week or two to catch up with myself, if I could stop everything for a week or two and find out where I'm at.' And I also think that this last concern is deeper and more honest."

Refusing to comply with the existing order and its constraints by managing one's illness in such a way that it becomes the equivalent of a strike against one's social role—that is, an active, voluntary, and even sought-for interruption—is tantamount to a legitimate way of escaping from, indeed rejecting, all professional, familial, and social responsibilities. Here illness is no longer only a defense but becomes an actual protest of the individual against society.

Sick Leave and the Management of the Body

It is in relation with industry, in the work place, that illness can be most clearly understood and interpreted as a real menace to the social order, for here it is liable to impair an industry's productive capacity. The health of the workers is a major issue at the level of power relations within industry, where it must be balanced, often at the cost of permanent compromise, against economic imperatives. Seen in this perspective, taking sick leave can be an individual's legitimate way of protesting against the exigencies of production. The sociologist Pierre Dubois goes so far as to consider it "a purposeful and active labor strategy, a form of action of the same nature as strikes and slowdowns."[22] Nonetheless, despite their "social" causes, occupational illnesses and work-related accidents remain individual health problems; in the same manner taking sick leave—granted that what is commonly called "absenteeism" constitutes a social problem—is first and foremost an individual means of managing the body and translates a whole set of interactions among working conditions, personal commitment to one's job, mastery over one's time, and states of corporal ill-being. "For the same illness," writes J. C. Sournia, "one person will feel terrible and take sick leave, while another will continue in his habitual occupations. Every individual also has his own conception of the social obligations involved in his work. If artisans, directors, managers, and foremen take less sick leave than unionized workers, it is because we have not yet found a way to *interest* all wage earners in their work."[23]

By becoming an issue in the contractual relations involving the individual and the State on the one hand, and the worker and his employer on the other, the matter of sick leave thus reveals the plasticity of the notion of illness. The existence of an institutionalized right to sick leave and compensation demands a straightforward decision in the face of a series of often ambiguous states, namely whether or not to take sick leave, whether or not to be "sick." A recent study[24] shows how in the work place the notion of illness and the decision to "take a break" are part of a complex set of considerations in which the more or less constricting nature of the worker's relations with the job and the possibility of modifying them play the most important role. The status of the individual also plays a role, as does the manner in which the sick leave will be judged, that is, the degree of confidence or suspicion with which the individual is viewed. Moreover, in each case, an implicit normative standard determines how much morbidity and discomfort, interfering with work without bringing it to a halt, is to be tolerated; a similar standard implicitly acknowledges each person's right to a permissible amount of sick leave. The traditional "capital of health" has thus been superseded today by a "fund of permissible sick leave," a kind of institutionalized safety valve designed to ease the constraints and exigencies of work. To some extent individuals are free to manage this fund as they see fit, sometimes independently of any symptoms. This is quite obvious in the statement of a female librarian, who said, "I have had little colds, stuff like that, but I don't stop working very easily, I don't like to; but if I do, I go all the way and take a week, *I give myself a week*."[25]

Sick leave can even be used to indicate discomfort with one's work, which in that case becomes a symbolic equivalent of illness. "When I am sick, I usually go to work," a young educator told Nicholas Dodier in an interview in 1982. In this young man's case it is not illness that keeps him from working and imposes inactivity; it is discomfort with his working situation that he manifests by making use of his right to sick leave. "If I take sick leave, it is because something has gone wrong in my work. When that happens I ask for sick leave to get some distance, to see if it can be worked out . . . I take sick leave to show that I don't agree, I use it as an argument."[26] Sick leave as a pretext becomes part of a combative attitude of protest; in making use of it, the young educator proclaims his right to control the constraints and the conditions of his work.

Illness and Social Protest

If we want to go beyond individual experiences and the reasons why individuals decide to stop working, we must investigate the times and the places in which the issue of illness has united and mobilized collectivities in protest movements against pathogenic or dangerous working conditions that have threatened the social order in the past. In the nineteenth century, as we have shown,[27] health was one of the workers' demands, and the struggle for shorter working hours was also a struggle against the effects of overwork. Following the promulgation of a social legislation at the end of the century, the struggle for better working conditions came to include the struggle for effective use of the new rights granted to the workers. Work-related accidents and the law of 1898 that provided for medical care and a pension for the injured worker became the central issues of these movements. The unions demanded that work-related accidents be certified as such by physicians of their choice, rather than by doctors in the pay of the industry. Some groups of left-wing medical practitioners participated in this movement, in particular those connected with the Syndicat de la Médecine Sociale after 1908. One can read, for example, in the February 1911 issue of their periodical *La Médecine sociale*: "The workers' right to channel the victims of work accidents toward certain physicians is a necessity for the working class in its struggle against the employer class . . . The labor unions have a duty to seek out those physicians who give them every guarantee of defending their rights and their interests." At the same time, however, physicians and unionized workers sought to state, also in this periodical, the problem of working conditions and health. Between 1920 and 1930, at the time of the debate over the creation of a system of social insurance, one also finds in the union publications some effort to steer the discussion toward the idea that public health and the health of the working class should be guaranteed through the institution of social insurances. One can read in the review of the 1929 Congress of the Confédération Generale du Travail (C.G.T.): "Social insurance is not, in our opinion, only an institution that will have to distribute services . . . it can become, if the working class as a whole wants it to be, the rational first step in our country of a vast, scientifically and methodically organized campaign for the defense of public health."[28] And, further on: "For us, the law concerning social insurance is essentially *a law for the protection of working-class health* or, stated better, of public health. It marks the active involvement of the working class in the country's health policy."[29]

Yet in actual fact, as the social laws became more encompassing, and as the medical profession was called upon to judge the right to sick leave, the problem of pathogenic working conditions was too often reduced to the problem of access to medical care and payments for services rendered; and these decisions were made by the physician. Moreover, the activities of the Committees of Health and Safety, which were established in each factory after World War II, were essentially restricted to problems of health and safety and did not afford any real input into the discussion of actual conditions of production.[30] It is worth noting, in fact, that both the wage earners and the union leaders are willing to grant the medical profession and the Social Security administration their role as experts and as guardians of health. In 1979 a garment worker, serving as the representative of his union in his firm's Committee of Health and Safety, said: "If Social Security were watching the working conditions, it would be good for the workers' health and for working people in general. Social Security should monitor the shifts in the work place and use medical specialists, who must know what kinds of shifts the workers can put up with, how long they can work without stopping." However, he was opposed to the intervention of a nonmedical expert: "One day a time-and-motion engineer showed up and started to clock me. It's simple, he could never get the same time twice. So I said, 'What does this have to do with medicine? Does he know a person's value? Is he a health professional?' "

In recent years, however, various groups issued from the Movement of May 1968 have developed actions designed to further radical objectives. In addition to denouncing work as a pathogenic factor, they also object to the "screen of medicine," its "neutralizing" function in the conflict between workers and employers. Such groups as the Comité d'Action Santé or Tankonalasanté* in France and the Heidelberg Socialist Patients' Collective (S.P.K.) in Germany set out to develop an aggressive concept that would turn illness into a revolutionary force, the site where the contradictions within society become visible.

*["Tant qu'on a la santé" ("As long as one has health").]

"Politicizing medicine," says Dr. Jean-Claude Polack, "is to find in each illness that which, despite the screen of medicine, protests against the social order and hence, once it becomes conscious, threatens it."[31] In the early 1970s the aim was to "use illness as a weapon," to cite the title of one of S.P.K.'s militant pamphlets.[32] This implies bringing the message to the place where the exploitative relationship is played out, where illness, as the militants of the S.P.K. put it, "objectively digs the grave of capitalism by weakening the labor force"; that is, to the work place.

This is also the perspective of the Comité d'Action Santé in France, which in February 1969 distributed at the gates of the Renault plant in Flins a tract denouncing the natural violence of capital and calling for a takeover in the interest of the workers' health. "We must change the working day. You are your own doctor. Take power in this factory and in society, and you will be in charge of your own lives ... You demand sick leave. Social Security takes care of it, but you can be sure that you will pay the bill in the end. Take power in the factory, make a revolution. It's healthier."

This radical position, which harked back to May 1968, was followed in the years around 1972 by a certain number of conflicts over work-related hazards within industry. With the support of physicians and members of the group Information Santé, miners in northern France acquired a better understanding of silicosis, and sanitation workers came to denounce their working conditions in the sewers. But the very symbol of this movement was the conflict that racked the Pennaroya Company. When strikes broke out simultaneously at its Saint-Denis and Lyon plants on 9 February 1972, a statement written by the workers and cosigned by the C.G.T. union representatives of Saint-Denis and Lyon denounced intolerable working conditions and the risks of lead poisoning, to which the workers were exposed because their job involved the manipulation of lead. The statement demanded, in particular, "the workers' control over the medical analyses."[33] In the course of the thirty-two-day strike, "documents supporting the workers' demands and information about the hazards to which they are exposed (lead poisoning, the legislation about the handling of lead in the work place, criticism of the regulations for preventing lead poisoning, and so forth) were published by a physicians' collective."[34] After the signing of the strike settlement, a *collective letter from the workers*, signed by the Lyon branch of the Confédération Française et Démocratique du Travail (C.F.D.T.) on 31 March 1972, reported on the first results of the action. "*In order to defend our health*, we have won the right to automatic communication of medical analyses after each medical examination. We have obtained the presence of a registered nurse in the factory during 40 hours per week. We have obtained a general inspection of the plant, with a view to deciding which installations are necessary to control smoke, dust, and poor lighting."[35]

These struggles over toxic hazards and occupational illnesses thus gave rise,

just as had been the case in the early years of the century, to a collaboration between physicians and labor unions. The "experts" decided to place their
professional knowledge at the disposal of the workers. In this manner, not only
illness itself but also its recognition became an issue within the industrial enterprise. In the view of those who denounce it as the result of working conditions and the logic of economic necessity, illness is neither inevitable nor an
individual concern. Nor is its identification only a matter for medical expertise, for those who suffer it know how to recognize its first manifestations and
to detect its warning signs. They themselves are capable of relating their own
experiences to the technical knowledge transmitted by the physicians. It is important that their input be taken into account and recognized independently of
the medical legitimacy that is called upon to sanction and authorize medical
services.

Yet one may wonder about the limits of such endeavors, considering that
these actions, along with subsequent protests against the employers' control
over sick leave, focused on the issue of the workers' appropriation of medical
knowledge and a redefinition of the relation between experts and lay people,
providers and receivers of medical care. The same position was taken by the
group that, under the leadership of Dr. Jean Carpentier, began in 1973 to pub-
lish *Tankonalasanté*. "If we want to use illness as a weapon with which to
change society," we read in the editorial of the second issue, "it is important to
fight, in word and deed, the separation between care-giver and care-receiver."
Similarly, the patients of the Socialist Patients' Collective of Heidelberg
directed the bulk of their criticism against the psychiatric establishment without breaking with medicine as a whole or going much further than questioning
the doctor-patient relationship.

No doubt this orientation is due in large part to the fact that these actions
were undertaken by or in collaboration with physicians. But as we have shown,
this is no coincidence, for as the arbiter of the right to sick leave the physician
is also, by the same token and even if he would prefer not to think about it, the
arbiter of health as a factor of production. As soon as this set of values is being
questioned, some physicians are bound to feel directly involved.

This situation once again reveals the ambiguity of the socialization of illness that resulted from the establishment of national health insurance and social legislation. The right to sick leave made illness a social issue, yet it has also
remained an individual right. We do know that the link between work and illness is inherent in the social relations of production, yet this link is expressed
as one individual's absence from work, a statement by another individual, and
an encounter that involves only these two persons. This may be one of the
main reasons why it has been difficult for these protests to merge with larger
movements and to bring about a greater control of the workers over their concrete working conditions. Indeed, the very emphasis on the individual implied

in medicalization may have the effect of a certain neutralization of social relations. The sick person defined as legitimately inactive, as entitled to sick leave and medical care, does have a specific status in society, but such a person cannot be a social activist.

11·

Providers and Receivers of Care: Medicine and the Sick

*T*he recognition of a right to illness, to which the individual gains access through his or her occupational activities, has defined a new status of the sick. In this process medicine is constantly involved. Medicine is still called upon to make the final decision in identifying and legitimizing illness. The physician is the necessary point of entry to the itinerary by which illness marks and reveals the social order. Illness as a social phenomenon must thus be understood in its twofold reference to work and to medicine.

There is no question that for all of us today recourse to the physician has become the immediate corollary of any state of illness. The physician, for his or her part, is obliged to provide "care" in all cases; even if the problem is minor and will in all probability cure itself; even if, on the contrary, the disorder is one of those against which modern medicine remains powerless. We have come to consider outlays for health and medical care as self-evident items in the national budget. Indeed, obtaining medical care has assumed the value of a moral obligation. "The good patient," we are told by Talcott Parsons, who in the 1950s formulated the notion of the "role of the patient,"[1] has the duty to look for competent medical help and to cooperate with the physician. Today, any reflection about the status of the sick must therefore begin with an analysis of the sick person's relations to medicine. How do the sick experience their illness in their relations with health-care institutions? In what ways does being taken in charge by medicine shape their identity? In asking these questions, we must keep in mind that medicine is not just one institution among others; Eliot Freidson has gone so far as to define it as the prototype of all contemporary social institutions.[2] The question that looms behind these first questions is therefore: In what ways does medicine today affect the experience of the individual's place in society?

The Slow Ascent of Medicine

This central importance of medicine in society is a recent phenomenon. The "receiver of care" – and by this we mean both the individual as the object of active and ineluctable medical intervention and the metaphorical crystallization of a relationship with modern society – is a thoroughly contemporary figure.

Combating illness, of course, is a timeless behavior. It is certainly not difficult to find in the past evidence for all kinds of endeavors to find help against illness. But these were long deployed in all directions before they were vested in the physician. Robert Muchembled[3] tells us that in the Western world, even in the late Middle Ages, the people of the countryside – where death was always threatening and where no physician was available – appealed almost exclusively to soothsayers and healers, whose practices were a close combination of magical and religious rituals. Healers were omnipresent in the countryside until the end of the sixteenth century. They faded from view in the seventeenth century – the period when sorcerers and especially witches were hunted and burned in France – only to resurface in the eighteenth century. For several hundred years the Church was adamant in its opposition to such people and endeavored to trace a dividing line between religion and superstition, between the appeal to God, which it presented as the only true hope of the sick, and magical practices. In the countryside, the physician was by and large uninvolved in the conflict between the priest and the healer.

In the cities by contrast, and especially at court, the physician was a well-known figure; in the fourteenth century, Froissart mentioned King Charles V's confidence in them: "Of all the people in the world, those whom he trusted most for his health were good masters of medicine, and these doctors very often comforted and pleased him, telling him that with their good prescriptions they would make him live naturally as long as would be sufficient."[4] Although one notes, in the course of centuries, the increasingly frequent presence of the physician at the bedside of the sick or the dying, the physician long remained a secondary figure. When Anne d'Autriche was dying, for instance, the function of the attending physicians amounted to little more than announcing the imminence of death.[5] The priest still occupied the entire space of illness and death. In the eighteenth century the physician began to assert himself, and Michel Vovelle tells us that as the grand ceremonial of death became more intimate "the confessor had to yield his place to the physician."[6] He cites as an example the presence of the physician, M. Tronchin, at the death of Mme de Custine, described by Mme de Genlis. "The night of the fourth day of her illness was dreadful. She sent for her confessor at two o'clock and at three she received extreme unction. This was the beginning of her fifth day; M. Tronchin, whom we had asked to be awakened, came at half past three."[7] One notices, however, that the priest was present before the doctor, just as he had been in the preceding century. But one does recognize an attitude close to our own in the reaction of the friends of Chateaubriand, who was ill in London in 1793. Concerned about his condition, they "dragged him from doctor to doctor," he tells us.[8] But as recourse to the physician became more common, it was accompanied, as a corollary no doubt of increasing dependence, by defiance and denigration. Montaigne, for example, never ceased to criticize medicine and physicians: "In medicine I greatly honour that glorious name, what it suggests, what it promises, so useful to mankind, but what it designates among us, I neither honour nor value."[9] For centuries, moreover, the image of medicine as transmitted by testimonies that have come down to us was usually one of ineffectiveness, and often one of outright brutality. In many of them we perceive the dread, only half-expressed, of those treatments that intensified the pain without improving the sufferer's chances of recovery. Here, for example, is the seventeenth-century account of the death of Saint François de Sales and the strange "butchery" to which his surgeons subjected him:

> Toward five in the evening, the physicians judged and resolved [that it was necessary] to use extreme means: that is why, having already applied a poultice of Spanish flies to his head, they twice thrust the tip of a red-hot iron into the nape of his neck, which he suffered with great patience, although he shed quantities of tears and, lifting up his shoulders very slightly, only uttered the sacred names of Jesus and Mary. And surely such remedies, and such butchery by the surgeons, made his death quite inevitable. But even more was done to him: for after they had applied the red-hot iron to his skull for the third time, they pulled off the poultice, which peeled off his outer skin and left him altogether without skin from the nape of the neck to the forehead, and in this state they thrust the iron so deeply into his head that thick smoke issued from it and that the skull was burned.[10]

In the last decades of the nineteenth century, however, medicine and the physician definitively came into their own. In 1892, following a long struggle,[11] a law was passed that gave the medical profession its full legitimacy and ensured its monopoly vis-à-vis the various kinds of healers who still existed in large numbers. In 1902 the passing of the Public Health Law also testified to society's faith in medicalization. In this manner the physician had become a respected notable who had a decent and often comfortable income, an enviable social status, and unquestioned influence in society at large. At the same time, his public image was being idealized, and focused in particular on his charity and devotion to duty.[12] Henceforth the physician was seen as one who tirelessly relieved suffering, comforted, and reassured. As the brutality of medical intervention faded from the collective imagery, the intrinsically helpful power of his very presence asserted itself.[13] "Responding to the patient's call," which was reassuring though far from always effective, was henceforth seen as the typical conduct of the practitioner.

Above all, the physician now embodied science and its power. He partook of it by an almost religious connection, so that the "ministry" of the physician-scholar became part of a popular set of unexamined notions concerning medicine. This view was the source of his power to establish norms. Confident in the values it incarnated, medicine henceforth claimed the right to state the rules by which society should abide. As early as the late eighteenth century, sanitarianism, which had analyzed the interrelations among health, the material environment, and social conditions, had tended quite naturally to enter the public arena in order to state the principles that make for a harmonious balance among these factors.

In 1833 Balzac already described, in the figure of Dr. Benassis in *The Country Doctor*, the connection between sanitary and social intervention. In the second half of the century, moreover, the physician entered the private space, that of sexuality and the family. Syphilis in particular was the occasion that permitted the practitioner to invade the areas of sex and the lineage.[14] Luc Boltanski has also analyzed the ways in which, around 1900, early childhood and its special requirements came under the control of medicine and have been governed by its rules ever since.[15] In the wake of the Pasteurian revolution, which afforded the physician the prestige of increased effectiveness and the certainty that the principles he incarnates are correct, advice gave way to orders. Society entered the *"age of medicine,"* which was announced some sixty years ago by Dr. Knock.[16] Today we are firmly entrenched in that age, for all of our practices involving the body in any way assume meaning in relation to medicine. "All of existence is medical," writes J. B. Pontalis, paraphrasing Jules Romains.[17]

Yet, paradoxically, it is the sick who have held out longest against the ascendancy of medicine. For a long time there were more ukases handed down by medicine than physicians who treated the sick. It is true that the number of practitioners, as well as the recourse to practitioners, increased.[18] Nonetheless, even between the two world wars, consulting a doctor was a fairly unusual step, a resource in cases of serious illness and dramatic situations rather than a routine form of behavior. The physicians themselves felt that the exercise of medicine should remain a rare and costly act, in the interest of upholding the prestige of the profession.[19] It was only in the wake of the organization of Social Security in 1945, and especially its progressive generalization in the following decades, that Dr. Knock's objective, "above all I want people to get medical care," was fully attained.[20] When he stated it in 1923, this wish was still far from becoming a reality. But today it has been fulfilled, for seeking medical help and thus being inducted into a "medical existence" has become the almost immediate reaction to the slightest malaise. In 1960 the attitude of a 31-year-old professor, who said, "I have no real fear of illness, I am not at all concerned with preserving my health," was already beginning to be atypical. It would be even more so today.

The Obligation to Seek Medical Help and to Get Well

Seeking medical care has, moreover, assumed the value of a norm. Our vocabulary henceforth includes the notion of the "good patient." All of us have a clear idea of what this means: "good patients" are those who take care of themselves. In 1960 a technician said: "When one is sick, one obviously tries to get better as soon as possible. Personally, I do everything I can, I try to do my utmost to be cured as quickly as possible." He added, "I would be a good patient, come to think of it." By contrast, twenty years later, a young female employee admitted that she was a "bad patient," "not in the sense that I complain," she specified, "but in the sense that I don't seriously take care of myself."

Within this framework, getting well has become the equivalent of an obligation. Although recovery is part of the medical model, it is uncertain and was long perceived as such. As Ambroise Paré said: "I dressed his wound, God cured him." Looking at our own time, the sociologist Rose Coser writes: "The good patient, as defined by society, is one who not only obeys the doctors and the nurses, but also recovers quickly and is able to resume his activities."[21] Getting well responds to the needs of society: in 1960 a young woman journalist put it this way: "Even under a communist regime one has the right to be sick. But one does not have the right to be useless to society; so once you are sick, the only thing you are absolutely asked to do is to get well." Recovery also calls upon the subject's will power and "desire to get well," which have become imperatives. Also in 1960, a 60-year-old agricultural engineer saw his return to health as a veritable moral duty: "It is a moral duty to recover one's health, the first duty to oneself and everyone else." This duty also implies "seeking help from those who can restore one's health, that is to say, the doctors. It seems to me that in this respect one must not count on oneself too much and trust those who are capable of getting one's health back." This man characterized himself as someone who frequently consulted doctors, trusted them, and was confident that they would make him well. Yet, he added, "one of the things one must have is self-confidence and confidence in one's own strength; it is much harder for people who give up to regain their health, and besides, they don't make the task of those who treat them any easier." What is expressed here is a different conception, one in which the modern notion of expert treatment allies itself with the very old theme of the individual as his own physician. Getting well demands obedience to the physician, but also will power and effort on the part of the sufferers, the mobilization of their own healing power.

In his notion of the "patient's role," Talcott Parsons has perfectly formulated this conception, which is entirely centered on the positive value of medicine and the recourse to medical care. He says that in modern society the individual has the right to be sick, and that those who are sick are exempted from their responsibilities, in particular the demands of production. Here Parsons's theory reflects the fact that illness has become part of the social space of work. The sick person is also entitled to help. But this help, as well as the legitimacy of the illness, will only be granted under the condition that the sick person "wants to get well," for this desire constitutes the most effective barrier against the temptation of deviance represented by illness and the secondary benefits that come with it. The other condition is that the sick person seek and follow competent medical advice. In Parsons's perspective—which was elaborated in the early 1950s; that is, at a time when medical techniques and institutions were developing rapidly—providing medical care thus constitutes the essential part of society's help to the sick person. Parsons makes the point that this care has replaced the family, whose role he sees as declining.[22] He also views medical supervision as entirely positive; to seek treatment more often and earlier can only be beneficial. Thus, medical treatment and medicine itself are presented here in the light of a flawless legitimacy.

In our interviews with certain persons, especially in 1960, we also encountered this total adherence to the positive value of medical treatment and the need to submit to it with complete docility. The already cited electronics technician said: "When you come right down to it, in order to get well it is necessary to go along with a treatment, and one is glad to take on this obligation in order to get well. Myself, anyway, when I know that I must do something to get well, I don't mind doing it. If someone doesn't want to go along with a treatment, that really amounts to wanting to commit suicide." Among the lower classes in particular, statements of entire confidence, pure and simple obedience to the doctor's orders, are quite common. Thus a 57-year-old road worker, hospitalized in 1972, told us: "So I went to the clinic of a doctor who, I think, is taking very good care of me. He knows what he is doing, he knows what my trouble is and I trust him. I really do. The doctor tells me, 'Here is what it is, and here is what must be done.' He tells me what to do, and I do it." The same total acceptance was shown by a 58-year-old retired railroad man, the victim of a heart attack, who was interviewed in 1980. "So far as I am concerned, whatever my cardiologist tells me, I do it, I don't make trouble . . . If they had told me, 'Mr. M., we'll have to operate on you, I would have said, 'Okay, all right, go ahead, if it has to be, let's do it.' I wouldn't have quibbled at all."

Many observations have shown that in the attitude of lower-class patients toward the physician class relations play a definite role. They perceive the physician, a member of the middle or upper-middle class, as "above themselves." "I don't like to bother these gentlemen too much . . . they are our superiors," said a 69-year-old retired female worker who was hospitalized in the 1960s. In 1972, the previously cited waitress who had cancer actually felt reassured that surgery and science were "above her": "My bother-in-law had an operation, a successful operation: it was perfect! They took out his stomach, a whole part of his spleen; he had the operation on a Friday, and just about two weeks later he was home. That's telling you that really there is something about surgery that is above us, and one must have confidence in everything that's above us . . . science sure is a great thing." This same perception underlies the reaction of a 41-year-old agricultural worker who, hospitalized in 1972 for an automobile accident, did not dare ask when his operation would take place: "After all, one can't bother the surgeons all the time, ask them every hour, 'Tell me this, tell me that.' One mustn't bother them because one knows what one has to do; either one is a doctor or one isn't."

Expertise and Professional Authority

"I'm no doctor," said the already cited road worker by way of explaining his docility. For his part, a 48-year-old architect, interviewed in 1971 after he suffered an attack of uremia, acknowledged that "one must have confidence . . . I am not a physician, I know absolutely nothing about this, so I trust him . . . the people who come to see me about building a house for them trust me, and so I trust the doctor." From these statements a new dimension emerges, namely the respect for professional authority, for the specialist's expertise. This authority is recognized both by the architect—himself a "professional"[23] and a depository of a specialized system of knowledge—and the road worker. The physician "knows"; he alone is in a position to state an opinion that can be considered the truth about the condition of the sick. The latter feel separated from the knowledge about their own bodies, but they believe that this knowledge is present in another person who, for that very reason, is authorized to speak and prescribe. The sick acknowledge themselves to be in the hands of others, objects of their knowledge and their action.

Specialized knowledge is thus attributed to the members of a "profession," which is thereby legitimized as the guarantor of health, the value that it is called upon to preserve or restore. This characteristic reality of present-day society is presented in the Parsonsian model as completely devoid of conflict; his vision matches that of the persons cited thus far. Recognizing their own ignorance and impotence, the sick confidently submit to a system of knowledge about whose content or legitimacy they have no doubts and which, they believe, is operating unambiguously for their good. Its existence makes it possible for them to get well and thus to regain their place in society.

Yet in the last decades other visions of professional authority and its role in industrial societies have come to the fore, and some of them are very polemical indeed. Ivan Illich[24] claims that it is not intrinsic ignorance or impotence, but rather the development of the modern medical establishment, that destroys the ability of individuals to interpret their condition and to react to it in an autonomous manner. Having become dependent on the specialized interventions that are practiced upon them, today's sick, far from benefiting from the specialist's actions or knowledge, lose confidence in their own recuperative powers and the biological adaptability of their organism. Dispossessed in this manner of their vital energy, the sick also lack the words and the notions they would need to express their anguish. Illich says that because the objective of medicine is the radical elimination of illness, infirmity, pain, and death, it has stripped these experiences, which had hitherto been essential in every society, of all positive value. Illness and death are reduced to a mishap and a failure. Far from being reintegrated into society, the sick person, "on strike against health," as Gérard Briche has put it,[25] has become a broken object continually in need of repair.

Which of these two conceptions is best suited to reflect the experience of the sick? How do today's sick feel about their relations with medicine? What can we say, on the basis of their discourse, about the effect of their dependence on an institution that has unquestionably become indispensable? Until now we have stressed the confidence and docility of certain persons, the total faith in the legitimacy of medicine that is postulated in the Parsonsian model. Yet one also encounters, at least as frequently, defiance or outright revolt against the hold of the professionals. In 1960, in fact, a 31-year-old engineer analyzed his evolution from blind confidence to a definitely guarded attitude toward the "specialists": "I used to think that if one is sick, why, one goes for treatment, there are specialists for that, in this case the doctor; there the individual is in good hands, and he trusts the practitioner. Now I have come to the conviction that *the people who are so-called specialists are just like everyone else*, and not gods, and that it is not at all sure that one will be lucky enough to get out of a hospital when one is sick . . . I no longer have unlimited confidence in the specialists."

More concretely, many persons are dissatisfied with a totally asymmetrical relationship, especially in the hospital setting. In their opinion, there is no justification for this asymmetry. One 54-year-old white-collar worker, hospitalized in 1972 for respiratory insufficiency, objected to the "paternalism" of this relationship: "What I don't like is the tone that the doctors or the medical personnel often use in dealing with the patients. This tone of *cheerful paternalism* that they often use, I can't stand it, even the words. He said to me, 'Well, are we waking up all right, Pops, how are you doing?' I think that's too much. I wouldn't dream of talking like that to anybody, it really shocks me."

"One is being infantilized," said a 25-year-old young woman hospitalized in 1980 for a case of gonorrhea complicated by salpingitis: "In the relations with the nurses, you just feel completely infantilized. Above all, don't try to speak about your feelings, or about your desires, or anything like that . . . just swallow your medications like a good girl, smile a lot, and especially don't think that you know what's good for you better than the nurse. That is to say: she always knows everything, *you must blindly obey her and not say anything* . . . just be there like a good girl."

In the last ten years this criticism of "medical power" has been expressed with particular virulence. But in 1960 already, a 32-year-old woman investigator spoke about her indignation in the same terms. "I had a blood count made in the hospital. When I asked for the result, I was told, 'We don't have the result.' I said, 'Well, I need to know, because it may be a reference for a future consultation.' But that doctor considered this a real scandal! Because I demanded an answer, because I placed myself on a kind of equal footing with him. He thought that was outrageous! A patient who stands up to a doctor in the hospital! Really, these doctors take themselves for superior beings and think that people must accept not knowing what is the matter with them!" Not knowing what is the matter, being faced with the doctor's silence or esoteric language, are sensitive points for everyone. It was difficult for an 18-year-old high-school student who suffered from a malformation of the esophagus and was hospitalized in 1972 for several surgical interventions. His problem was particularly painful, for he perceived himself as the anonymous object of barbaric interventions without understanding the precise reasons for them.

> I have had a malformation of the esophagus from birth, but it was only noticed a year ago, and that is why I have been dragged from hospital to hospital in the last year . . . I am disoriented and no longer know what is going on . . . They are doing something here, they are doing something there, they take you over there, they don't tell you when you'll get out, they don't tell you what's the matter with you, they give you tests, they don't tell you the results; *in short, one is a number among others*, an item in a register. The doctors tell you what they want to tell you . . . They don't answer any questions, it really gets to you. And if they want to explain something in detail, they use words that one can't understand . . . And also it's incredible, the stuff they can do to you, the experiments, the tests, I would never have believed that it was possible: they stick probes down through your mouth, rigid iron tubes, without local or general anaesthesia, and then they clean you out like a chimney. Or else they bore holes in your abdominal wall and look inside with some kind of binoculars.

As we pointed out before, questioning and denigrating the physicians was not invented yesterday. Montaigne, for example, already objected to the medical profession's propensity to extend its field of intervention too far: "Physicians are not content to have the control of sickness; they make the healthy sick, in order to make sure that there is no escape from their authority at any time."[26] In the eighteenth century Rousseau derided their dogmatism: "Physicians and philosophers ... only admit that to be true which they are able to explain, and make their understanding the measure of what is possible. These gentlemen understood nothing about my complaint: therefore I was not ill at all; for of course doctors knew everything."[27] Today, given the importance of medicine and science in modern society, the great value attached to health, and the patients' intense desire to get well, this conflict has reached its highest point and takes the form of an essential ambivalence. It would of course be absurd to construct some kind of balance sheet listing the expressions of rebellion and those of blind confidence concerning medicine or to seek to decide which of these attitudes is prevalent; we simply must accept them together as unresolved opposites. The fact is that we recognize as necessary that which we also refuse; we question the medical norms even as we conform to them. In 1960 a female translator, suffering cruelly from rheumatism, highlighted the discordance between the sufferer's and the physician's objectives in these terms: "By and large, modern physicians use their patients a bit like guinea pigs, they record. That is interesting for their files or a paper that someone is going to give. That's perfectly all right, I am not saying that these things should not be studied, but at the time of a consultation, a sick person has the right to demand attention ... The sick are there to be helped, and the doctors don't even have the decency to hide from them that what interests them *is another case to be put into a file.*" Yet this woman also said, soon thereafter: "You know, for all the bad things I say about the doctors, when I am sick, the first thing I do is to call the doctor, and if he doesn't come right away I am furious, because I do need the doctors' opinion, whether they are right or not." "When you get into this situation, you do need them," the young high-school student who was interviewed in the hospital in 1972 also said between two recriminations.

This ambivalence is not irrational, it is inherent in the sick person's difficult situation. Yet it may well be that its significance goes beyond the problem of being taken in charge by medicine; one wonders whether it is not the prototype of a certain relationship to society, and whether the "sick," groping to find their way, are not among the exemplary figures of our time. For the fact is that the "powers" with which we are confronted today are much less likely than they were in the past to take the form of a brutal imposition of massive constraints, and much more likely to produce norms and even images of ourselves and our needs, so that it appears "natural" and "for our own good" to conform. As individuals we are caught in this dilemma, torn between our personal vision and this very evident model of ourselves, which we partially interiorize and partially reject.

Professionals and Lay People: Conflicting Perspectives

This mechanism is indeed needed to create the physician's "dominance," which is founded both on the objectivity of science and the legitimacy of "professional" status. Eliot Freidson analyzed this mechanism before Ivan Illich; his analysis is much more precise, though less polemical in tone.[28] According to Freidson, the conflict of "perspectives" is inherent in the encounter between the professional and the lay person, for the professionals, secure in the autonomy and the legitimacy they have acquired in the practice of their task, tend to define in their own terms the nature of the problem faced by those who are at once their clients and the objects, at times even the raw material, of their work. The professionals also want to be sure that they themselves determine the nature and the extent of the service they are ready to render to others. In their dealings with these professionals, the sick or "lay people" realize that their view of their own problem does not count for much, and that their needs, as they perceive them, are being ignored. Conflict is thus bound to arise between two visions of illness and the response it demands, although both of them — the physician's and the lay person's — are socially constructed. Usually, however, the physician's vision prevails, and the very manner in which the sufferer states the problem is dismissed.

This tendency is becoming accentuated today as the specialization that defines the field of the physician's intervention becomes more and more narrow and thus increasingly ignores the total reality perceived by the patient. Yet, as early as 1886, at a time when the legitimacy of medicine was beginning to be recognized throughout Europe, Tolstoy expressed this phenomenon perfectly in "The Death of Ivan Ilyich." Ivan Ilyich, a Russian magistrate, concerned about his health, goes to see a famous practitioner: "There was only one question Ivan Ilyich wanted answered: was his condition dangerous or not. But the doctor ignored this question as irrelevant."[29] Yet the magistrate, having abandoned his own professional prestige and become an ordinary "layman," insists: " 'I suppose you are used to having your patients ask you foolish questions, but, in general, would you call my illness dangerous or not?' The doctor shot him a severe look over his glasses, as if to say: 'If you do not restrict yourself to the questions already allowed, prisoner, I shall be compelled to have you put out of the court.' "[30]

It is clear, therefore, that the sick person is neither fundamentally passive nor really active, neither entirely docile and trusting nor totally in revolt. Aware that it is necessary to have recourse to the professional, yet far from blind confidence, convinced both of the professionals' usefulness and their deficiencies, the sick almost always compromise, often use devious means, and sometimes succeed in negotiating. Seen in this perspective, the most perfect apparent docility is often no more than a mask that hides various strategies by which the sick attempt to preserve or to reconquer a certain control over their situation. Such a strategy can go hand in hand, for instance, with a totally impersonal stance, in which the sick person assesses the quality and the limits of the services provided. In 1960, the previously cited translator spoke about her consultation with a very well-known rheumatologist: "We talked, and he prescribed certain massage treatments, as he does for everyone. I could see that this was not appropriate for my case, it was just routine. It is done because it has been noticed that it makes people feel better, but I don't think that he understands very well what it is doing. I was sitting across from him, and *I almost felt sorry for him*. I didn't ask him too many questions, because he doesn't know any more than I do." One would be mistaken to see in that phrase, "he doesn't know any more than I do," only the expression of exasperation. In protracted illnesses, the sick often do come to possess a "knowledge of their own," made up of assimilated medical notions combined with the daily observation of their own state and the effects of treatments received; most of the time, however, this knowledge is ignored or denied by the physician.[31] Yet on this basis the sick are sometimes able to evaluate their physicians' performance very perceptively. Interviewed in 1979, a 45-year-old woman, the wife of an engineer and head of a health-care consumers' association, spoke about her experience, ten years earlier, also with a rheumatic condition. She had perfectly perceived the conflicts brewing within the medical team involved with her case:

> I realized that the professor at the hospital's rheumatology clinic and his assistant did not agree about my case. I myself appeared to them like some stupid little thing when they examined me in my little velvet dressing gown. There they were, discussing the case, and I could see that lots of things were going on, that one did not tell the whole truth to the other. *But I could follow, I understood the terms . . . and I said to myself, "Why, they are just messing each other up."* The assistant did not want to tell his boss that he did not agree with him at all. The boss was developing some far-out ideas about my case, but the assistant gave me the treatment . . . I realized it and I was wondering what I was doing in the middle of this.

Though aware of the conflict, she did not know how to extricate herself and was therefore delighted that a long stay abroad provided the occasion for changing doctors. "I was very glad to get out of this, because I didn't know how to handle it." And, she added, "this is probably why I am now working with an association."

At times, docility is part of assuming a role. The conformism of the lower classes, which, as we pointed out, is an aspect of class relations within society, does not necessarily mean full and wholehearted consent. For the already cited agricultural worker, the hospital where one goes "because one has to" is still a kind of prison.[32] "Hospitals," he said simply, "I am not too fond of them, I don't like it there, because one is not in prison, maybe, but almost." Being a docile patient appeared to him as the only possible attitude; the patient, just like the prison inmate, has to adopt a prescribed role.

For others, who are better able to master their relations with an institution that is not quite as strange to them, a show of docility is often a strategy for obtaining the best possible service. "One must be patient"—rather than "I am patient"—said, for example, a 50-year-old industrial executive who, during his stay in the hospital, thought that this was the price to be paid for "having everything go smoothly." "I think that one has to be patient when one is in the hospital, that is one of the important conditions. One must be patient and make up one's mind to have confidence in the treatments one is given. Those who are not patient are having a very hard time; for one thing, they antagonize the nurses . . . whereas, if you are patient, everything goes smoothly." In the same manner, confidence in the treatments may well represent a wager by which the sick person attempts to beat the odds in this difficult situation, rather than the sign of absolute faith in the possibilities of medicine and the action of the physicians.

The Strategies of the Sick

We do not intend to review here the multiple ways in which people seek medical help in the course of their illnesses. A large number of variables is involved here, including personal and family history, the social and geographical origin of the individual, the intrinsic nature of the care available, the sick person's information about it, and so forth. What we do want to show is that the sick person's attitude is governed by a logic of its own, which, although completely different from that of the professionals, is by no means devoid of rationality. In their difficult relationship with an institution of whose power they are well aware, the sick—just like all of us in our endeavor to come to terms with the established order—attempt to preserve, if need be by duplicity, some measure of mastery over the situation.

It would be interesting to find out, however, in which cases this ambiguous situation allows for more open negotiations resulting in a more symmetrical relationship. A great many studies, concerning both France and the English-speaking world, have shown that social class, and the level of education that is related to it, is the crucial variable in this respect. When it comes to illness and its treatment, people of the "lower" classes exhibit a set of attitudes (reluctance to perceive themselves as "sick," less attention to symptoms, lack of information about treatments available) that makes them less likely to use the existing professional system in an active and purposeful manner. Various studies of health-care consumption[33] confirm these systematic differences and show the existence of more or less strict "channeling," by which the members of the lower classes are shunted off into the least prestigious sectors of the health-care system.[34] Members of the middle and upper classes, on the other hand, by dint of their proximity to the members of the medical profession in terms of class and social values, their educational level, and their greater control over the problems of everyday life, are better able — and increasingly so in the last few years — to master the social space of medicine and to negotiate actively with the professionals, thereby escaping the "alienation" and the "passivity" that can result from a situation of illness.

Today, middle-class people who are ill usually know what type of practitioner they want to consult. Thus, in 1978, a young female professor wanted to go "directly to the specialist." "Three months ago, I found myself with a severe case of acne on my face, which is something that had never happened to me, even as an adolescent, and so I went to a dermatologist, who has been treating me for two months now. I certainly wouldn't wait, there is no use letting these things drag on, I would rather try to go to a specialist." Sometimes middle-class patients are even able to influence decisions concerning their treatment. One example is the 40-year-old wife of an executive in Bordeaux, who in 1980 asked her physician for a medical treatment, rather than a surgical intervention, and obtained it. "One of my neighbors had had the same thing that I had, and she did not have an operation . . . I had been operated on once before for intestinal occlusion, that was at the time of my first attack, when I was sent to the clinic and operated on. When I had the second occlusion, I remembered my neighbor, and I asked the doctor, 'Couldn't one try to unblock me, rather than operating?' That's why I was sent to this department of the hospital, and they told me that they would do everything they could to unblock me." Once her demand had been recognized as valid, she established excellent relations with the professionals; above all — and this is rare enough to be stressed — the patient was very satisfied with the information she was given: "I would ask questions and *they would answer me very well* every time I wanted to know something from the nurses or the doctors . . . Professor B. gave me a very good explanation of what is meant by intestinal attachments."[35]

In 1979, a young director of research in a marketing research firm told us how she had gone about choosing the hospital department where she would undergo a surgical intervention for a detached retina. Upon learning that an operation would be necessary, she felt overwhelmed at first. "I felt absolutely at the mercy of an expert's decision to make me go to a hospital about whose value in terms of surgery I knew nothing. That scared me just a bit." But she pulled herself together and went to see two other practitioners, who confirmed the necessity of an intervention. At that point, she said, "My problem was to find a department with a surgeon who knows what he is doing in case of a detached retina." She therefore solicited the advice of physicians, but her search for information was active and systematic, and she tried to evaluate the advice she was given. "So I first tried to find out about the X hospital . . . it was considered all right, by and large, and then I wanted to know if it wouldn't be better to go to Z hospital . . . All that in a half-day, it was not easy, because it was an emergency. They seemed to tell me that it didn't matter, that what really counted was the surgeon anyway, the surgeon and the intern. Well, I quite agreed with that, and so I said, 'Yes, but who?' Now that meant trouble, and I even believe that the professor almost slammed the door in my face; he was really annoyed that I asked him for names . . . he was visibly bothered." Yet she insisted. "In fact, it was the assistants who helped me out, because they know this milieu very well, and they told me, 'This guy is pretty good, and the surgeon of that team is N., who is very good.' So we talked about it, and perhaps because I was young and because they sort of liked me, and because I was standing up for myself—*after all, there is no reason to give up one's status as a person just because one is sick*—anyway, they told me, 'If you go to X hospital and if you get this surgeon, it's okay, it'll be fine, he is young and very good.' " In dealing with the hospital system, this young woman thus deployed the behavior of a knowledgable consumer who, before making a decision, tried to compare the available products according to various criteria. Her dialogue with the professionals was based on this premise, and the professionals were willing to participate in it.

Today such behavior has become part of a general "consumerism" characteristic of what is sometimes called the "new middle classes." In certain cases, however, it is the seriousness of an illness that prompts the sick to engage in such active negotiations and enables them to face a possible conflict with the physician for which nothing in their earlier attitudes had prepared them. In 1960, a 50-year-old employee, Mme G., who was suffering from breast cancer, reported on her sometimes dramatic negotiations with the medical profession. She had made some difficult choices. It began, she said, "as it usually does, with a lump in the breast. But the doctor didn't believe it, he told me, 'It doesn't mean anything.' And so I kept this lump for eighteen months. I was losing weight, I was all worn out, and so I absolutely wanted to know what was the matter with me." When the cancer was finally recognized, the doctor urged an immediate operation, but she refused: "I categorically refused. I did not think that this was the way to do it and I was furious with the doctor, a nice fellow otherwise, who had told me, 'This lump doesn't mean anything' and who suddenly one day declares, 'Tonight, and I don't mean tomorrow, we are going to do the operation.' I said, 'No indeed, you should have thought of it earlier.' " One can of course—and she knows this—question the wisdom of her refusal; but she does accept the risk, and among the reasons she gives for it one discerns her desire to know and to keep some control over her difficult situation. "I know this sounds crazy, but in my opinion having a breast removed is a terrible thing for a woman. It's really stupid, because I am alone and I don't show myself in public except when I'm dressed. I don't know why, but this is something that has scared me very, very much. I said to myself, 'All right, I'll first find out what this is about, and I won't do just anything.' "

Treated subsequently by a physician who "is not for the operation" and who began an x-ray treatment, Mme G. asked to be told the truth. "The doctor told me the truth because he could see that I had to know it. I told him, 'I have a little girl, I am alone, *I want to know the truth*: Do I have two months, six months, a year? . . ?' " On the day of the interview, three years later, she still showed the same lucidity: "The rough moments come every time I go to see Dr. M. to ask him what my situation is. Every time before I see him I am sick for three days, wondering, 'What is he going to tell me?' I know that he won't lie to me. I think that he would say, 'Well, dear, I think we'll have to go for another treatment,' and if he said that, I would know very well what it means . . . So you see, I am pretty scared, I really am, everybody is; one is scared, but one lives with it."

Yet before the ordeal of her cancer, Mme G. was the very model of the passive patient. "Before I had cancer, I blindly went along with the doctors. I have been operated on, I don't know how many times, because the doctor said, 'We have to operate on this.' And I didn't get a second opinion, because I believed in my doctors. And suddenly, because they wanted to remove a breast, I didn't want to go along, I categorically refused the operation because I didn't know whether that would cure me." The seriousness of the problem she had to face, her desire not to be left out of the decisions concerning her—"I want to know what is being done to me, I am here," she kept saying in various forms—had given her the courage to make that difficult choice. Because she saw her situation as a struggle, and because of her desire to "treat her illness with respect" as she put it, she had recourse, in addition to x-ray treatments and chemotherapy, to parallel therapies. "I tried some unusual things, though I did not see Professor Solomidès; one hears a lot about him, but I did not go to see him, I didn't have the nerve. I really think that the most serious thing I have tried was the *cazoledan* from Germany, and I also saw homeopathic physicians, who gave me very old medications, such as *giscor*, which is the mistle of the ancients. It used to be considered a universal remedy in the past, and it did me a lot of good." Not that she believed in magic that would bring about a miraculous cure; she only wanted to try everything. "When one is in this condition, one has to try everything," she said simply. It is difficult to dismiss the question she then asked the interviewer: "Don't you think that if you had such a thing, or if this happened to someone in your family, you would try just about anything? I think you would!"

Recourse to Parallel Therapies

In the eyes of medicine, the search for alternative therapies, not to mention the appeal to healers, can only be a behavior tainted with irrationality, since in its foundations and its logic it is entirely different from the recourse to medical treatment. Reality is infinitely more complex. To begin with, it is quite clear that although a fair number of persons told us that they had consulted homeopaths, used plant-based therapies, and seen mesmerizers, bonesetters, or various kinds of healers, most of them stated that they refuse to do "just anything." Mme G. may have said that she was determined to "try everything" and that she did consult several homeopaths; yet, as we have seen, she did not "have the nerve" to go to see Dr. Solomidès. She also refused to see clairvoyants or healers. "I had around me many friends who regularly saw healers, clairvoyants also, which is something I have never done in my life. I have no desire to do that."

Often the sufferers set a limit for themselves, a point beyond which they will not go in a quest of whose uncertain or hazardous character they are aware. For these people, however far they may stray, "medicine" thus remains the model of reference. Nonetheless, such conduct has its own rationale, to a far greater extent at any rate than the physicians believe. In 1972, a 35-year-old nurse, who had suffered a fall resulting in a persistent pain that was not relieved by treatments, did not hesitate to consult a bonesetter. "They often hurt you very much, because they probe, they feel with their fingers, and then, all of a sudden, they say, 'Don't move,' and—here you go!—they pull . . . I know that many people are incredulous, but *when one is hurt and feels that they are going to help you, I think one will go back*. Besides, I won't see just anybody; this one, if the trouble is not in his domain, he tells me so. 'This is not for me,' he'll say, 'Go to see your regular physician.' For people who go to see a charlatan, the important thing is to believe; but here that's not the case, because one can see how it is done."

Indeed, for many people the recourse to parallel therapies is not necessarily incompatible with classical medical treatment. It often happens, in particular, that the sufferer, realizing the ineffectiveness of such unorthodox endeavors, returns to regular medicine. The high-school student suffering from a malformation of the esophagus, whose discourse certainly came closer to wide-eyed confidence in the magic powers of a healer than anything we heard, finally recognized that in his case, despite his reticences, it was necessary to return to the hospital for an operation. "I can say that I tried everything before I had the operation, I went to see a healer, a mesmerizer, I also went to see an acupuncturist, but in the end I had to go for the operation. *That mesmerizer was really something*: I have seen him do mesmeric passes over someone, and I have seen him doing lots of passes over roses. He holds a rose in his hand for ten minutes, and the rose stays fresh forever. *It is miraculous.* But on me, he tried, but he couldn't do anything, because it was a malformation and not an illness."

Faced with the failure of scientific medicine — for in practice the recourse to "something else" takes place in that context — sufferers often state the hope that it may be possible to approach the ill with which they are confronted in a manner different from that of classical medicine. "I have turned to paramedicine because I thought that there must be something else in life than morphine and the lancet," said Mme G., for example. Such language is not heard, as one might expect, from the most uneducated people but, on the contrary, from some of the most sophisticated. In 1960 a young intellectual, the son of a physician, said, "Even though I had the very best of care, *I have to a large extent lost confidence in medicine,* in fact in the exact sciences in general. When I got over my ulcer and then came down with rheumatism, I was very tempted to go to see a healer whose address had been given to me, but I didn't do it, out of respect for my father." The case of Dr. Allendy is therefore particularly significant, for he decoded his ill on three levels: that of classical medicine, that of psychoanalysis, and also that of astrology, shifting without apparent difficulty from one perspective, one language, to the other. By contrast, a 76-year-old cleaning woman, interviewed in 1972, stated with deep conviction that "science" alone, despite the limits that she herself had discovered, is the only possible recourse. In connection with her rheumatism, she said: "The doctors say, 'Science is working for you, but it has not yet found a way to cure rheumatism.' Science is working all right, but I have the feeling that it will have a hard time finding a cure for this. It's like cancer, it's hard to treat . . . Some people go to see healers; I wouldn't do that, I wouldn't trust them. I wouldn't go to see a healer when even science doesn't have a cure . . . passing a hand over you like that, in the spot [where it hurts], in order to cure you, I don't believe in that, I believe in science."

The concept of a "different approach" is often founded on the very deeply rooted and almost universally shared idea of the body's power to heal itself. Many of these sick believe that this power is neglected, even destroyed, by scientific medicine, and that its limited effectiveness stems from this fact. The young man who admitted to "being tempted to see a healer" made a distinction between the effect of medical treatments and what he believed to be the action of the healer. "I have the impression that the treatments and medications so weakened me that it all took terribly long. The illness went on and on because the body was exhausted and poisoned by the medications." He felt that the healer, on the contrary, can reinforce a spontaneous capacity for healing: "I suppose that these are people who feel the ill health of others very keenly, feel it in their fibers, their muscles, their guts, sensing exactly what is going on in the sick person's body, and that they are able, by touch or by thought, to bring about a certain relaxation in the affected part of that person's body, or to give him enough vitality and enough confidence to get better."

In 1960 as well, a 46-year-old technician, in speaking of homeopathy, developed in a particularly striking manner the idea of an autonomous struggle on the part of the organism, and the individual's participation in improving his or her condition. "Homeopathy means to fight illness with equal arms; with allopathy, one doesn't fight, one considers oneself defeated from the start, takes a foreign agent and brings it into the body, where it tends to attenuate the trouble or to make it disappear . . . but only for a time, because it often returns . . . it takes very little effort, whereas with homeopathy, one has to make a real effort, for the body is struggling at the same time . . . Homeopathy involves the individual more deeply than allopathy. Homeopathy demands a certain self-discipline, whereas the other is just a quick fix." The body, in other words, can be "its own physician." This idea, incidentally, was an inspiration to the journalist Norman Cousins several years ago, when he suffered a case of rheumatoid spondylitis that did not respond to any of the classic treatments. Cousins decided to treat himself by ingesting high doses of ascorbic acid and by cultivating his "will to get well," which he kept up by laughter: for several months he watched several comic films every day. Whether by spontaneous remission or as a result of this unusual treatment, Norman Cousins is for the moment "cured."[36]

These persons' recourse to different forms of parallel therapy, then, is not the manifestation of blind faith but, rather, motivated by the same desire to fight their illness and to manage their condition which we saw at work in their relations with medicine. More generally, one can assert that many people who in serious and uncertain cases go in for unorthodox therapies do not exhibit a different attitude toward these than toward orthodox medicine. Conscious of the risks they run and of the slender possibilities they are offered, but determined to attempt something, they "act as if."[37] Determined to fight, they take this step as a gamble that does not exclude doubt or skepticism. But their situation is usually such that any gamble seems hazardous, whether it involves a healer or official medicine.

This was, for example, the case of a taxi driver interviewed in 1980, who had been suffering from multiple sclerosis for many years. He described his experience with a physician who applied a resolutely unorthodox therapy: "He cured with plants, so it was . . . a bit . . . special. The plants were encased in asbestos, with a string attached to it, and one tied this around the waist and taped some to the back with adhesive tape; there was also water, and finally a preparation from the pharmacy, which one had to rub on the legs." He discontinued this treatment after a few months because, he admitted, "I didn't see any improvement." Yet, when asked to make a judgment of such practices, he refused to condemn them categorically: "If I were asked, I would say yes, it's not

bad; it didn't do anything for me, but perhaps it will do something for others."
He was thinking about seeing a healer. "That's the only thing I haven't done,
I think, so far; but perhaps one day I will do it, because I say to myself, 'One
never knows, perhaps this will be like an electric system for me, perhaps I'll
have a reaction' . . . Because, come right down to it, there were moments when
this did happen to me; all of a sudden, without knowing how or why, I would
walk as if nothing at all were wrong with me, as if I had never been sick . . .
it lasted perhaps five minutes or so, but I was running around normally . . . so
I make a connection between that and the healer."

To this man, for all his skepticism, such an attempt appears to be the only
reasonable conduct. His attitude toward official medicine is the same, for he
regularly sees a physician. He only gets angry when a doctor demands absolute
faith, which he considers irrational, in the progress of science. "Every time I
met a new doctor, he would say to me, 'Well, this is a disease that we'll easily
defeat in the next 3 or 4 years, they're just about ready to find . .'. The last time
he started up again, and so I said, 'I've been hearing this song for 10 years . . .
I have come to see you because you have to give me medications, because that's
all there is. Encouragement is all very nice, but I don't believe in what you are
telling me. I believe in your therapy without really believing in it' . . . but in
fact . . . and anyway, that's all there is, and so I go with it."

12·

From Self-help to the Duty to Be Healthy

*T*oday, as chronic illnesses are becoming increasingly frequent, we witness the emergence of the "new sick," who negotiate with medicine in a very specific manner. In these cases, which are typical of today's pathology, modern medicine proves its power, for complex but readily routinized therapeutic means are now able to keep alive people who in the past would have been condemned. But here medicine also encounters its limits, and when that happens, the Parsonsian concept of the "role played by the sick" becomes totally inappropriate, because even if the chronically ill seek medical help and strictly conform to the physician's prescriptions, they cannot hope to get well. Such persons must develop a new mode of relating to illness and to medicine, and this involves, first of all, recognizing the inadequacy of the very powerful "idea of being cured."

This idea, however, is being replaced by another notion, that of managing an illness. This is the basis of the concept of the "new sick," new, that is, with respect to their relations with the professionals and their knowledge and techniques, and, through them, with the entire network of their social relations. "Instead of adopting the blithe notion of being cured, which is often an empty promise, I made the choice of managing my illness,"[1] wrote Gérard Briche in 1979. A journalist writing for *L'Impatient*, who suffered since 1960 from an "acute disseminated lupus erythematosus," Briche analyzed in his "hospital diary of a lupus" the steps by which he had arrived at this conception of illness and of being sick. This new conception has enabled him, despite the seriousness of his condition and only after many dramatic episodes, to recapture a positive self-image. Among the chronically ill, few as yet are able to carry this notion of managing an illness to its logical conclusion and to accept themselves in this new role. This type of itinerary is still rare, to be sure, but it is no longer absolutely unique, and therefore definitely significant.

Managing One's Illness

This is not a matter of adopting an idyllic vision, for to discover that one has a chronic and incurable illness is, like finding out that one has cancer, a profoundly traumatic experience. In 1981 a 51-year-old woman, who had had diabetes for 21 years, still remembered her shock upon being told about her condition by her physician father: "I didn't even know what diabetes was, no idea, when my father told me, 'You know, we've found out something very unfortunate, you have a glycemia level of 3 g. 30.' I said, 'But you are going to cure me, Papa.' So he very gently made me understand that he would not cure me. Of course this was a horrendous shock . . . Whatever they say, and every diabetic will tell you this, it is an awful shock. Life will never be the same, never again." This shock has to do not only with knowing that one will be sick for life, limited in one's possibilities, and threatened in one's body—all the chronically ill evoke their anxiety about a possible aggravation of their condition or complications and the probability of a shortened life—but also with knowing that one will have to have treatments at all times and accept the constraints that this involves. Interviewed in 1972, a 40-year-old working-class mother of several children was diabetic and insulin-dependent and therefore had to follow a diet and needed daily insulin injections. She remembered the first shot she gave herself, as most diabetics do: "The first shot I wanted to do all by myself; I cried and cried . . . saying, 'I'll have to give myself shots like this for the rest of my life.' "

Yet, more or less quickly, more or less completely, the sick come to terms. "Afterward one gets used to it; if it has to be, it has to be," the same woman continued. Another 40-year-old woman, suffering from Addison's disease, another chronic condition that implies regular treatments, also said: "I have had this illness for about 10 years, and I had to get acclimatized to it . . . so I got used to living with it for the rest of my days; I am not saying that I am happy about it, but I am used to it." The 50-year-old diabetic, after describing her initial shock, then assessed her situation in terms that were not altogether negative. "It can be done, first of all because it's a matter of life and death . . . and besides, one does have a feeling of victory: after all, one does manage to stay alive and . . . I mean one is a better person than before, one is more courageous, in fact *one knows oneself*, it means a whole lot to know oneself physically and physiologically. That is definitely an enrichment, it's a kind of philosophy . . . not the burnt-child philosophy of one who is beaten, no, but a constructive philosophy, I think."

"One knows oneself," this woman said. And indeed, for all these chronically ill, "managing one's illness" is first of all a matter of getting to know it, acquiring a body of knowledge. Another Parisian diabetic, a 31-year-old secretary, explained: "With diabetes, one has to learn a lot of things, all at the same time

. . . I very quickly learned to take care of myself, to measure the doses of insulin myself, to do a little cooking, it was very hard for three to six months, but after that I very quickly managed to recover my independence." The housekeeper suffering from Addison's disease showed us how on the basis of this knowledge some of the sick—and this is the crucial fact—adjust their own treatments and thereby partially control their condition. "It is an illness that I have learned to know myself. One has to, because one is condemned to drag something around all one's life, and one has to know what it is that one drags around. This is very important, because in this way one is better able to sense one's reactions, *one can react when something goes wrong*. I tell myself, 'All right, next time I won't do this,' or else, 'How about that, I reacted like this, so perhaps by taking more or less of this, or perhaps by doing something else, I'll get some improvement.' "

Paradoxically, then, the chronically ill, obliged though they are to follow an uninterrupted course of treatment, are able to escape the absolute authority of the physician and to recover a certain independence. The same patient continued: "One can't always run after the doctor for every little snag; if you know that you have to increase the dose of a medication, you don't need anybody to tell you so." This knowledge, and the independence it affords, are a matter of necessity, for usually the chronically ill are determined to manage both a serious illness and a "normal" life. Thanks to their treatments, they are not hospitalized, except for short periods. Very often they work and lead a family life. They therefore necessarily elude the continuous control of the physician and of medicine, which is the very essence of acute illness, yet they must treat their condition every day, sometimes in a most complex manner. "One can't go to see the doctor every time one has to have a dose of insulin, we have to adapt to this ourselves, and they have to delegate their responsibilities to us . . . this treatment is in my hands, and I am treating myself," says the oldest of the diabetic women. In this manner the sick cease to be "receivers of care" and become "providers of care"; by providing treatments for themselves, they engage in "self-help."

At this point, the logic of medicine is offset by another logic, that of life, work, leisure, and human relations—a "social" logic as opposed to a "medical" one. Many of the chronically ill must make a choice between strict adherence to their therapy, which, though best suited to ensure their physiological equilibrium, entails very serious constraints in their day-to-day life, and better integration in social life achieved by the relaxation of the therapy, but at the cost of a threat to their present or future physical integrity.[2] Depending on the case and the circumstances, behaviors will vary, but the crucial fact is that the choice must be made concretely, and daily, not by the physician alone, but also by the sufferer. The diabetic housewife interviewed in 1972 adhered to a strict diet, which led her to curtail her social life: "I am on a weighed diet; I have to weigh everything I eat, and I can't ever go off it, because then I couldn't record it . . . so when one goes somewhere, it's rather embarrassing because people fix a meal and one has to refuse . . . so now, going out . . . I don't do it much."

The young secretary whom we interviewed in 1981 negotiated in a much more supple fashion. She clearly stated the alternative with which she was faced:

> One has to know what one wants, either to be halfway balanced with few constraints, or else accepting a great deal of constraint and be well-balanced. I myself have gone through both states: until two years ago, I only had one insulin shot a day, which gave me a rather poor balance, because with just one shot in the morning, if I made a mistake in my diet at noon, it took me until the next day to make up for my mistake. But then, after a while, my doctor made me understand that two shots would really be better for me. Well, it took me six months to make up my mind because, after all, . . . it's just one more constraint.

It is clear, then, that the physician did not impose anything upon her and that she hesitated for a long time to adopt this modification of her therapy. This young woman obviously did not want the "social logic" of her condition to yield to the "medical logic" and its exigencies. "I do not want to cut myself off from the world. I know people who are much stricter than I am about their diet, and who never make an exception, but these people never go out . . . I don't think this is a good way. One must try, after all, to stay in touch with reality; I could of course take much better care of myself if I never permitted myself any excess . . . but *if all I get is three extra days at the end of my life, it isn't worth it.*" "It is very important not to let oneself be gobbled up by one's diabetes when one has the feeling that there are more important things," the 52-year-old woman said. But the secretary immediately indicated the limits of the liberties she accorded herself: "When I say that I permit myself some excesses, I don't of course do it every week, only occasionally."

Kidney patients undergoing hemodialysis treatments at home are confronted with choices of the same kind. They too can modulate their treatments to allow for exigencies of their social life; for instance, by deciding to lengthen the interval between dialysis sessions when traveling. Yet the account of a 41-year-old technician gives us the measure of the constraints implied by this practice, as well as of the need for knowledge demanded by the sick person's condition. "I have come to the point where I can go on vacation without dialysis for as many as six days, but I need a week to get ready. First I have two days of dialysis, one right after the other, and these are twelve-hour sessions.[3] In this way one gets thoroughly cleaned out, one shouldn't have more than 0.3 g. of urea per liter of blood. And besides, one goes on a diet and one doesn't get very tired, because that too causes urea. The diet is very strict: no milk, no meat, no eggs, no salt, and at the end of six days I haven't gained any weight. But I do feel the acetone, and my blood pressure is up."

This example reminds us that it would be disingenuous to claim that all of the "self-provider's" problems are solved. Living with a chronic illness—even if one is able, like the persons we cite here, to master its management—is a most trying experience. It is trying, first of all, in the physical sense. All of these sufferers, whether they be kidney patients in dialysis or diabetics, are more or less frequently subject to different kinds of physical mishaps, some of which, like a diabetic coma, are extremely frightening. "Deep down," says the lower-class housewife, "I am always afraid that something will happen to me; sometimes, when I go into a coma, I say to myself: 'It's quite possible that I won't wake up,' even though I'm always told that it isn't fatal, but then . . . there is always that fear." Mentally, some persons find it very difficult to be responsible for their own treatment. Thus, many kidney patients refuse to undergo dialysis at home—"no hospital in the house"[4]—and do not want to saddle either themselves or their family with this burden. In the case of diabetes as well, the permanent effort to remain in control, and the constant need for self-discipline, are the main difficulties facing patients who treat themselves. The young secretary acknowledged: "Always, *always having to pay attention*, that . . . is something that people have trouble accepting. *This is the thing that's hard to learn*, because the shots . . . I am always worried, but I do it. The analyses are not hard to do, but what is so constraining is that one has to pay attention at all times." The older diabetic also said, "That is why we who are sick are so tired, because we always have to gather up our will power to do the things that have to be done, and that one couldn't deal with if one let oneself go."

Self-help, Knowledge, and Medical Techniques

For these patients the "knowledge of the sick" thus gives rise to a different way of life and to a veritable "subculture." Even more than specific knowledge, such a way of life implies the definition of personal norms, an aptitude for negotiating with the illness and adjusting to it emotionally, as well as the ability to make choices and to carry them out in concrete acts. Attentive observation of oneself and one's symptoms is not new in itself. Montaigne, for instance, in his *Journal d'un voyage en Italie*, which he kept while taking the waters there, noted from day to day the effects of the water on his health. These extraordinarily detailed observations often caused him to modify his treatment without paying much attention to the medical prescriptions; he wrote, for example:

> On Wednesday, early in the morning, I again drank of that water, being in great discomfort from the little effect I had felt the day before; for although I had moved my bowels immediately upon taking it, I attributed this to the

medicine of the day before, since not one drop of the water I made came from that of the spa. On Wednesday I took seven glasses measured by the pound, which was at least twice as much as what I had taken on the other day, and I believe that I had never taken as much at one time. It gave me a great desire to sweat, which I did not want to encourage, having often been told that this is not the effect I need; and like on the other day I kept to my room, sometimes walking around and sometimes resting. The water came out, for the most part, from behind and caused me to have several loose bowel movements, without any effort. I feel that it was not good for me to have this kind of a purge, for the water, finding that nature was moving toward the back, was incited to follow the same direction even though, on account of my kidneys, I should have wished it to go to the front; and so I decided that the next time I take the waters I should prepare myself by fasting the day before.[5]

But of course in the case of the sixteenth-century writer, this extremely careful self-observation and the resulting modification of the treatment were related to the deficiencies of a medicine that was generally considered ineffective by cultivated people such as Montaigne. For today's sufferers, by contrast, the transition to a personal management of an illness implies a new way of relating to a physician and a medicine considered to be the only legitimate repositories of the right to diagnose and treat illness. Through this conduct, self-treating patients assert their right to adopt a specific discourse about their sick body and proclaim the effectiveness of taking autonomous charge of their condition. In so doing, they state not only the possibility but indeed the value of a different vision of illness: the patient, no longer a passive recipient, thus enters into a new relationship with professional expertise. This being the case, it is perhaps no exaggeration to say that today's self-treating patient appears to be a figure of a new type in our cultural universe. Yet an essential role was played in this development by two factors, both of them related to medicine. One is the recourse to sophisticated techniques, which physicians were able to teach their patients as initially experimental procedures became routinized; the other is the existence of a collective form of dealing with illness in "patients' self-help groups," which were also originally brought into being by physicians with a view to motivating patients to learn these difficult procedures. The autonomy of the self-treating patient was thus wrested from medicine; yet initially it was delegated to the patient by medicine itself.

Here the role played by technology is of paramount importance. The kidney patients who undergo dialysis at home, in particular, often express their pride in having learned to master a difficult therapy. The already cited technician calculated: "I have now been doing my own dialysis for 7 years, that comes to more than 900 dialyses, 960 and some . . . in fact, I record all the dialyses I do and their results in a notebook."

Yet learning abstract notions and complex manipulations is not the only aspect of this switch from the role of receiver to that of giver of care. Even more important is the fact that the sufferers' action has a direct bearing on their bodies and sometimes their most vital organs. This surely means to break out of the rule by which the physician alone had access to the sick body. "It really is a very intense medical treatment, it's no joking matter, after all, one manipulates the blood," says a 40-year-old shopkeeper. A 36-year-old salesman analyzes the patient's literally vital stake in the hemodialysis session, as well as the quality of the effort he is called upon to make: "One really has one's life in one's hands, when it comes to asepsis, to the rinsing of the blood disks, or the treatment itself . . . the machine is very advanced, it has an alarm system that keeps track at all times of the different constants one must watch, but . . . one has to pay attention, one is really responsible for one's life . . . one's life in one's hands, everyone has it . . . but not to this degree . . . three times a week, if I make a mistake, that can be the end of me." Then he continues: "At the hospital you are in the hands of nurses, of doctors, you are entirely entrusted to them, they are responsible, but then, that is their job, but you yourself *become responsible even though this is not necessarily your job* . . . I have never studied medicine, I have never studied nursing, but practically I now have the same responsibility for myself."

The knowledge of the sick and their mastery of a technology thus lead them to question the traditional allotment of roles between the patient and the physician and to abolish the distance that usually separates the professional from the lay person. Some of these sick feel that this appropriation, far from being just a temporary expedient, is totally to their advantage. They consider their own proficiency in performing the treatment superior to that of the professionals. The previously cited shopkeeper asserts: "I feel much safer having my dialysis here [at home] than at the hospital. And I don't think that this is just a notion I have; it isn't safe at the hospital, there are incidents and even accidents there all the time. But not at home, I think at home one is more careful, and one works more slowly."

A railroad employee also says: "Medically speaking, the treatment is not as good [at the hospital] as it is at home . . . for the simple reason that if my wife puts in the needle, she knows my arm perfectly . . . the nurse cannot possibly know fifty arms as well as my wife knows mine." In the diary of his lupus, Gérard Briche admits: "One of the small achievements of which I am proud is that I taught the night nurse something useful, namely to give abdominal injections under the skin, rather than into the abdominal muscle."[6]

Some sick persons have decided to acquire, through systematic and specialized reading, actual medical knowledge. The 50-year-old diabetic woman whom we have already cited several times said: "Fortunately, I am lucky that I am interested in this; I find medicine really exciting, you can see that I am reading books, treatises on anatomo-pathology." Gérard Briche, for his part, hesitated for a long time to "make the leap"; if he was reluctant, he thinks, to "learn the language of the professionals, thereby placing myself on their own turf, it was no doubt because I was afraid that I could not be both of these antagonistic figures, the patient and the physician."[7] But then, he wrote in 1979, "I have been reading and gathering information for a year now. I now know enough to be able to judge my past conduct and also that of the physicians."[8] But this is not the most important point; for if some of the sick go so far as to consider their knowledge "superior" to that of the professionals, it is precisely because of their situation. Medical knowledge, they claim, is always limited by the exteriority of the physician's point of view; but the sick who practice self-treatment realize that it is their turn. "The only one who is in the place is the sick person. He has no weapon, he is pretty nearly crippled, but his strength consists of being within the walls," writes Gérard Briche.[9] "Even a very competent physician does not know what a hypoglycemia is, he cannot feel it," said the diabetic secretary. A 40-year-old female kidney patient, working as a researcher in a ministry, said essentially the same thing about the sudden drop in blood pressure that can occur during hemodialysis: "The nurses, however kind they may be, cannot realize what such a drop is, they have never had one."

Patients and Physicians: A New Relationship?

Many of the sick thus assert that they have been able to elaborate, with a subtlety that no professional can muster, an understanding of their condition that comes to them from both inside and outside. This understanding, they claim, is individualized, adapted to their person and to the exigencies of their life. It is on this basis that they succeed, despite great difficulties, in reconciling the "medical logic" with the "social logic" of illness. Seen in this perspective, the relationship between patient and physician becomes infinitely complex. In the case of diabetes and kidney conditions, all the sufferers recognize that their new-found identity as the "new sick" came into being in the wake of a transfer of knowledge and a delegation of responsibility by the physician. "I was well taught . . . the doctor whom I used to see was quite pedagogical, he guided me very well," said the diabetic secretary, for example. But this is only the first stage. Subsequently, certain physicians accept the reality of their patients' own knowledge in this matter; when this happens, the latter finally feel recognized as complete persons. "In my dermatology department at X hospital, they are now willing to listen to me," writes Gérard Briche.[10] "They tell me that I am taking good care of myself," the 52-year-old woman said, pleased. She even described a virtual reversal of roles between herself and her diabetes specialist. "To be a diabetes specialist is not a very gratifying job; first of all, he is not the boss, the patients often contradict him, saying, 'Oh no, I am sorry, but this is not it, it's not what you are saying, it's that.' We know more about ourselves than he knows about us, even if he has followed us for years, that's quite obvious. And therefore the diabetes specialist must adapt to what we are doing."

But, this woman continues, "some take it better than others; I must say that mine does not always react very well, because he doesn't think one has the right to do that . . . But they have to, they have to adapt." In short, here the physician is faced with the problem to which Gérard Briche devoted his entire book; that is, the matter of sharing decisions with the patient.

Yet one wonders whether this attitude spells an end to the need for, and dependence on, the physician. The same diabetic interrupted the detailed account of her negotiations with her illnesses without the involvement of the physician and admitted that "if there is a tragic episode, then of course yes, one must see him right away." A 53-year-old woman, the wife of a military man, who performed hemodialysis at home, spoke of the comfort it gave her to know that recourse to professional help was always possible. "If something goes wrong, one calls up and one right away gets a technician to fix the generator or the [artificial] kidney, or one gets to a doctor who gives advice if one has an accident, a leaking of the blood or something . . . and if it were really serious, they would come and get you in an ambulance . . . so it's really of the utmost importance to feel that there is a backup." Even Gérard Briche admits that "one must be honest enough to recognize that the sick person's intervention in his illness has its limits."[11] In fact, even in cases of open conflict, which are not glossed over in such more egalitarian relationships, self-treating patients realize that, whatever their grievances, they cannot do without medicine and physicians. Following a rather sharp altercation with the medical team that had been treating him for years, Gérard Briche observes: "If I followed my reasoning about this present matter to its logical conclusion, I would leave the hospital and its medical team with which I cannot collaborate, but where would I go?"[12]

At the same time, one is struck by the warmth and the closeness of the ties that some patients establish with a medical team, especially in cases where the treatment is still in the experimental stage. These ties are totally different from the affective neutrality that, in principle, informs the doctor-patient relationship. As early as 1959, the American sociologist Renée Fox had analyzed what she called the "red carpet treatment"[13] accorded by the physicians to certain very seriously ill patients undergoing experimental therapies in one of the most prestigious Boston hospitals. In these cases, where the outcome of the therapy was extremely uncertain, the physicians, aware of the constraints and the suffering with which they burdened the almost certainly condemned patients, established ties of friendship and partnership with them, and at the same time also raised them to the status of "medical superstars." Having an emotional investment in these very personal relationships, the physicians kept the patients informed of every detail of their treatment, shared many decisions with them, and finally celebrated the courage of these extraordinary patients when they published their findings about a case in scientific journals.[14]

In 1974 in France, hemodialysis, which today has become a routine procedure, did not of course have the same dramatic character. Nonetheless it was still a fairly unusual therapy, which made patients and professionals feel that they were involved in an innovative and adventurous undertaking and created ties of affection that can be read, for instance, in the words of the military wife cited above. Performing the treatment at home at the time of the interview, she evoked her relations with the medical team that had performed her dialysis at the hospital for several years and then taught her to treat herself at home. "I feel at home with all the doctors and all the nurses; we embrace, and when I go to the hospital, the lady who trained me, Madame V., and Monsieur P., we all hug each other. *They are all glad to see me and I would also like to go there more often.* Once I told them, 'It would be nice to spend a week with you,' because I do like to return there." Gérard Briche as well, although his book is one long critique of hospital life and the relations with the medical profession, nevertheless says: "I love the hospital . . . paradoxically, I like life in the hospital, especially when dawn and the new day bring an exhilarating sense of hope for life."[15]

The diabetic secretary, for her part, agreed to stay in the hospital forty-eight hours longer than necessary for the test she had to undergo in order to participate as a volunteer (!) in a trying experiment concerning the development of an artificial pancreas. "It was physically very hard, but I was very, very well informed about what was going on, how it was working, what they were trying to do. So, really, I was lucky to be hospitalized just at that moment, because it was interesting—except that I was completely exhausted, because for forty-eight hours one does not get any sleep, I couldn't move, my arms were stuck full of needles, and I was tired to begin with . . . but it was very interesting, and I had a chance to learn lots of things." The close ties that patients of this type establish with the medical milieu profoundly affect their identity. Even while insisting on their hard-won independence from medicine, these self-treating patients may find it interesting, indeed satisfying, to be seen as privileged objects of medicine. Jealously guarding their autonomy, they are nonetheless willing to accept being defined as a "beautiful case," choice material for medical procedures. Even Gérard Briche, just before he left the hospital, went so far as to send a bottle of champagne to the medical team in charge of his case, "with my calling card inscribed: 'Presented for the inauguration of an experimental cortisone treatment by the first resident guinea pig.'"[16] The clearest expression of this internalizing of a patient's value as an object of medicine—albeit always interspersed with the will to negotiate and manage the illness autonomously—was given by the 50-year-old diabetic woman, who also suffered from several other illnesses. "I was an extremely interesting subject for observation," she reported with a certain pride in speaking of one of the many episodes of her medical history. "At the time they used to send my blood to London, I mean I was the guinea pig, my case was studied several times, and all of that was published in reviews." Even more significant is the sentence with which she concluded the exposé of her case: "So that's the history of my illnesses, which I find really exciting; *I think I am interesting* . . . I mean it . . . and if it came to that, I would be interested in the fifth illness."

Self-help Groups

The collective dimension, membership in a "self-help group" or patients' association, is the second characteristic that marks the originality of these self-treating patients and makes them a new phenomenon in our culture. In France these groups have tended to spread in the last few years; in 1981 they founded a National Federation of Health Care Users, but they are still relatively few in number. In the United States and in various northern European countries, by contrast, the "mutual aid" or "self-help" movement[17] has already developed to a considerable extent. A conference on this topic, held in Copenhagen in 1981 by the World Health Organization (W.H.O.),[18] has established that in the United States, "self-help groups" have been constituted in connection with the two hundred most frequent illnesses, handicaps, and disorders, and that fourteen to fifteen million persons belong to them. In England, one can count about two hundred groups or associations. Everywhere their members meet for colloquia and conferences. At Rennes, a French meeting was organized in November 1981 by the review *Autrement*; in Illinois, meetings about different themes were held in July 1980 and November 1981;[19] "Health Days" were organized in Hamburg from 30 September to 4 October 1981. A specialized literature has come into being;[20] annual reports are published and reviewed by information centers. The W.H.O. is interested in them, and scholars want to study them. Surely, this is a new social phenomenon. Does it mark the birth of a new social movement?

Before investigating this question one must ask, however, what membership in a self-help group or patients' association means to the individual. Throughout this book we have again and again analyzed the collective dimension of illness as the characteristic of being sick in the past. But this dimension was related to the nature of the diseases of the past, which struck down large numbers of people at once. Today's efforts, by contrast, aim to develop a collective way of coping with being sick and to break the isolation that becomes the lot of one sick person surrounded by people who have been spared. "In the beginning one is truly cut off, one feels completely different from everyone else . . . the healthy cannot understand the sick, one really belongs to a world apart," says the ministerial researcher, for example. The desire to break out of their loneliness, to make contact with others, is at the core of the motivation of all those who join a patients' group. The taxi driver suffering from multiple sclerosis whom we have cited at length in chapter 11 diligently goes to his association's monthly meetings: "It's a way to meet people, to be on common ground, and to have a bit of distraction." In his case, however, the implication is not very strong; the association, he says, is a kind of senior citizens club that provides entertainment. Moreover, in comparing himself with the other sufferers on these occasions, he feels that the differences are greater than the similarities. "I know that for me this is a way of realizing that I am not the only one in this situation, and in fact, when I look at the others, I find that I am not doing so badly after 15 years with this disease. When all is said and done, I have done rather well."

But most of these sick have a more intense emotional commitment to the group, dominated by the desire to derive comfort from merging into the "great family" of fellow-sufferers. The previously mentioned military wife evoked the reunions of the group of patients who had met during the training sessions for dialysis at home: "We are always glad to meet with the former patients with whom we had the training, we get together for a little meal, there are also outings—I haven't had a chance to go yet, because my husband was too busy— but it seems it was great, really extraordinary to get together with other patients . . . *we really are a big family,* and that's very good because in the beginning one really needs support."

The ministerial researcher stresses the similarity of the experiences of the sick, which are inaccessible to anyone else and in themselves make for congeniality and comprehension. "A kind of congeniality springs up among the sick; if there is someone who is sick in the same way you are, who may feel as you do, you understand each other, it's only normal; where one usually is, people may like you as much as you please, they can't put themselves in someone else's shoes . . . while with someone who is sick, one can get together, one is experiencing the same thing. That's what it is."

"There is a solidarity among sick people because they are having the same troubles," she also said. This notion gives rise to an attitude of mutual help and more active support. It is this attitude that informs, for example, the association "Vivre comme avant" [Living As Before], created in France in 1975 by women who have undergone breast removal for cancer and make hospital visits to other women who have recently experienced that operation. In 1980, a 58-year-old member of the association said that the point was "to bring them some friendly help, to make them feel better, to *show them that one can live with this,* that one does live with it, and also to give them a lot of small pointers about things one needs to know when one is lying there, all worried, in bed, wondering, 'How am I going to get along?' " "We give them," she continued, "a booklet containing all kinds of indications about what one must and must not do . . . and we leave with them what is called a 'façade,' that is, a Dacron-filled bag they can put into their bra, so that it won't show. We also give them addresses where they can find prostheses."

This association helps women who are still reeling under the double shock of discovering their cancer and undergoing the operation to meet others who had the operation several years ago. The association, however, defines itself as a "movement providing sympathy, comfort, and example" and refuses to deal with medical matters. "We do not talk about medicine, we do not know anything about it, we are not physicians," said the spokeswoman whom we interviewed. A completely different attitude is adopted by the members of groups for whom mutual help in dealing with medical matters, problems arising from their self-treatment, and the day-to-day management of their illness is paramount. A 35-year-old woman undergoing hemodialysis at home with the help of her husband told us how her association functioned in her town in southern France. "We sometimes telephone each other when there is a problem, and we try to help out as best we can. It may be a matter of fixing the machine or anything else, and then we help out. For instance, Monsieur X. changed his needles, and the doctor told him: 'When you see Y. (this woman's husband) tell him to show you how to do it.' My husband went to his house, put in the needles, and showed him."

Such help is sometimes provided in more dramatic circumstances and can even become a substitute for appeal to the physician. "One day, Monsieur X. called us at three in the morning because his punctures were bleeding and he was hemorrhaging. And his wife, thinking that she was doing the right thing, wiped off the blood instead of tightening the needles and trying to fill in the spaces, and the wiping made it bleed even more. So at three in the morning the two of us went over to help them. We did the best we could. We did call the doctor, though, and he told us, 'You are doing the right thing, just keep going.' So we managed it; there is a brotherhood among all dialysis patients."

The 52-year-old diabetic woman explained how participation in the group enabled her to acquire personal autonomy and to break the extreme dependence, a veritable "umbilical cord," by which she was tied to her sister. Suffering from a dangerous case of diabetes and threatened by frequent nocturnal comas, she had lived for years in immediate proximity to her sister, who subjected her to constant "mothering." Gradually, and thanks to support from the group, she had acquired sufficient self-confidence to break this dependence and to establish a more flexible system, a network of friends who telephone at fixed times to find out how she is. Today, she says, "I do have a network of people who are watching out for me, but it is as unrestrictive as possible, both for the people who are watching me and for myself."

For this woman, then, the association to which she belongs — an offshoot of the Association Française des Diabétiques created with the intent of reflecting and studying *"the diabetic's psychosociological problems"*[21] — constitutes one of the essential means of gaining autonomy and managing her illness. "This has changed my life," she says, and "the meetings of the group are a top priority for me." She absolutely rejects the image of a social and leisure-oriented club. "Some people came but never came back; the group did not grab them . . . Why? Some come because they want to be mothered a bit, or perhaps they are looking for cooking recipes . . and others think that it is there to organize outings for diabetics. Not at all; if we do organize an outing, fine, to celebrate our anniversary perhaps, or else we invite one another to our homes, because we have made friends, but it is nothing like a travel or leisure-time agency . . . not at all. Actually, it's a bit austere, no question about it; this group is not for fun and games, but so interesting."

A Positive Identity

For these severely ill people, the group is thus a means of confirming their decision to treat themselves. In exchanging information with others, they increase and assert their own. In this manner they reinforce the mastery over their condition and, more importantly, strengthen the positive identity they have forged for themselves. This is not an easy thing to do; and although the persons we interviewed often spoke of their pride in having become what they are, they also told us that in order to achieve it they had to overcome the often rather unpleasant image reflected by the rest of the world. As sick people, they are painfully aware of their solitude; as the sick of a new type, they often realize that they frighten others. The self-treating patient appears to others to be engaged in a mysterious and somewhat disturbing enterprise. Sometimes the treatment itself is frightening. The military wife who underwent her dialysis at home told us about the reactions of her friends and relations when she proposed they "come and watch." *"I tried to invite friends to come, but they are all scared.* They say, 'Oh no! We don't like to see blood. Oh gee, if I see blood, I pass right out.' I told them, 'No, come and see me some night anyway, so you can see what it's like.' But not many came."

For outsiders, the fact that the sick themselves, outside of the presence of medicine, manipulate and apply sophisticated techniques to their own bodies is probably the most disturbing aspect of all this; the sick perceive this feeling of strangeness they create in others perfectly well. One person who also underwent dialysis at home, a 42-year-old salesman, said: "For some people who see this from the outside, and who don't know what hemodialysis is, *we are acrobats;* yes, acrobats, I mean for people who are not familiar with this kind of treatment. Several times I have seen friends' or relatives' eyes pop out of their heads when they heard, not in any detail, but simply that I am having the treatment here, at home." In such cases it is the function of the group to show all the members that they are not alone in their disturbing strangeness. "The first time I went to the group," said the 50-year-old diabetic woman, "I had the impression that I was meeting Martians, and I too was a Martian . . . discovering other Martians like that breaks our loneliness."

Often this discovery can help the sick person to elaborate a positive identity. This makes us understand the double, and apparently contradictory, statement that we so often heard in the course of our interviews. "I am not a sick person," many of our informants said, by which they meant—aside from the invisible nature of their physical condition, which we have analyzed in connection with the image of illness today—their continuing social integration, especially through work.[22] "We who are sick," they nonetheless would say a few minutes later, often with a certain pride. For under the new dispensation, belonging to the "world of the sick" signifies not only that one has taken charge of managing one's body but also that one has established a relationship of familiarity, even mastery, with science and technology, entities whose symbolic importance in our society is a well-known fact. It can also signify that one has established a partnership, or even an adversarial relationship, with one of the most prestigious experts, the physician.

In this last case the sick person's identity becomes openly "offensive,"[23] and here some of the sick stress the dimension of protest, the antiestablishment perspective of their various endeavors. Yet in France, with the exception of some groups of cancer patients who, painfully aware of the limits of medicine, have turned to parallel means,[24] patients' associations rarely have the deliberately "alternative" character they have in Germany, for example; they usually remain within the context of official medicine. All of them, however, do not do this in the same manner. The case of diabetes is typical. The Association Française de Diabétologie was founded at the instigation of physicians, yet two of the diabetics whom we interviewed belong to a group that came into being owing to a near-break, or at least a divergence, with it. This type of group wishes to function in complete independence from the medical profession. "We absolutely do not permit physicians to attend," said the previously mentioned 50-year-old diabetic. Yet the patients do want to make their voices heard; the same woman continued: "We do attend colloquia and seminars; not long ago we went to the diabetology meetings and N. spoke up. She stressed the fact that it is pretty sad that we had to wait until 1981 before they looked into the living experience of the diabetic. But I do think that now the physicians are beginning to listen to us."

The young secretary is not as optimistic about the possible influence of the knowledge of the sick on medical conceptions. "We have noticed symptoms of which you never hear in the books, and after we discussed them in the group we mentioned them to the physician; when you do that, he thinks you want to teach him his job, and he takes it more or less well; but there are others who listen to you and who say, 'How about that . . .' *but one can never find out whether they retain it as an idea* and whether they maybe bring it up at some international colloquium – there is no way of knowing that." She did, however, describe a very positive experience in one hospital's department of childhood diabetology:[25] "At N., for example, we were very well received by a professor who completely agreed; he called a meeting, asking all his students and the hospital staff, and he invited two members of the group so that these people could hear from us both as members of the group and as diabetics; well, of course, the students have no experience at all, so they had lots of questions to ask; the hospital staff had experience with children, and so they wanted to know what would become of them when they grow up, okay . . . all those who took part in this found it very interesting."

Communication with the professionals and the endeavor to make the voice of the sick part of constituted medical knowledge, moreover, are not the only activities pursued by this group. It also tries, for instance, to obtain reimbursement by Social Security for products and tests not yet recognized by that agency. In this respect, these groups deliberately go beyond their demands for recognition of a "subculture of the sick" or the affirmation of the legitimacy of a lay discourse. Rather, they attempt to act as agents for the collectivity,[26] as partners in the management of the health-care system.

This was also the idea expressed by Gérard Briche, who, in speaking of the need for groups of patients who can pool their experiences in order to "help each other to intervene positively in the healing enterprise,"[27] also stresses their "public-health and social role," "their involvement in the choice of public-health options."[28] Such groups, he also says, "if they proved their viability, would soon become consumers' unions. Having first served to establish communication among patients suffering from the same condition and to facilitate exchanges with other groups, they would enlarge their audience and take in people who are not ill but convinced of the socio-political importance of health, as well as physicians who share their ideas. They would thus become a power capable of standing up to the corporate powers."[29] In this manner "patients' groups" take up the concerns of the consumers' and users' movements, which have their roots outside the medical field and are part of the larger protest movement against the modern consumer society, a movement that came into being in France in the wake of May 1968.

"Health-care Users"

These movements have embarked upon a general critique of the type of production pursued by the industrial societies, their "waste" and their "conspicuous consumption," which in the realm of health takes the form of "overuse" of medication. The ecological movement in particular has stressed the invasive character of technology and chemical pollution and has attempted to promote the notion and the use of practices that can easily be mastered by human beings and come about "naturally." In the area of health-care consumption, these different trends have given rise to a wide gamut of practices and organizations. To cite only a few: the increase in the number of health-food stores selling "healthy" and "natural" foods; the renewed interest in homeopathy and acupuncture, in addition to other kinds of so-called "gentle" medicines; the rising popularity of such practices as iridology [observation of changes in the iris], aromatotheraphy [theraphy based on aromatic substances], phytotherapy [therapy based on plants]; the publication of studies and tests of medical products and services in reviews such as *Que Choisir* and *Cinquante mille consommateurs*; the considerable success of Dr. Pradal's *Guide des médicaments les plus courants* [*Guide to the Most Common Medications*];[30] and the opening of the first "fitness center" at Tours in 1972, followed by a number of others. All these initiatives aim to facilitate the general public's access to knowledge and hope to make a dent in the power that the professionals derive from the monopolization of knowledge.

Not all social categories, however, have become involved in this trend. Indeed, the practices advocated by these movements are clearly part of the logic that informs the life style of the upper-middle classes. Academics, executives, and technicians, for example, attach great importance to all phenomena of consumption, whether it be in the area of food, culture, or medicine — and it appears that the level of "medicalization" is particularly high among the members of this social category.[31] M. Wieviorka has shown that "*consumer action* functions in two distinct ways, with the first at times reinforcing the second."[32] On the one hand, scandals serve to sensitize public opinion to the general themes of consumer action and to show the usefulness of the organizations devoted to this work; on the other hand, decidedly less popular efforts are being made to provide information and definitions about the "alternative" consumption practices of this new petty bourgeoisie. *L'Impatient: Mensuel de défense et d'information des consommateurs de soins médicaux* [*The Inpatient: A Monthly Publication for the Defense and Information of Health-care Users*] partakes of this double schema, as its subtitle indicates. In its first issue it promised not only to provide health-care users with information about the various existing associations, about their rights and ways to enforce them, but also to "denounce the abuses and scandals at the patients' expense, about which the press is usually too delicate to speak."[33] Yet a few years later its editor, P. Clermont, was to write: "We felt that we had to oppose this excessive medicalization. But to settle for verbal denunciation of abuses and mystifications did not seem sufficient. In order to provide real resistance against this encroachment, we had to anchor it in new practices; *in short, we wanted to provide people with concrete means of taking their health into their own hands*, of refusing to resign to the 'specialists who will handle everything.' That is why we have turned to noninstitutionalized kinds of medicine."[34] Unorthodox cancer therapies, vegetarianism, yoga, homeopathy, healers, "natural" medications, and antigymnastics were some of the themes treated in depth by *L'Impatient*.

The search for "a different way," the desire to live "alternatively," was indeed almost always the main aspiration of those nonsick people interviewed who in 1979–80 belonged to a health group or association, frequented a fitness center, and, in a larger sense, shared the perspective of a protest movement against "medical power." To be sure, in some cases a specific initiative may be sparked by an objective problem; the director of a public cultural center in Paris and president of a health organization, for example, evoked the fact that the community became aware of the lack of medical facilities in an old Parisian neighborhood. "All around the neighborhood we have long had several associations interested in health issues . . . and the question came up again when the nuns who ran the dispensary decided to quit, that's when we had the idea of getting in touch with some doctors." But these associations adopted an "alternative" stance from the outset and meant to define a different mode of physician-user relationship. "And besides, we wanted to do things differently, so the associations tried to set up a medical practice staffed with physicians chosen by them. That of course is exactly the opposite of what is usually done . . . in our association this was one thing everyone totally agreed with: we wanted to find docs who were willing to play the game that way." In fact, more than a year after this practice has opened, the association still keeps an eye on "its" physicians in a manner from which the idea of control is not altogether absent. "We discuss the way they work with our docs, without exercising control of course, but if it got too shitty, we would tell them that something is wrong."

Similarly, it was the poor health of her small children that led the young wife of an executive living in a "new town" in the Paris area to create a health group. But here again, the problem was part of this couple's larger aspirations, for they wanted to live "alternatively" in a "new town." The young woman analyzed the motives that led her and her husband to this choice. "We had thought about it: we came here because this was a 'new town,' because we thought we would find something different and would be able to run things in town ourselves." The health group, which began as a women's discussion group and eventually sought to work with the D.D.A.S.S. [Direction Départementale de L'Action Sanitaire et Sociale] and the municipality, is an outcome of this desire to "run things." "We wrote a paper outlining what we wanted for the new town and presented it to our elected representatives. We said that in our new town we wanted the availability of alternative medical services, preventive medicine, third-party insurance, a gentle medicine . . . we wanted a municipal health center run by a salaried physician, where the user also has some input into the management."

In this case, however, the group's action failed to lead to any concrete results, and the young woman subsequently limited her ambitions to solving the problem of her children's health. She found the solution in a form of "alternative medicine," homeopathy. In the end, "doing things differently" was possible only on the individual level. This was also the case for a 40-year-old female speech therapist, a member of several associations, whom we interviewed in 1979. "First I changed doctors, and after a while I wanted to change medicines. And when I took one of my children, who had sinusitis, to a homeopath-acupuncturist, I truly felt that I was burning my bridges to lots of things, and I said to myself, 'All right, I have made a choice that is almost irreversible; not irreversible perhaps, but important.'" The same search for alternative ways motivated a young woman who decided to have a child differently. For the birth of her child she therefore chose "Les Lilas."[35] "'Les Lilas' is a place where you can have your baby just about any way you like." "Besides," she continued, "I had made up my mind that I wasn't about to have my kid at the hospital or any other maternity clinic."

In these last cases the search for alternatives is quite different from the behavior of the sick evoked in chapter 11, for the sick, faced with the uncertainty of a serious illness and adopting an attitude in which taking a chance is a matter of anguish and hope, are trying "something else" without really breaking with official medicine. In the case of the healthy, alternatives and rupture are sought for their own sake. They are carried out, moreover, by way of compromise or alliance — although this also happens in patients' groups — between individual conduct and collective action. The individual is sustained by a group, but the motivation for the individual conduct usually remains individual; it is a matter of defeating "my" illness, improving the conditions of "my" health. Groups of "health-care users" are frequently the expression of a collective focus on individual concerns.

This paradox is, in fact, openly asserted as part of the ideological, even properly political, dimension to which certain members of these groups aspire. Health is political precisely because it is an individual concern, writes, in essence, Gérard Briche — who has traveled the entire length of the road leading from the alienated "patient" to "self-treatment" and militancy — in an article suggestively entitled "At the Crossroads of Solitude and Politics."[36] In 1979 a 33-year-old traveling salesman also explained how his assiduous participation in the activities of the fitness center in the 10th arrondissement [of Paris] tied in with his definition of politics; the body and health — in other words, individual realities "that are everybody's concern" — are truly the domain of politics. "There is something ideological underneath ... something almost purely political, namely action taken by the neighborhood ... so that's the first thing. But there is another angle, and that is communicating in a different way ... but, in fact, to me all of this comes to the same thing; there is no difference between political action in the sense of parties and power relations in the everyday sense . . . to my mind, the redefinition of human relations starts with the fitness center. There it is!" Like several others, this man analyzed his career as a political militant: "I am one of these guys of '68 who have had trouble since then . . . who, after having gone through a period when they were into it up to their necks, began to realize that they had had it with doing all this crap, with running all kinds of stuff like political parties and organizations."

From the anonymous victim of epidemics as collective scourges, from the traditional image of the alienated and passive "patient" to the "self-provider of medical care" as a new cultural figure, to the "health-care user" as a collective actor in the public-health system, and finally to the militant for whom the body is the basis of a new political action, the "sick person" appears to have traveled a long way, about which a number of questions must be asked. In fact, we are convinced that today's sick, except in acute episodes and at the immediate approach of death, are rarely totally passive. These "new sick" relate to knowledge and expertise in a manner that is a new phenomenon in our culture; for it does appear that the health-care users' and consumers' movements act as partners in the collective interplay of forces concerned with the problems of health.

Nonetheless, we must not permit ourselves to be taken in by the discourse of these various actors and in each case attempt to delineate its limits. These limits have already clearly appeared in the case of the "self-help" groups. There is no denying the importance or the sometimes tragic dimension of what is at stake for the members of such groups; it reflects the reality and the intrinsic loneliness of death. It also seems incontestable to us that the sick person's individual body becomes the focal point of actions involving certain ordering principles of social life. New kinds of knowledge are elaborated, points of view that compete with hitherto accepted views are expressed; moreover, very small but significant changes are wrought in the distribution of social roles and in the "microphysics of power." Nonetheless, the "new sick" always have to return to medicine at one time or another.

A particularly interesting aspect of these movements is their properly political dimension. It is true that they practice a militancy of a new type, which has been related to the emergence of a "new middle class."[37] Yet, at present, the health-care users' movement is losing momentum; a new impetus does not seem to be in sight. As early as 1979–80, the few militants whom we interviewed spoke of "stinging failures" in connection with their efforts to go beyond the most habitual channels of action. The fitness centers hardly amount to more than meeting grounds for a homogeneous group of people, members of the middle class who are already sensitized to health issues.

Even more importantly, one must examine the meaning of the categories by which the members of these groups define their action, above all the opposition between "individual" and "private" concerns—the body, health, and illness are part of them—and "public" and "collective" concerns, as the very definition of the terrain for true political action. Does not every "private" concern have its social dimension? It is rather astonishing, incidentally, to observe the reversal that has occurred at the level of language over the last fifteen years: in 1968, many people asserted that there is no such thing as a "private" concern, because everything is political. In the early 1980s, there is a great deal of emphasis on "private" concerns, which are a priori, and sometimes in an incantatory discourse, invested with political meaning.

The extent to which the practices of certain of these groups constitute a "break" is also problematical. However innovative they may be culturally,[38] it is difficult to see such groups as a potential challenge to the State and to society. Moreover, they do, for the most part, seem to express the perfectly legitimate but by no means revolutionary desire to obtain above all a better quality of medical services. And finally, as we learned in certain of our interviews, the desire for autonomy and self-reliance often exists side by side, and in a most ambiguous fashion, with demands for the development of public services and State responsibility.

In addition, one may wonder whether the effort to achieve a "demedicalization," which is central to all these groups, does not have its ambiguities as well. Paradoxically, it can go hand in hand with an extreme concern for all questions of health, which has become the supreme value, a reference that goes far beyond the realm of the organic and is accepted as the most apposite metaphor of the good life and of happiness.

The shift is clearly evident in the thinking of Gérard Briche, who writes: "In learning about their pathological destiny and then becoming aware that they can take a direct role in organizing and shaping the attitudes of health policies, the new sick can become activists or messengers in the task of building a global conception of health taken as a primary moral value of our civilization."[39] The pursuit of a demedicalization of social institutions can thus go hand in hand with what has been called a "new health-consciousness," a "healthism" in the system of values with which not everyone will agree. This attitude was expressed, for instance, by the young traveling salesman who frequents a fitness center, and who said: "Health is everything for me, it is primordial, and I live for it." Participation in the fitness center, he continued, "has to do with responsibility, responsibility for oneself." In this case, health and the body are still the objects of a vision dominated by moral criteria.

The Duty to Be Healthy

Today this type of concept joins a public discourse initiated by the medical profession and, especially, by high administrators and politicians. This discourse stresses the role of individual behavior in the triggering of illness and the maintenance of health. "Your health is your business" has become the leitmotif of these efforts to inculcate personal responsibility for the management of health through the adoption of rational forms of behavior.

The objectives of this discourse are ambiguous. On the one hand, the findings of epidemiological surveys on which it is based show not only the risks associated with certain pathogenic forms of behavior but also the limits of the effectiveness of medicine. On the other hand, the official discourse clearly reflects the desire to reduce health-related expenses, a fact that, albeit implicitly, gives rise to a redefinition of the "right to health." Until now, this right meant the reduction of the inequality of access to medical care; in order to treat illness, which was considered unforeseeable, it was important to develop the means of recourse to the medical infrastructure. Today, the "right to health" implies that every individual must be made responsible for his or her health and must learn to adopt rational behavior in dealing with the pathogenic effects of modern life. Health education is the means to achieve this objective.

It is this perspective that, as early as 1966, informed the introductory report of the Ninth International Congress of Medical Psychology written by a team of public-health physicians. The task of the medical profession, it read, "is to bring about a change in day-to-day behavior, to create a new style of life, and almost, if we dared, a new morality. The aims of such an education would include sound child-rearing practices, a balanced life style, rational dietary habits, the elimination or reduction of the consumption of certain modern toxic substances such as tobacco or alcohol . . . for it will be necessary to bring about a true psychological change."[40] A few years later, the modification of individual behavior had become a privileged strategy for improving health, as the economist V. Fuchs wrote in 1972: "It is becoming increasingly evident that many health problems are related to individual behavior. In the absence of dramatic breakthroughs in medical science the greatest potential for improving health is through changes in what people do and do not do for themselves."[41]

In Quebec, this strategy has assumed the dimensions of a veritable health policy. The duty to be healthy tends to replace the right to illness. The sociologist Marc Renaud has analyzed the manner in which all our experiences and our most ordinary behaviors can be reevaluated and reoriented in relation with this notion of health.

> If we are to believe the government propaganda and the practices of professional groups that are championing the cause of prevention, the "good citizen" of the 1980s will be defined by a series of health-related criteria. On getting up in the morning, this good citizen weighs himself and then eats the balanced breakfast recommended by the nutritionists. At work, he avoids

tense situations, refuses the cigarettes his colleagues offer (or, better yet, becomes a militant opponent of smoking), takes a good hour for his noon meal, during which he watches his calories and does not take any alcohol, and if he should become hungry in midafternoon, he takes a piece of fruit instead of buying something greasy or sweet from the vending machine. On his way home from work, where he is careful to fasten his seat belt and not to get upset in traffic jams, he stops at an exercise center at least every other day to do his jogging. His balanced evening meal consists of meat, fish, vegetables, and fresh fruit. Before going to sleep for at least eight hours, he listens to soft music and does the relaxation exercises he has been taught. From time to time he undergoes the screening tests appropriate to his case recommended by his physician, who has a complete file of his family's health history.[42]

There is no doubt that in France, even more than in Quebec, many individuals and entire social groups have largely resisted conforming to this new image of the "best of all possible worlds." Certain of these preoccupations have nonetheless come to be interiorized, all the more easily because they are supported by reminiscences of a traditional moral discourse; this is the discourse which, as we have seen, has been woven around the notion of biological transgression and which, even in the absence of any specific menace such as syphilis, always uses the body as one of the privileged loci of the norm.

Today we still encounter, as we did in 1960, statements in which "abuses" and "excesses" are condemned, not only because of their organic consequences but also for strictly ethical reasons. In 1960, a postal employee said with disapproval: "Animals are less subject to illness than humans; animals do not go in for excesses as much; humans commit a lot of abuses, animals are satisfied with what they need; humans have a craving for profit, a craving for everything, they're afraid of not enjoying themselves enough." In 1979, a 41-year-old female worker still expressed the opinion that prevention is an integral part of a moral way of life: "Prevention is also how people act in their homes, in their life. *Preventing illness is to manage properly*, to pay attention to lots of things. If one is careful to save, not to spend too much, one must also know how to watch one's health." But it was a Tunisian worker who, also in 1979, expressed better than anyone a normative conception of the "duty to be healthy": "Everyone does the best they can to be in good health and stay that way, because *being in poor health is not proper for human beings*. The one who is often sick, there is something wrong with him, his buddies look at him in a funny way, but on the other hand, the one who is in good health, he is esteemed by everyone, and respected."

Among members of the middle classes — where, incidentally, the ideology of the "duty to be well" is most pervasive — this language is, to be sure, less narrowly normative. Here this new ethic attempts to reconcile two contradictory affirmations, namely the value of the norm and the need for constraints on the one hand, and individual expression and personal growth on the other. Health is an exigency of society, it calls for effort and discipline, but it is also the means to achieve the individual's free personal "self-realization." An ascetic ideal goes hand in hand with the pursuit of personal liberation and pleasure. Depending on the individual, one or the other pole predominates in the discourse. Effort and even asceticism are paramount in the young teacher, interviewed in 1979, whose entire life was organized around his health: "One must avoid tobacco, one must avoid alcohol, one must eat whole-grain cereals, one must cut back on fats and, especially, cut out meat. Now we know what is wrong, what is bad in our diet, and I know all about it, and so I eat very modestly: cereals, un-processed of course, whole-grain bread, cold-pressed virgin olive oil, sea salt, brown sugar, and no coffee, no stimulants, and when my friends come to see me no cigarettes, no wine, apple juice. *In this way one prevents illness and builds one's health* by acting on the body." By contrast, also in 1979, a 48-year-old secretary, although she called herself "vigilant," took "chances" in the name of pleasure and personal freedom. "Health is a matter of personal vigilance. After all, one is free, everyone does as he pleases and therefore takes or does not take chances. For example, if I feel like eating something that is not permitted or that is not good for me but that I want very much, *well, I do it at my own risk.* Thank God, I still have that freedom, but I know what I'm doing. You see, I am aware of what I can and what I cannot do, and I take my chances with cigarettes, because I do smoke."

Certain people, however, forcefully reject these efforts at inculcating responsibility. Also in 1979, a female employee in a public administration balked: "These people are really funny, you mustn't smoke, you mustn't drink; but after all, one smokes because one is upset, one drinks when one is a bit depressed, and then it becomes a vicious circle. As far as I am concerned, I know that the more I get upset, the more I smoke; the more I get depressed, the more I drink. As soon as you relax you see that you smoke less, drink a lot less, and are less upset. So I think it's crazy to tell people, 'Don't smoke so much'; it would be better to tell them, 'Don't work so much.'" A postal employee, for her part, insists that the true responsibility lies elsewhere: "I don't like their way of making people feel guilty by telling them, 'You yourself are responsible for this or that,' when it isn't true and when they try to make them believe it in order to hide the real and much more important responsibilities from them. As individuals we can try and refuse to buy all this filthy, chemically produced junk, but the industries that produce all this chemical and unnatural stuff, their responsibilities are a whole lot more important."

It is probably no coincidence that in the context of this conflict several persons proposed the idea that our health-related behavior constitutes more than a moral—namely a legal—obligation. In 1979, a 43-year-old worker asserted:

"Every year people should be requested by registered letter, and under penalty of a fine, to spend a day at the hospital, where they would be given a checkup. That would already turn up certain things." A young academic, for her part, regretted that medical supervision was not more strictly required at her work place, and said that she would like to be "constrained." "I think that medical checkups should be mandatory in the work place, and indeed for everyone. *It should be mandatory.* I know that in the 3 years I have worked in the same place, I have not had a thorough mandatory checkup. My colleagues had a chest x-ray, but I didn't even do that . . . It was my own fault, I just didn't feel like going out to Bondy on my day off. So that is why I wish it were mandatory for me." Such an appeal to the law and the authority of the State no doubt reflects a certain disillusionment with the kind of preventive medicine that is practiced in the work place or in the schools, which is considered inadequate or poorly implemented. But does it not also testify to a conflict between the awareness of a "duty to be healthy"—coupled with guilt feelings toward society, since health care is costly—and the perception of the difficulties involved in mastering one's own behavior in a rational manner? Can this dilemma be resolved by the imposition of an obligation?

The fact that we recognize the "duty to be healthy" as a potential new ideology does not mean that we preach the rejection of any movement that seeks to make individuals or groups aware of their responsibility for their health, any more than the abandonment of efforts at health education or attempts to control the expenditures for public-health measures whose effectiveness is by no means always certain. Nonetheless, it is well to keep in mind that so far there is no proof that health education and the awareness of individual responsibility have made a decisive difference.

Moreover, it is also necessary to be explicit about the ambiguities that almost necessarily mark the road from the "passive patient" to the "responsible health-care user." If health becomes a central value for which each individual feels accountable, then not being in good health can become a serious offense for which the victim will be blamed, according to Robert Crawford's analysis, which has become famous in English-speaking countries.[43] But this is to forget, among other things, that all of us do not have the same strengths and the same resources for keeping control of our behavior. In industrial societies, it is very likely that the members of the middle classes—who are facing less dangerous risks to begin with and are already sensitized to health problems—will always be in the best position to make full use of public information campaigns designed to enhance the individual's rational management of his or her health-related behavior.

It is also to forget that as long as equality of access to health care, indeed to health itself—for the life of a manual laborer is still on the average eight years shorter than that of an executive—is far from achieved, attributing the major part of the responsibility for illness to individual behavior and by the same token concealing its social determinants is certainly not an innocent mistake. It is to forget, finally, that illness is also a reality reflecting the malaise of the individual's relationship with the environment and with society, and that this malaise demands more than the use of behavioral orthopedics.

Conclusion

*T*hroughout this book, we have seen the emergence, and then the transformation, of the figure of the sick person. We do not wish to recapitulate here the various stages of this evolution, but we do want to stress once again the extent to which each society has "its sick." The sick person is a social figure in at least two respects. We know that a period's dominant pathology decisively shapes the experience of illness and the condition of the sick. In this sense, illness is related to society by its nature and its distribution, which vary according to the period and the society. Moreover, the condition and the identity of the sick—the place that is assigned to them in the social space and in the collective consciousness—fit into the value system of each society, the body of knowledge it develops, and the caretaking institutions it puts into place.

Yet in this historical evolution, we are struck by the apparent permanence of certain notions, among them the ancient idea of fate, which we still find formulated today. But the space in which it operates has become considerably smaller; today it is rarely invoked by anyone but the gravely ill at the threshold of death, for whom it constitutes a last and fragile rampart against the onslaught of anguish. We must not permit this apparent continuity to mask the profound evolution of our attitudes, which today are firmly oriented toward action and the mastery of biological fate.

In the past, moreover, fate was collective; today, by contrast, this idea is relevant to individuals, who must face their suffering alone. This same shift, beneath an apparent continuity, can also be discerned in the set of notions of "sin," "fault," and "responsibility," which throughout the ages has never failed to come into play when illness has struck. A normative dimension is always associated with biological misfortune, but its formulation and its specific functioning vary with the vision of the world in which these notions are embedded. In the religious vision, "sin" as the origin of illness marked the human race as a whole. Today, "responsibility" for his or her physical condition falls upon the individual, even if health is seen as an asset for society as a whole.

In these two cases, and indeed throughout this book, we have seen how the matter of illness and the sick gave rise to a shift in the interrelations among the collectivity, the individual, and society. In the past, illness was collective in the sense that it affected people in large numbers and brought turmoil at the scale of the city, sometimes even the province or the entire continent. Yet illness and the condition of the sick were also linked to a transcendent order that had nothing to do with social relations. In this context, there was little need to identify the sick as such, and indeed we usually see them portrayed either as dying or as sinners. Today, by contrast, illness affects specific individuals in their private environment, yet we have come to feel as a matter of course that *being ill has become a social condition*, and that illness restructures our relations with what we call society. We have shown the important role played in this evolution by the linking of "illness" and "work" in a single legal framework and by the enactment of a social legislation that was itself related to industrialization and the development of wage labor.

It may also be useful to reflect on this advent of the *sick individual* with a specific *social status* as part of the development of the modern concept of "the individual," a concept which, in the view of Louis Dumont for example, is related to the constitution of economics as an autonomous domain and to the emergence of society as an end in itself, no longer subject to a divine will beyond human volition.[1] In earlier societies the collectivity was everything, and without it the individual was not thinkable; yet it was rarely conceived of in terms of its own functioning, being considered only as the reflection of a transcendent order. The notion of the individual thus came into being in conjunction with the emerging awareness of the rules that inform the relations of individuals among themselves and with social organization. And indeed it is in this context that, from the nineteenth century onward, we can observe the emergence of the sick person as an individual. The conditions granted to this figure serve to reveal the interplay of the principal social rules, for the sick came to be defined, in particular, by their legitimate exemption from one of the most fundamental rules, the duty to participate in work and production.

In addition, however, this particular dimension of today's sick person as an "individual" also expresses other aspects of our relations with society. Social conditions are always "indicted" in the very widely held conception of illness as produced by the "way of life" of a society that "harms" nature, our nature, which is intrinsically "healthy." This concept reflects the conflicted, indeed negative, representations that inform our relationship with a society dominated by urbanization and industrialization. In this scheme of things illness becomes a metaphor for a society that harms the individual in his or her very body; and the sick person becomes its exemplary victim. This may well be one of the themes that has most clearly perpetuated itself—albeit in varying degrees and formulations[2]—in our collective thinking since the end of the eighteenth century.

Today these ideas, which are expressed at great length in everyday discourse, not only constitute one of the ideological foundations of such phenomena as the various ecological movements, but are also the basis for the rejection of modern medicine on the part of certain sick persons.[3] In this last case, their concepts of illness mark a return to a neo-Hippocratic theory, which holds that the individual's "nature," its "resistance," and its fundamental "health" constitute the essential weapon against the aggression of society, compounded by medical intervention. Sufferers who in this spirit attempt to avail themselves of alternative therapeutics not only combat their illness but also, and simultaneously, oppose modern society, which legitimizes medicine and expresses itself through it. This makes it clear to us that today *medicine itself, and not illness, has become a metaphor* and that, in the last twenty years in particular, medicine has become the focal point of certain of our most fundamental questions concerning the future for which our society is headed.

The development of institutionalized medicine over the last two hundred years, along with the linkage between illness and work, is no doubt one of the most decisive factors to shape the condition of today's sick. Medicine gives that condition its specific content, and it has been one of the purposes of this book to show how the relations with medicine of the sick—whether traditional or "new"—are prototypical of social relations that are almost always fraught with conflict. Correlatively, the increased scope and power of institutionalized medicine—whose most important aspects are scientific advances and the movement toward specialization and professionalization—have come to be seen by many as exemplary trends of our social evolution. If we often read this development as a sign of the power of medicine, we read it even more often as a sign of the constraints and dangers it poses.

One can see an example of this attitude in the development of the debates about the social and ethical implications of medicine that have sprung up in recent years in connection with new medical techniques such as the various resuscitation and life-sustaining practices by artificial means and genetic engineering. In this manner our doubts about the evolution of science—and we are all aware of the essential role of science for the future of our societies—are projected onto medicine and biology. The dilemmas crystallizing around a medical activism that has become incomparably more vigorous than ever before, and around experiments that call into question our very notions of life, death, the individual, and biological descent,[4] have a direct impact on the social and ethical choices that must be made in applying these new techniques. The issue of the reciprocal rights of the physician and the patient or health-care user with respect to euthanasia or the various possibilities of genetic inter-

8. Ibid., 78.

9. Giovanni Boccaccio, *The Decameron*, trans. Mark Musa and Peter Bondanella (New York: Mentor Books, 1982), 12.

10. Pepys, *Diary*, 2:279.

11. Daniel Defoe, *A Journal of the Plague Year*, ed. Anthony Burgess and Christopher Bristol (London: Penguin Books, 1981), 174.

12. Sue, *Le Juif errant*, 79.

13. In Sendrail, *Histoire culturelle de la maladie*, 338.

14. Daniel Panzac, "La Peste à Smyrne au XVIIIe siècle," *Annales, E.S.C.* 28 (1973): 1071–93.

15. Maxime Ducamp, *Paris, ses organes, ses fonctions et sa vie dans la seconde moitié du XIXe siècle* (Paris: Hachette, 1894), 142–43.

16. Benassar writes: "What was the frame of mind of the plague victims? What was their dominant feeling? . . . This is the great gap in our knowledge; we have nothing that would permit us to get *inside* this frame of mind and these feelings, for we do not have a diary or an 'account book' kept by a sick person, someone who was likely to die. I write this in the singular, but I wish we had it in the plural" (B. Benassar, *Recherches sur les grandes épidémies dans le nord de l'Espagne a la fin du XVIe siècle* [Paris: S.V.P.E.N., 1969], 80).

17. Boccaccio, *Decameron*, 8, 9.

18. Daniel Defoe (who however, as we pointed out, was not an eyewitness) makes us hear the voice and the reaction to his exclusion of one plague victim, the man who unexpectedly calls on a family of London bourgeois because he is going to "die tomorrow night." Seeing the terror of the family, "the poor distempered man," who, Defoe says, was "as well diseased in his brain as in his body, stood still like one astonished. At length he turns around: 'Ay,' says he, with all the seeming calmness imaginable, 'is it so with you all? Are you all disturbed at me? Why, then I'll e'en go home and die there' " (*A Journal of the Plague Year*, 174).

19. Erckmann-Chatrian, *Histoire d'un paysan* (Paris: J. J. Pauvert, 1962), 1:17.

20. Benassar, *Recherches sur les grandes épidémies*, 23.

21. Bartolomé de Las Casas, *Très Brève Relation de la destruction des Indes* (1552) (Paris: Maspero, 1974), 84.

22. Michel Vovelle, "Preface," in Dominique Cier, *Scènes de la vie marseillaise pendant la peste de 1720* (Le Paradou: Editions Actes-Sud, 1979).

23. Pepys, *Diary* 2:265, 307.

24. Martin Nadaud, *Léonard maçon de la Creuse* (Paris: Maspero, 1976), 63–64.

25. Defoe, *A Journal of the Plague Year*, 28.

26. Marshal de Castellane, *Journal (1804–62)* (Paris: Plon-Nourrit, 1895), 502, cited in R. Baehrel, "La Haine de classe en temps d'épidémie," *Annales, E.S.C.* 7 (1952): 351–60, 354.

27. Cited in Baehrel, "La Haine de classe," 354.

28. Ibid., 536.

29. Ibid., 356.

30. Charles de Mertens, *Traité de la peste* (Paris: Didot, 1784).

31. Cited in Baehrel, "La Haine de classe," 356–59.

32. Cited in J. N. Biraben, *Les Hommes et la peste en France et dans les pays Européens et méditerranéens* (Paris: Mouton, 1976), 2:83.

33. Froissart, *La Guerre de cent ans*, ed. Andrée Duby (Paris: U.G.E., 1964).

34. Defoe, *A Journal of the Plague Year*, 50.

35. Ibid., 42. In the Middle East as well, people tried to defend themselves against the scourge by magical practices which were often the popular version of religious practices. In particular, many of the prayers and formulas recited against the plague were

based on verses of the Koran. Cf. M. W. Dodd, *The Black Death in the Middle East* (Princeton: Princeton University Press, 1977).

36. Biraben, *Les Hommes et la peste*, 2:18.

37. Defoe, *A Journal of the Plague Year*, 71.

38. Cf. M. D. Grmek, "Préliminaires d'une étude historique des maladies," *Annales, E.S.C.* 24 (1969): 1476–83.

39. To this day there are still two major theories concerning the origin of syphilis. One is the "Columbian theory," which holds that the disease was brought to Europe in March 1493 by Christopher Columbus's sailors returning from the Antilles. The other, or "unitary theory," claims that this disease had existed everywhere since prehistoric times but had been confused with other affections such as leprosy. The supporters of this theory also note the kinship of the disease with other, nonvenerial forms of treponematosis like the "pian" or "pinta" that are found in Latin America.

40. *Libellus Joseph Grumpeckii, de mentalugra, alias morbo gallico* (n.p., n.d.), translated [into French] in 1884. We thank Claude Quetel for bringing this text to our attention.

41. Albert de Queux de Saint-Hilaire, ed., *Oeuvres complètes d'Eustache Deschamps* (Paris, 1887), 5:27–28, Ballade DCCCLIII.

42. André Martin, ed., *Journal de L'Estoile pour le règne de Henri IV*, vol. 2, *1601–9* (Paris: Gallimard, 1958), 50.

43. Pierre Decourcelle, *Les Deux Gosses* (Paris: Jules Rouff & Co., 1896), 138.

44. *Journal de L'Estoile*, 53, 124, 297, 338.

45. J. P. Goubert, *Malades et médecins en Bretagne (1770–1790)* (Paris: Klincksieck, 1974), 343

46. Ibid., 318.

47. François Lebrun, *Les Hommes et la mort en Anjou aux XVIIe et XVIIIe siècles* (Paris: Flammarion, 1975).

48. F. Destaing and A. Blaise, "Le Général Typhus," *La nouvelle Presse médicale* (1976): 45–48.

49. This is, for example, the opinion of William H. McNeil, *Plagues and Peoples* (New York: Anchor Books, 1976), 194.

50. Lebrun, *Les Hommes et la mort*, 123.

51. Ibid., 114.

52. For a very long time mortality remained particularly high among children put out to wetnurses (and this was a widespread practice). Thus of the 13,830 Parisian infants put out to wetnurses in the provinces in 1885, 27.5 percent died before the age of 1. Cited by G. Jacquemet, "Les Maladies populaires dans le Paris de la fin du XIXe siècle," *Recherches*, special issue "L'Haleine des faubourgs," no. 29 (December 1977): 349–64. For the difference in infant mortality among popular and middle classes in late nineteenth-century Paris, cf. F. Pelloutier, *La Vie ouvrière en France* (reprint, Paris: Maspero, 1975), 257–59.

53. Lebrun, *Les Hommes et la mort*, 134.

54. Ibid., 315.

55. See, for example, the works of Philippe Ariès and Michel Vovelle, as well as the already cited work of François Lebrun.

56. Robert Debré, *L'Honneur de vivre* (Paris: Hermann & Stock, 1974), 253.

57. Maurice Genevoix, *Trente Mille Jours* (Paris: Seuil, 1980), 38.

58. Léon Frapié, *La Maternelle* (1904; reprint, Paris: Livre de Poche, Albin Michel), 173.

59. Charles Marie de La Condamine, "Mémoire sur l'inoculation de la petite-vérole" (Paper delivered at the public meeting of the Académie des Sciences, Paris, 24 April 1754) (Paris: Dunand, 1754), 95.

60. Chateaubriand, *Mémoires d'outre-tombe*, 336.
61. Ibid., 344.
62. Ibid., 345.
63. Honoré de Balzac, *Le Curé de village* (Paris: Editions Fernand Hazan), 48.
64. Marie Bashkirtseff, *Journal*, 1st ed. (Paris: Fasquelle, 1887), 1:11.
65. Erckmann-Chatrian, *Histoire d'un paysan*, 2:477.
66. Ibid., 482–84.
67. She wrote to one of her friends, Sarah Chiswell, on 1 April 1717: "A propos of distempers, I am going to tell you a thing that I am sure will make you wish yourself here. The small-pox, so fatal and so general amongst us, is here entirely harmless by the invention of *engrafting*, which is the term they give it. There is a set of old women who make it their business to perform the operation every autumn, in the month of September, when the great heat is abated. People send to one another to know if any of their family has a mind to have the small-pox; they make parties for this purpose, and when they are met (commonly fifteen or sixteen together), the old woman comes with a nut-shell full of the matter of the best sort of small-pox, and asks what veins you please to have opened. She immediately rips open that you offer her with a large needle (which gives you no more than a common scratch) and puts into the vein as much venom as can lie upon the head of her needle, and after binds up the little wound with a hollow bit of shell" (Moy W. Thomas, ed., *The Letters and Works of Lady Mary Wortley Montagu*, 2 vols. [London, 1893], 1:308).
68. Cf. N. D. Jewson, "The Disappearance of the Sick-man from Medical Cosmology," *Sociology* 10, no. 2 (1976): 225–44.

2. From Consumption to Tuberculosis

1. Phthisis, or pulmonary consumption, is not of course the only form of tuberculosis. For the Middle Ages the frequency of "king's evil" or "scrofula," which were long considered specific disease entities, is well known. The single entity "tuberculosis" became known only at the end of the seventeenth century and was firmly established by Laennec. But the natural history of this disease shows the increasing predominance of its pulmonary form, phthisis. In addition, its long-term chronic forms gradually tended to become more prevalent than its acute forms, such as the sadly celebrated "galloping consumption."
2. These amounted to more than 500 for 100,000 inhabitants according to René Dubos, *L'Homme et l'adaptation au milieu* (Paris: Payot, 1973), 162.
3. "Among the causes that trigger pulmonary consumption I do not know anything more certain than the passion of sadness, especially if it is deep and lasting" (René Laennec, *Traité de l'auscultation médiate*, facsimile of the 1826 ed. [Paris: Masson, 1927], vol. 2, chap. 1, art. 4). Even today many physicians and analysts still look for psychic factors when dealing with tuberculosis.
4. During the first half of the century consumption—and indeed physical frailty in general—was positively fashionable. By the end of the century this attitude changed. Marie Bashkirtseff alludes to this in her diary in 1883: "It seems that at one time consumption was fashionable and that lots of people tried to appear and believed they were consumptive. Oh! If only it were imagination!" she wrote sadly, thinking of her own case (Bashkirtseff, *Journal*, 396 [cited chap. 1, n.64]). In her autobiography, published in 1977, Agatha Christie also mentions the favor in which "delicate health" was held in the nineteenth century; in her youth she herself perceived the aftermath of this attitude. She tells us how around 1910, when physical frailty had ceased to be an asset, her grandmother still adhered to the values of her own youth and tried to persuade her granddaughter's suitors that the young girl was "delicate": "Often, when I was eighteen, one

of my swains would say anxiously to me: 'Are you sure you won't catch a chill? Your grandmother told me how delicate you are!' Indignantly I would protest the rude health I had always enjoyed, and the anxious face would clear. 'But why does your grandmother say you're delicate?' I had to explain that Grannie was doing her loyal best to make me sound interesting" (Agatha Christie, *An Autobiography* [New York: Dodd & Mead, 1977], 36).

5. Franz Kafka, *Briefe an Milena*, ed. Jürgen Born and Michael Miller (Frankfurt am Main: Samuel Fischer Verlag, 1983), 10.

6. Thomas Mann, *The Magic Mountain*, trans. Helen Lowe-Porter (New York: Alfred A. Knopf, 1929).

7. This expression is used by I. Grellet and C. Kruse, *Histoires de la tuberculose: Les Fièvres de l'âme, 1800–1940* (Paris: Ramsey, 1983).

8. Cf., for example, the practitioners' manual by P. Pruvost, *La Tuberculose pulmonaire, tuberculeuse des séreuses* (Paris: Doin, 1927).

9. Cf. J. Delarue, *La Tuberculose*, Collection "Que sais-je" (Paris: P.U.F., 1972). In 1910, mortality in France was 275 per 100,000 inhabitants. It was still 89 per 100,000 in 1947, but had declined to 36 per 100,000 in 1953.

10. A. Boudard, *L'Hôpital, une hostobiographie* (Paris: La Table Ronde, 1972), 53.

11. On this point see, for example, Dubos, *L'Homme et l'adaptation au milieu*, 225–26.

12. Kafka, *Briefe an Milena*, 6.

13. A poster from the early years of the century reads: "Two Scourges: The *Boche* [i.e., the Germans] and Tuberculosis."

14. F. David, *Les Monstres invisibles ou les maladies microbiennes selon Pasteur* (Arras, 1897), cited in Grellet and Kruse, *Histoires de la tuberculose*.

15. P. Filassier, *De Quelques Causes de décès à Paris de 1893 à 1912* (Paris: Préfecture de la Seine, 1913). Cited in J. Jacquemet, "Médecine et maladies populaires dans le Paris de la fin du XIXe siècle," *L'Haleine des faubourgs, Recherches* (1978): 359.

16. Decourcelle, *Les Deux Gosses*, 616 (cited chap. 1, n.43).

17. Ibid., 620.

18. Victor Hugo, *Les Misérables* (Paris: Cercle du Bibliophile, 1963), pt. 4, p. 253.

19. Ibid., 258.

20. On this point, cf. A. Cottereau, "La Tuberculose: Maladie urbaine ou maladie de l'usure au travail?" *Sociologie du travail* (1978): 192–224.

21. Léon Bonneff and Maurice Bonneff, *La Vie tragique des travailleurs* (Paris: Jules Rouff & Co., n.d.), 17–18.

22. Ibid., 11.

23. F. Pelloutier and M. Pelloutier, *La Vie ouvrière en France* (Paris: C. Reinwald, Schleicher Frères, 1900; Paris: Maspero, 1975), 159.

24. Ibid., 256.

25. On this point see the recently published medical dissertation by V. Segalen, *Les Cliniciens ès lettres* (1902) (Paris: Editions Fata Morgana, 1980).

26. As indicated by Daudet's diary, *La Doulou* (Paris: Fasquelle, 1931).

27. Cited by Segalen, *Les Cliniciens*, 97.

28. "The novel henceforth calls for the study and the obligations of Science," the Goncourt brothers wrote in the preface to *Germinie Lacerteux* (Paris, 1864).

29. Michel Foucault, *Naissance de la clinique* (Paris: P.U.F., 1963), 198. [English translation by A. M. Sheridan Smith, *Birth of the Clinic* (New York: Random House, 1973).]

30. Cf. Jewson, "The Disappearance of the Sick-man" (cited chap. 1, n.68).

31. For an analysis similar to ours of mental illness, cf. G. Lanteri-Laura, "La Chronicité dans la psychiatrie française moderne," *Annales, E.S.C.* 26 (1973): 548–68.

32. This is the sense of the "sanitary file" established in Paris in 1894.

33. For the professionalization of the physician, cf. the studies by Jacques Léonard, in particular *La France médicale au XIXe siècle*, Collection "Archives" (Paris: Gallimard-Julliard, 1978).

34. Frapié, *La Maternelle*, 156 (cited chap. 1, n.58).

35. On this point, cf. Cottereau, "La Tuberculose," 192–224.

36. In *Una Vita violenta* [*A Violent Life*], written in the late 1950s, P.-P. Pasolini still tells the story of a revolt accompanied by a strike of hospitalized tuberculosis patients, which led to a confrontation with the police in an Italian hospital. The conflict is clearly presented as a class struggle.

37. Franz Kafka, *Briefe, 1902–1924*, ed. Max Brod (New York: Schocken Books, 1958), 159.

38. Bashkirtseff, *Journal*, 195 (cited chap. 1, n.64).

39. Kafka, *Briefe*, 177.

40. Ibid., 171.

41. Ibid., 441.

42. Bashkirtseff, *Journal*, 330–31. Author's italics.

43. Ibid., 167.

44. Kafka, *Briefe*, 160.

45. Ibid., 161.

46. Ibid., 242.

47. Ibid., 265.

48. Ibid., 180.

49. J. Middleton Murry, ed., *Journal of Katherine Mansfield*, definitive ed. (London: Constable & Co., 1962), 295–96.

50. "Dear Robert, I only give you the medical aspect, everything else is too complicated, but this — and that is its only advantage — has a most pleasing simplicity" (Kafka, *Briefe*, 479).

51. Kafka, *Briefe an Milena*, 6.

52. Mansfield, *Journal*, 207.

53. Ibid., 139.

54. Ibid., 149.

55. Ibid., 298.

56. Bashkirtseff, *Journal*, 427. Author's italics.

57. Kafka, *Briefe*, 304.

58. Mansfield, *Journal*, 137.

59. Ibid., 129. Author's italics.

60. Bashkirtseff, *Journal*, 264.

61. Ibid., 228.

62. Mansfield, *Journal*, 332.

63. Ibid., 333.

64. Ibid.

65. Ibid., 238.

66. Ibid.

67. Ibid., 333.

3. Registers of Memory and Forgetting

1. Jean Reverzy, *Oeuvres* (Paris: Flammarion, 1977), 17–168.

2. Cholera has by no means disappeared from the globe. On 25 September 1979, the French newspaper *Le Monde* reported that, according to an epidemiological study of the

World Health Organization, sixteen African and fourteen Asian countries are affected by this disease.

3. Interview in *Une Histoire de la médecine*, television film by Marc Ferro and Jean-Paul Aron, 1978, pt. 1.

4. Ibid.

5. Ibid.

6. Giono, *Le Hussard sur le toit*; Camus, *The Plague*; Thomas Mann, *Death in Venice*; Pagnol, *Les Pestiférés*. Among more recent works one can also cite the science-fiction novel jointly written by a journalist and an epidemiologist who directs the office of preventive medicine of New York City. This book by G. Cravens and J.-S. Marr, *The Black Death* (New York: E. P. Dutton, 1977), describes a sudden outbreak of the plague in Manhattan.

7. Antonin Artaud, *Le Théâtre et son double* (Paris: Gallimard, 1938), 31. [English text: Mary Caroline Richards, trans., *The Theater and Its Double* (New York: Grove Press, 1959), 30.]

8. Artaud, *Theater and Its Double*, 33.

9. Cf. chap. 5 below.

10. Albert Camus, *The Plague*, trans. Gilbert Stuart (New York: Alfred A. Knopf, 1948), 278.

11. Among the literary texts in which leprosy appears one can cite Paul Claudel's *L'Annonce faite à Marie* [translated as *The Tidings Brought to Mary*] and Flaubert's *Saint-Julien l'hospitalier*.

12. Cf. Claire Brisset, "Six Maladies tropicales à vaincre," *Le Monde*, 5 November 1980, 15.

13. Genevoix, *Trente Mille Jours*, 37 (cited chap. 1, n.57).

14. Grellet and Kruse, *Histoires de la tuberculose* (cited chap. 2, n.7).

15. "A day will come, soon perhaps, when human beings will know of illness only the pleasant feeling of no longer being threatened by it." Cited by Dr. P. Mainguy, *La Médecine à la Belle Epoque* (Paris: Editions France-Empire, 1981), 13.

4. The Illnesses of Modern Life

1. *Le Monde*, 27 January 1982. Since the day when we wrote these lines, this phenomenon has assumed considerable scope. It is known today as AIDS.

2. See, in particular, Cottereau, "La Tuberculose" (cited chap. 2, n.20).

3. H. Hatzfeld, *Du Paupérisme à la Sécurité Sociale: 1850–1940* (Paris: A. Colin, 1971), 32.

4. Irving Kenneth Zola, "Healthism and Disabling Medicalization," in I. Illich et al., *Disabling Professions* (London: Marion Boyers, 1977).

5. Marc Renaud, "Les Réformes québécoises de la santé ou les aventures d'un Etat narcissique," in L. Bozzini et al., *Médecine et société, Les années 80* (Laval, Quebec: Editions Cooperatives Albert Saint-Martin, 1981), 530.

6. I. K. Zola, "A Question of Invalidity," in *Santé, médecine et sociologie*, C.N.R.S. (Paris: I.N.S.E.R.M., 1978), 269.

7. Michel Vovelle, *Mourir autrefois, attitudes collectives devant la mort aux XVIIe et XVIIIe siècles*, Collection "Archives" (Paris: Gallimard-Julliard, 1974), chap. 4.

8. *Journal de la vie de S.A.S. la Duchesse d'Orléans douairière* by Abbé E. Delille, her private secretary (Paris: J.-J. Blaise, 1882), 185ff.

9. The first cancer hospital in France was founded in 1774, thanks to a donation made by a priest of the cathedral of Reims, J. Godinot, who bequeathed a considerable sum for the construction of a cancer hospital. Cf. R. Ledoux Lebard, *La Lutte contre le cancer* (Paris: Masson, 1906).

10. Cited by Sontag, *Illness as Metaphor*, 10 (cited introduction, n.1).

11. See G. Jacquemet, "Les Maladies populaires," 350 (cited chap. 1, n.52).

12. Cited by Sontag, *Illness as Metaphor*, 6.

13. André Gide, *Journal, 1889–1939* (Paris: Edition de la Pléiade), 1204 (30 March 1934).

14. Pascal Percq, "Le Dernier Combat du ministre Ségard," *Les Nouvelles Littéraires* (February 1981): 22.

15. *La Santé publique et l'épidémiologie* (Paris: I.N.S.E.R.M., 1982), 23.

16. Various types of data concerning morbidity are available at this time: (1) the discharge diagnoses of hospital patients, including in case of death, are gathered by the research department of the Ministry of Public Health, although no statistics are available for private hospitals; (2) information gathered by a marketing firm from a panel of physicians in private practice about their patients' pathologies; (3) since 1951–52 a few departments have been keeping statistics on the incidence of cancer, and in 1971 I.N.S.E.R.M. created a united national agency to study cancer morbidity and mortality throughout France; and (4) article L 23 of the National Health Insurance Plan makes it possible to identify beneficiaries receiving compensation for prolonged illness.

17. *Annuaire des statistiques sanitaires et sociales 1981*, Ministère de la Solidarité Nationale, Ministère de la Santé (Documentation française, 1982), 50. However, these findings cannot be considered totally accurate, because specialized cancer centers are not taken into account.

18. For the methodological problems involved in measuring morbidity, see E. Lévy et al., *Economie du système de santé* (Paris: Dunod, 1975).

19. G. Desplanques, *La Mortalité des adultes suivant le milieu social, 1955–1971*, Les Collections de l'I.N.S.E.E., D/44 (1976), 61.

20. M. H. Bouvier and N. Varnoux, "Cancers et catégories socio-professionelles," in *La Santé publique et l'épidémiologie* (Paris: Les Editions de l'I.N.S.E.R.M., 1982), 25.

21. Letter of 17 May 1849, cited in *Balzac et la médecine de son temps*. Catalogue of the exposition organized by the city of Paris, 5 May–29 August 1976.

22. See, however, chap. 6 below.

23. *Données sociales* (Paris: Editions de l'I.N.S.E.E., 1981), 153.

24. This term should be understood to include *apprentices*, *laborers*, *specialized* and *skilled* workers. Cf. *Statistiques technologiques d'accidents du travail, année 1979* (Paris: C.N.A.M.T.S., 1981), 17.

25. Ibid.

26. Georg Walther Groddeck, *Le Livre du ça* (Paris: Gallimard, 1963), 132. [Originally published in German in 1923. English text: *The Book of the It*, intro. Ashley Montagu (New York: New American Library, 1961).]

27. Wilhelm Reich, *La Biopathie du cancer* (Paris: Payot, 1975), 198. [English text: *The Cancer Biopathy*, trans. Andrew White with Mary Higgins and Chester M. Raphael (New York: Farrar, Straus & Giroux, 1973).]

28. Ibid., 188–89 (in French ed.).

29. Leo Tolstoy, "The Death of Ivan Ilyich," in *Short Masterpieces by Tolstoy*, trans. Margaret Wettlin (New York: Dell Publishing Co., 1963).

30. Fritz Zorn, *Mars*, trans. Robert Kimber and Rita Kimber (New York: Alfred A. Knopf, 1982), 118.

31. Ibid., 121.

32. Ibid.

33. Sontag, *Illness as Metaphor*.

34. "Rompre le secret," *Antenne 2*, 31 May 1982.

5. From the Body Horrible to the Space of Disease

1. Cf., for example, M. M. Lock, "L'Homme machine et l'homme microcosme: L'Approche occidentale et l'approche japonaise des soins médicaux," *Annales, E.S.C.* 35 (1980): 1116–36.

2. Boccaccio, *Decameron*, 6–7 (cited chap. 1, n.9).

3. Cited by M. Coudurié and F. Rebuffat, *Marseille, ville morte* (Marseille: M. Garçon, 1968), 82.

4. Artaud, *The Theater and Its Double*, 19–20 (cited chap. 3, n.7).

5. Defoe, *A Journal of the Plague Year*, 94 (cited chap. 1, n.11).

6. Thucydides, *The Peloponnesian War*, ed. and trans. B. Jowett (Oxford: Clarendon Press, 1881), 2:125–26.

7. Defoe, *A Journal of the Plague Year*, 75.

8. Geoffrey de Villehardouin and Jean de Joinville, *Chronicles of the Crusades*, trans. and intro. M.R.B. Shaw (Baltimore: Penguin Books, 1963), 237.

9. Abbé Pocque, ed., *Les Miracles de la Sainte Vierge*, trans. Gautier de Coincy (Paris: Parmantier Didron, 1858), intro., 138.

10. Cited by Vovelle in *Mourir autrefois*, 47–48 (cited chap. 4, n.7).

11. Bibliothèque de l'Arsenal, fonds Bastille 57–83. These testimonies and the following were found by Daniel Vidal in the course of his research for *Miracles et convulsions au XVIIIe siècle* (Paris: P.U.F., 1986). We thank him for bringing them to our attention.

12. Ibid.

13. Carré de Montgeron, *La Vérité des miracles opérés par l'intercession de Mr Paris et autres appelans, démontrés contre Mr L'Archevêque de Sens* (Paris, 1737–41), vol. 2.

14. Bibliothèque de l'Arsenal, *Huitième Recueil des miracles opérés sur le tombeau et par l'intermédiaire de Mr de Paris, diacre* (Paris, 1734).

15. Bibliothèque de l'Arsenal, "Abrégé de la vie de Mr Levier, prêtre habitué de la paroisse de Saint-Leu," *Nouvelles ecclésiastiques* (29 November 1734).

16. de Villehardouin and de Joinville, *Chronicles of the Crusades*, 109.

17. Defoe, *A Journal of the Plague Year*, 99.

18. *Journal de L'Estoile*, 3:91 (cited chap. 1, n.42).

19. Ibid., 2:161.

20. Cited by J. Revel and J.-P. Peter, "Le Corps, l'homme malade et son histoire," in J. Le Goff and P. Nora, eds., *Faire de l'histoire: Nouveaux Objets* (Paris: Gallimard, 1974), 178.

21. Cited by Vovelle, *Mourir autrefois*, 90.

22. Bibliothèque de l'Arsenal, Carré de Montgeron, *La Vérité des miracles*, 107.

23. *Troisième Recueil des miracles opérés au tombeau et par l'intermédiaire de Mr de Paris* (Paris, 1792).

24. *Huitième Recueil des miracles*, 107.

25. Yvonne Verdier, *Façons de dire, façons de faire, la laveuse, la cuisinière, la couturière* (Paris: Gallimard, 1979), 43–44.

26. Pocque, ed., *Les Miracles de la Sainte Vierge.*

27. *Troisième Recueil des miracles*, 109.

28. E. de Goncourt and J. de Goncourt, *Journal, 1851–63* (Paris: Fasquelle-Flammarion, 1956), 1:876.

29. Charles-Louis Philippe, *Bubu de Montparnasse* (Paris: Fasquelle, 1905), 86.

30. E. de Goncourt and J. de Goncourt, *La Femme au XVIIIe siècle*, Collection "Champs" (Paris: Flammarion, 1982), 55.

31. Balzac, *Le Curé de village*, 48–49 (cited chap. 1, n.63).

32. J. Starobinski, "Preface," in Segalen, *Les Cliniciens ès lettres* (cited chap. 2, n.25).

33. Honoré de Balzac, *Oeuvres complètes*, vol. 5, *Ferragus* (Paris: Pléiade Edition), 103.
34. Emile Zola, *Oeuvres complètes*, vol. 2, *Nana* (Paris: Pléiade Edition), 1485.
35. Thomas Mann, *The Magic Mountain*, 5 (cited chap. 2, n.6).
36. Kafka, *Briefe*, 318 (cited chap. 2, n.37).
37. Mansfield, *Journal*, 129 (cited chap. 2, n.49).
38. Kafka, *Briefe*, 478.
39. Honoré de Balzac, *Oeuvres complètes*, vol. 11, *La Peau de chagrin* (Paris: Pléiade Edition), 220. [English text: *The Wild Ass's Skin*, trans. Mary Ellen Marriage (New York: Macmillan, 1901).]
40. Kafka, *Briefe*.
41. Balzac, *La Peau de chagrin*, 245.
42. Bashkirtseff, *Journal*, 169 (cited chap. 1, n.64).
43. Bonneff and Bonneff, *La Vie tragique des travailleurs*, 9 (cited chap. 2, n.21).
44. Cf. chap. 1 above.
45. Dr. René Allendy, *Journal d'un médecin malade* (Paris: Editions du Piranha, 1980), 21.
46. Ibid., 62.
47. The medical literature about hemodialysis points out that this treatment is betrayed by little more than a slightly waxy complexion of the skin.
48. Daudet, *La Doulou* (cited chap. 2, n.26). This diary was only published thirty years after the writer's death.
49. Ibid., 39.
50. Ibid., 40.
51. Ibid., 46.
52. Alexander Solzhenitsyn, *Cancer Ward*, trans. Nicholas Bethel and David Burg (New York: Modern Library, n.d.), 78.
53. Madame de Sévigné, *Lettres*, to Mme de Grignan, 16 November 1688, cited by Vovelle, *Mourir autrefois*, 98.
54. Jean-Jacques Rousseau, *The Confessions* (New York: Modern Library, n.d.), 256.
55. J.-C. Guyot et al., "L'Hospitalisation, le malade et le médecin traitant" (Bordeaux: Université de Bordeaux II, 1981), 219.
56. Ginette Raimbault and Radmilla Zygouris, *Corps de souffrance, corps de savoir* (Paris: Editions l'Age d'homme, 1976), chap. 5, 97ff.
57. Rheumatoid polyarthritis, thyroiditis, hepatitis.

6. From Causes to Meaning

1. Walther Riese, *La Pensée causale en médecine* (Paris: P.U.F., 1950), 1.
2. Foucault, *The Birth of the Clinic*, chap. 1 (cited chap. 2, n.29).
3. Michel Foucault, *Madness and Civilization: A History of Insanity in the Age of Reason*, trans. Richard Howard (New York: Random House, 1967), 262 (in French ed.).
4. Ibid., 270 (in French ed.).
5. H. E. Sigerist, *A History of Medicine* (New York: Oxford University Press, 1951).
6. G. M. Foster, "Disease Etiologies in Non-Western Medical Systems," *American Anthropologist* 78 (1976): 773–82.
7. Cf., for example, Jean-Pierre Goubert, "L'Art de guérir: Médecine savante et médecine populaire dans la France de 1790," *Annales, E.S.C.* 32 (1977): 908–26.
8. *The Essays of Montaigne*, trans. George B. Ives, 4 vols. (Cambridge, Mass.: Harvard University Press, 1925), vol. 4, bk. 3, chap. 13, p. 329.

9. Cf., for example, J. P. Peter, "Les Mots et les objets de la maladie," *Revue historique* 499 (1971): 13–38; J. P. Desaive et al., *Médecins, climat et épidémies à la fin du XVIIIe siècle* (Paris: Mouton, 1972).

10. *Journal de L'Estoile*, 183 (cited chap. 1, n.42).

11. Ibid., 376.

12. Ibid., 513.

13. Benassar, *Recherches sur les grandes épidémies*, 41 (cited chap. 1, n.16).

14. *The Letters and Works of Lady Mary Wortley Montagu* (cited chap. 1, n.67).

15. Louis-Sébastien Mercier, *Le Tableau de Paris*, ed. Jeffry Kaplow (Paris: Maspero, 1979), 39.

16. Charlotte Brontë, *Jane Eyre*, ed. Jane Jack and Margaret Smith (Oxford: Clarendon Press, 1969), 89.

17. Cf. Jean Ehrard, "La Peste et l'idée de contagion," *Annales, E.S.C.* 12 (1957): 46–59.

18. Boccaccio, *Decameron*, 6 (cited chap. 1, n.9).

19. *Journal de L'Estoile*, 513.

20. Ibid., 183.

21. *Essays of Montaigne*, vol. 4, bk. 3, chap. 12, p. 267.

22. *Journal de L'Estoile*, 113.

23. Bibliothèque de l'Arsenal, fonds Bastille 6884. This document was brought to our attention by Daniel Vidal.

24. Cf. Ehrard, "La Peste et l'idée de contagion."

25. Cited by Marc Augé, *Théorie des pouvoirs et idéologie* (Paris: Hermann, 1975).

26. Arthur Rimbaud, "Correspondance," *Oeuvres complètes* (Paris: Pléiade Edition, 1972), 494.

27. On this point, cf. Herzlich, *Santé et maladie*, pt. 1 (cited introduction, n.5).

28. Mercier, *Le Tableau de Paris*, 1:6–7, cited by Daniel Roche in *Le Peuple de Paris: Essai sur la culture populaire au XVIIIe siècle* (Paris: Aubier-Montaigne, 1981), 51.

29. Lebrun, *Les Hommes et la mort*, 188 (cited chap. 1, n.47).

30. See, for example, *Traité des maladies les plus fréquentes et des remèdes propres à les guérir* par M. Helvetius, conseiller du Roi, Médecin Inspecteur Général des Hôpitaux des Flandres (A Paris chez la Veuve Mercier, rue Saint-Jacques, 1739).

31. Benassar, *Recherches sur les grandes épidémies*, 45.

32. Cited in Lebrun, *Les Hommes et la mort*, 276.

33. Cf. chap. 3 above.

34. Maurice Bonneff, *Didier, homme du peuple* (Paris: Payot, 1914), 289.

35. Cf. M. Grmek, "Arnaud de Villeneuve et la médecine du travail," *Yperman, Bulletin de la Société belge d'histoire de la médecine* 8 (1961).

36. See M. Valentin, *Travail des hommes et savants oubliés: Histoire de la médecine du travail, de la sécurité et de l'ergonomie* (Paris: Docis, 1978), 23ff. and 85ff.

37. Cf. Ibid., 79ff. Cf. also Arlette Farge, "Work-Related Diseases of Artisans in Eighteenth-Century France," in R. Forster and O. Ranum, eds., *Medicine and Society in France* (Baltimore: Johns Hopkins University Press, 1980), 89–103.

38. It should be stressed, however, that rather than work and the social relations that it implies, it was the more encompassing notion of "misery" that was the common denominator of the hygienists' preoccupations.

39. Mercier, *Le Tableau de Paris*, 150.

40. Ibid., 151.

41. M. Reberioux, "L'Ouvrière," in J. P. Aron, ed., *Misérable et glorieuse: La femme au XIXe siècle* (Paris: Fayard, 1980), 59–78.

42. Quoted by A. Faure and J. Rancière in *La Parole ouvrière* (18 October 1976): 83.

43. Cited by A. Trempé, *Les Luttes des ouvriers mineurs français pour la création des caisses de retraite au XIXe siècle*, Colloquium "Développement et effets sociaux des politiques de la vieillesse dans les pays industrialisés," Paris, July 1981, proceedings to be published by Russell Sage Publishers.

44. Cited by A. Cottereau in the introduction to D. Poulot, *Le Sublime* (1870), new ed. (Paris: Maspero, 1980), note 23–24.

45. Cf. chap. 3 above.

46. Léon Bonneff and Maurice Bonneff, *Les Métiers qui tuent: Enquête auprès des syndicats ouvriers sur les maladies professionnelles* (Paris: Bibliographie sociale, n.d.), 108; authors' italics.

47. Cf. chap. 10 below.

48. Cited in Roche, *Le Peuple de Paris*, 49.

49. John Powles, "On the Limitations of Modern Medicine," *Science, Medicine and Man* 1 (1973): 1–30.

50. Ibid., 12.

51. Lewis Thomas, "Medicine in America," *TV Guide*, December 1977, 25–26, cited in the introduction to Bozzini et al., *Médecine et société* (cited chap. 4, n.5).

52. Cf. chap. 4 above.

53. Franz Kafka, *Letters to Felice*, trans. James Stern and Elisabeth Duckworth, ed. Erich Heller and Jürgen Born (New York: Schocken Books, 1973), 544–55.

54. *Journal de l'Estoile*, 464.

55. J.-P. Aron, *Misérable et glorieuse, la femme au XIXe siècle* (Paris: Fayard, 1980), 15.

56. J.-P. Aron, *Essais d'épistémologie biologique* (Paris: Christian Bourgeois, 1969), 187–203.

57. *The Essays of Montaigne*, vol. 3, bk. 2, chap. 37, pp. 199–200.

58. Frapié, *La Maternelle*, 119 (cited chap. 1, n.58).

59. In the 1960s the antialcoholic slogan "When the parents tipple the child will be a cripple" [quand les parents boivent les enfants trinquent] had a certain popular appeal.

60. Henrik Ibsen, *Ghosts*, trans. K. Jurgenson and Robert Schenkkan (New York: Avon Books, 1972).

61. *Essays of Montaigne*, vol. 2, bk. 2, chap. 12, p. 251.

62. René Descartes, *Oeuvres et lettres* (Paris: Edition de la Pléiade), 1178.

63. *Journal de L'Estoile*, 98.

64. H. de Balzac, *Lettres à Madame de Hanska* (Paris: Les Bibliophiles de l'Originale, 1971), 3:407.

65. Rousseau, *Confessions*, 255 (cited chap. 5, n.54).

66. Cf. chap. 3 above.

67. Marcel Proust, *Correspondance*, ed. P. Kolb (Paris: Plon, 1905), 5:88.

68. Allendy, *Journal d'un médecin malade*, 67 (cited chap. 5, n.45).

69. Cf. chap. 4 above.

7. Fate or Disease without the Sick

1. Henry B. Wheatley, ed., *The Diary of Samuel Pepys*, vols. 7–8, *1667–1669* (London: Bell Co., 1924), 313.

2. It seems likely that this view of rabies contributed greatly to the symbolic importance of Pasteur's discoveries.

3. *Journal de L'Estoile*, 133 (cited chap. 1, n.42).

4. Ibid., 108.

5. Cited by Lebrun, *Les Hommes et la mort*, 314 (cited chap. 1, n.47).

6. Cf. chap. 12 below.

7. Cf. Herzlich, *Santé et maladie*, chap. 2 (cited introduction, n.5).

8. The Burden of Sin: Sinners and Penitents

1. Epistle to the Romans, V.12.
2. Cited in McNeil, *Plagues and Peoples*, 108–9 (cited chap. 1, n.49).
3. Cited by Hillebrand and Gilbrin, "Les Fièvres romantiques" in Sendrail, *Histoire culturelle de la maladie*, 395 (cited chap. 1, n.2).
4. Blaise Pascal, *Prière pour le bon usage des maladies* (Paris: Editions à l'Enfant Poète, 1946), 110.
5. Ibid., 114.
6. Ibid., 115.
7. Ibid., 119.
8. Ibid.
9. *Journal de L'Estoile*, 187 (cited chap. 1, n.42).
10. Delille, *Journal de la vie de S.A.S. la Duchesse d'Orléans douairière*, 193 (cited chap. 4, n.8).
11. Cited in F. Jeanson, *Montaigne par lui-même*, Collection "Ecrivains de toujours" (Paris: Seuil, 1954), 79.
12. Brontë, *Jane Eyre* (cited chap. 6, n.16).
13. Many manuals teaching the art of preparing for death testify to this concern. Cf. Daniel Roche, "La Mémoire de la mort," *Annales, E.S.C.* 23 (1976): 76–119. F. Lebrun (*Les Hommes et la mort* [cited chap. 1, n.47]) also reminds us how important it was to the peasants to have a priest available, so that he could bring them the last sacraments.
14. *Journal de l'Estoile*, 163.
15. Ibid., 187.
16. Ibid., 163.
17. Ibid., 213.
18. Ibid.
19. Ibid.
20. Ibid., 464.
21. For this point, and for this entire set of problems, cf. Lebrun's *Les Hommes et la mort*, chaps. 11 and 12.
22. Lebrun, *Les Hommes et la mort*, 295.
23. Robert Muchembled, *La Sorcière au village (XVe–XVIIIe siècle)* (Paris: Gallimard), 42.
24. According to the expression used by Vovelle in *Mourir autrefois* (cited chap. 4, n.7).
25. Vovelle, *Mourir autrefois*, chap. 4, "Le grand cérémonial," 79–116.
26. Ibid., 89ff.
27. Ibid., 89.
28. Ibid.
29. Ibid., 91–92.
30. Ibid., 92.
31. Ibid., 94.
32. Ibid., 95.
33. Ibid., 101.
34. Ibid.
35. Ibid., 102.
36. Bashkirtseff, *Journal*, 330 (cited chap. 1, n.64).
37. Author's italics.
38. Author's italics.
39. Mansfield, *Journal*, 228–29 (cited chap. 2, n.49).
40. In the literature of the nineteenth century one can observe the appearance of a melodramatic but laicized version of punishment through illness. Here it is no longer

God but a human avenger who administers the punishment to the wicked. Balzac provides the first example of this in *La Cousine Bette*, where the Brazilian Montes contracts an "exotic illness" (syphilis perhaps?) and transmits it to the horrible Mme Marneffe, who dies of it. Subsequently some of the most famous popular novels used exactly the same schema. In *Les Nouveaux Mystères de Paris* by Aurelian Scholl, the plot is designed to strike terror into the reader's heart: there is a duel in which the "avenger" wounds the "wicked" character, who must be punished with a sword dipped in the blood of a rabid dog. The wounded man contracts rabies and the avenger strangles him with impunity according to the time-honored practice.

41. Zorn, *Mars*, 121 (cited chap. 4, n.30).
42. Ibid., 118; cf. chap. 4 above.

9. The Damaged Individual: The Flawed Body

1. Proust, *Correspondance*, 5:111 (cited chap. 6, n. 67).
2. Samuel Butler's book was based on the coverage of a trial for theft in the contemporary press, but he "replaced" the offense with illness.
3. G. de Molinari, *La Viriculture* (Paris: Guillaumin, 1897), 50, cited in L. Murard and P. Zylberman, "La Cité eugénique," in *L'Haleine des faubourgs, Recherches*, 429 (cited chap. 2, n.15).
4. Reissued by Editions J. J. Pauvert (Paris, 1964).
5. Ibid., 86.
6. Ibid., 93.
7. Ibid., 99–110.
8. Ibid., 123–24.
9. J.-K. Huysmans, *A rebours* (1884) (Paris: Garnier-Flammarion, 1978), 137.
10. Ibid., 139.
11. P. W. Lasowski, *Syphilis* (Paris: Gallimard, 1982).
12. On this point see the article by A. Corbin, "Le Péril vénérien et le discours médical," in *L'Haleine des faubourgs*, 245–83.
13. Theodore Zeldin, *France 1848–1945: Ambition and Love* (New York: Oxford University Press, 1979).
14. Corbin, "Le Péril vénérien," 251–53.
15. Emile Duclaux, *L'Hygiène sociale* (Paris: Félix Alcan, 1902), 253.
16. This was the title of a lecture given by Dr. Emile Coudert to the Société de Prophylaxie Sanitaire et Morale, published in 1904 by the Librairie Jules Rousset.
17. Daudet, *La Doulou*, 78 (cited chap. 2, n.26). The title *La Doulou* appears to be a contraction of *douleur* [pain] and *Lamalou*.
18. Daudet, *La Doulou*, 27.
19. Ibid., 41.
20. Cf. chap. 5 above.
21. Daudet, *La Doulou*, 31.
22. Ibid., 54.
23. Ibid., 60.
24. Ibid., 55.
25. E. de Goncourt and J. de Goncourt, *Journal* (1870), 553.
26. Ibid., 561.
27. Ibid., 558–59.
28. Ibid., 554.
29. Huysmans, *A Rebours*, 137.
30. Cited by Corbin, "Le Péril vénérien," 245–83.
31. Ibid., 249.

32. Eugène Brieux, *Les Avariés* (Paris: Stock, 1902), 56–57.

33. Among the best known are A. Couvreur, *Les Mancenilles* (Paris: Plon, 1900), and P. Bru, *L'Insexuée* (1903).

34. Brieux, *Les Avariés*, 187.

35. Ibid., 187–88.

36. Duclaux, *L'Hygiène sociale*, 246.

37. Ibid., 245.

38. Ibid., 248.

39. Ibid., 263.

40. Ibid.

41. Brieux, *Les Avariés*, 261.

42. Cited by Lasowski, *Syphilis*, 12.

43. Goncourt and Goncourt, *Journal*, 1:876.

44. Brieux, *Les Avariés*, 11ff.

45. Philippe, *Bubu de Montparnasse*, 168 (cited chap. 5, n.29).

46. Daudet, *La Doulou*, 41.

47. Cited by Lasowski, *Syphilis*, 12.

48. Ibid.

49. Cf. chap. 5 above.

50. Philippe, *Bubu de Montparnasse*, 85–86.

51. Ibid., 96–97.

52. Anita Rind, "Les Maladies vénériennes: Informer et déculpabiliser," *Le Monde*, 22 December 1976, 15.

53. A study published in 1958 (Sicard de Plauzolles, *Les Maladies vénériennes: Leur Danger actuel et permanent* [Paris, 1958]) clearly shows their decline and the break in the curves of incidence in the 1940s, brought about by the therapeutical use of antibiotics. There was, for example, a decline from more than 15,000 cases of fully developed contagious syphilis in 1945 to fewer than 2,000 in 1951. But by 1956 the curve began to show a slight rising trend (1,156 cases in 1955, 1,452 in 1956) and this phenomenon became accentuated beginning in the 1960s. Today it is estimated that throughout Europe the incidence of "sexually transmissible diseases" is increasing by 10 to 15 percent per year.

54. Cf. above, note 45.

10. From Inactivity to the Right to Illness

1. Guy Perrin, "Pour une théorie sociologique de la sécurité sociale dans les sociétés industrielles," *Revue française de sociologie* 8 (1967): 302.

2. Ibid., 303.

3. Ibid.

4. Cf. also J. J. Dupeyroux, *Sécurité Sociale*, 5th ed. (Paris: Dalloz, 1973), 30–31.

5. Perrin, "Pour une théorie sociologique," 303.

6. David Wallace Carrithers, ed., *"The Spirit of Laws" by Montesquieu: A Compendium of the First English Edition* (Berkeley and Los Angeles: University of California Press, 1977), 316–17.

7. Mercier, *Le Tableau de Paris*, 42 (cited chap. 6, n.15).

8. Cited by Perrin, "Pour une théorie sociologique," 303, and by Dupeyroux, *Sécurité Sociale*, 31.

9. Hatzfeld, *Du Paupérisme à la Sécurité Sociale*, 193 (cited chap. 4, n.3).

10. Friedrich Nietzsche, *The Genealogy of Morals*, trans. Horace B. Samuel (Edinburgh: T. N. Foulis, 1910), 68–69.

11. Hatzfeld, *Paupérisme*, 26.

12. Karl Marx, *The Class Struggle in France, 1848–50* (New York: International Publishers, 1934).

13. Hatzfeld, *Paupérisme*, 188.

14. Ibid., 327.

15. Cited by Dupeyroux, *Sécurité Sociale*, 257.

16. Bonneff, *Didier, homme du peuple*, 288–91 (cited chap. 6, n.34).

17. For further discussion, see Rémi Lenoir, "La Notion d'accident du travail: Un Enjeu de luttes," *Actes de la recherche en sciences sociales* 32/33 (1980): 77–78.

18. Allendy, *Journal d'un médecin malade*, 62 (cited chap. 5, n.45).

19. Ibid., 67.

20. Chateaubriand, *Mémoires d'outre-tombe*, 345 (cited chap. 1, n.6).

21. Gide, *Journal 1889–1939*, 998 (cited chap. 4, n.13).

22. Pierre Dubois, "L'Absentéisme ouvrier dans l'industrie," *Revue française des affaires sociales* (April–June 1977): 35.

23. J. C. Sournia, *Ces Malades qu'on fabrique* (Paris: Le Seuil, 1977), 11. Author's italics.

24. N. Dodier, "La Maladie et le lieu du travail," Mémoire D.E.A. de sociologie [Diplôme d'Etudes Approfondies], Ecole des Hautes Etudes en Sciences Sociales, Paris, June 1982.

25. Cited in ibid., 208.

26. Ibid., 102.

27. Cf. chap. 6 above.

28. Musée Social, Paris, "Rapport sur les assurances sociales" (1929), 208.

29. Ibid., 209.

30. Nonetheless, the Auroux Law of 1982 opened new perspectives by modifying these committees and enlarging their competences.

31. J.-C. Pollack, *La Médecine du capital* (Paris: Maspero, 1971), 9.

32. S.P.K., *Faire de la maladie une arme* (Paris: Editions Champ Libre, 1973).

33. Anselme, "La Grève de Pennaroya," in *Quatre Grèves significatives*, preface by F. Krumnow, C.F.D.T (Paris: Editions Epi, 1972), 161.

34. Ibid., 72.

35. Ibid., 144; italics in original.

11. Providers and Receivers of Care: Medicine and the Sick

1. Talcott Parsons, "Structure sociale et processus dynamique: Le Cas de la médecine moderne," in F. Bourricaud, ed. and trans., *Eléments pour une sociologie de l'action* (Paris: Plon, 1955), 197–238.

2. Eliot Freidson, *The Profession of Medicine: A Study of the Sociology of Applied Knowledge* (New York: Dodd & Mead, 1970).

3. Muchembled, *La Sorcière au village* (cited chap. 8, n.23).

4. Froissart, *Chroniques, mémoires et autres documents*, ed. Jean Yanoski (Paris: Firmin-Didot, 1886), 197–98.

5. Cf. Vovelle, *Mourir autrefois*, chap. 4, "Le grand cérémonial" (cited chap. 4, n.7).

6. Ibid., 190.

7. Madame de Genlis, *Mémoires inédites sur le XVIIIe siècle et la révolution française depuis 1756 jusqu'à nos jours* (Paris: Ladvocat, 1825), vol. 1, bk. 2, pp. 49ff. Cited by Vovelle, *Mourir autrefois*, 189.

8. Chateaubriand, *Mémoires d'outre-tombe*, 353 (cited chap.1, n.6).

9. Montaigne, *Essays*, vol. 3, bk. 2, chap. 37, p. 203 (cited chap. 6, n.8).

10. From M. Henry-Coüannier, *Saint François de Sales et ses amitiés* (Paris, 1962), cited by Vovelle, *Mourir autrefois*, 50.

11. On this point, cf. the work of J. Léonard; for example, *La Médecine entre les pouvoirs et les savoirs* (Paris: Aubier-Montaigne, 1981).

12. Various authors (among them J. Léonard) have shown the existence of a non-negligible medical philanthropy, but the theme of the "poor people's doctor" goes far beyond the often limited and calculating charity of most practitioners.

13. By the end of the nineteenth century the figure of the doctor who spends long hours at the patient's bedside and reassures the family by his mere presence appears in literature. Cf. for example Zola, *Une Page d'amour* (1878; Paris: Garnier-Flammarion, 1973), 52ff.

14. Cf. chap. 9 above.

15. Luc Boltanski, *Prime Education et morale de classe*, Collection "Cahiers du Centre de Sociologie Européenne" (Paris: Mouton, 1969).

16. Jules Romains, *Knock, ou le triomphe de la médecine*, play in three acts (1923), Collection "Folio" (Paris: Gallimard).

17. J. B. Pontalis, "Une Idée incurable," *Nouvelle Revue de psychanalyse*, special issue "L'Idée de guérison" (Spring 1978): 6. Jules Romains had written: "Give me a few thousand neutral, indeterminate individuals. My role is to determine them, to bring them into a medical existence."

18. For the period before the surveys of "medical consumption" conducted in 1960, we have very few data on this point, except with regard to the number of practitioners. Despite some differences of opinion among investigators, one can agree on a figure of 15,000 physicians [in France] in 1900; actually, their number declined somewhat between 1870 (16,000) and 1900 (according to J. Léonard, *La Médecine entre les pouvoirs et les savoirs*). Their number was 20,700 in 1921, according to a census of the interior ministry, 25,000 in 1931, and 28,600 in 1938 (according to F. Mace-Kemp, "La Profession médicale, sa situation économique et sociale en France de 1920 à 1940" [Law thesis, Paris, 1958]). J. Léonard also gives some indications concerning the development of *hospital* care at the end of the nineteenth century; between 1871 and 1911 the number of hospital establishments increased by 30 percent, that of hospitalizations by 39 percent, and that of patients treated by 31 percent (*La Médecine entre les pouvoirs*, 303). Another indication is the fact that the number of participants in mutual insurance groups rose from 850,000 in 1870 to two million in 1898 (Léonard, 306).

19. This is shown, for example, in the debates that occupied the medical profession at the time when the Social Insurance Laws were being enacted in 1928–30. The physicians were concerned above all about the banalization of medical care that would ensue if it were available to everyone—and therefore poorly paid—and debated at length about the potential "abuses" of widespread recourse to the physician.

20. Romains, *Knock*, 59.

21. Rose L. Coser, "Un chez-soi hors de chez soi," in C. Herzlich, *Médecin, maladie, société* (Paris: Mouton, 1970), 74.

22. Cf. T. Parsons and R. C. Fox, "Illness, Therapy, and the Modern Urban American Family," *Journal of Social Issues* 8 (1952): 31–44.

23. The sociological literature on the notion of "profession" is considerable, but we use it here in the sense given by Eliot Freidson, *The Profession of Medicine*; that is, as competence attributed to an individual on the basis of a specialized system of knowledge and the fully autonomous exercise of a social activity (such as medicine or law) by the members of a group to which society has delegated this activity.

24. Ivan Illich, *Medical Nemesis: The Expropriation of Health* (New York: Pantheon Books, 1976).

25. Gérard Briche, *Furriculum Vitae: Chronique hospitalière d'un lupus* (Paris: Imprimerie Soucher, 1979), 333.

26. Montaigne, *Essays*, vol. 3, bk. 2, chap. 37, p. 204.

27. Rousseau, *Confessions,* 267–68 (cited chap. 5, n.54).

28. Eliot Freidson, *The Profession of Medicine,* and *Professional Dominance* (New York: Atherton, 1970).

29. Tolstoy, "The Death of Ivan Ilyich," 249–50 (cited chap. 4, n.29).

30. Ibid.

31. Many years ago, an American study already showed this constant tendency on the part of the physicians to underestimate their patients' information: L. Pratt et al., "Physicians' Views on the Level of Medical Information among Patients," *American Journal of Public Health* 47 (1957): 1277–83.

32. This must be seen as the vestige of a long history. We know that for a long time, following the creation of the general hospital in the seventeenth century, the hospital was for the poor a place of confinement and supervision rather than a therapeutic institution. We find many traces of their terror in the writings of the past, even under the pen of bourgeois writers. On the eve of the French Revolution, Louis-Sébastien Mercier wrote: "Oh the cruel charity that is practiced by our hospitals! Fatal succor, false and baneful lure! Death here is a hundred times more sad and dreadful than if the indigent met it under his own roof, left to himself and to nature! The house of God indeed! How do they dare call it thus! The contempt for humanity seems to add to the ills one suffers there" (*Le Tableau de Paris,* 214 [cited chap. 6, n.15]). In 1930 we can read in André Gide's *Journal* that, for the poor, the hospital is still a place of abuse and ill treatment. "Em and Mlle Zaglad are talking about hospitals and the scandalous abuses that take place there, of the bad food for the patients, of unfair promotions, of favoritism and the frequent blackmail to which orderlies and nurses subject the unfortunate patients. But by criticizing these abuses, one would play into the hands of the leftist parties, and that is why so many keep quiet. Meanwhile, this *terror of the hospital* that one encounters so often among ordinary people, seems alas!, only too justified" (*Journal,* 985 [cited chap. 4, n.13]).

This terror is very real in working-class testimonies, for example in this anonymous text, written around 1850 by a militant worker, which speaks about what death is like at the "hospice": "If he dies, it is here that the worker's fate is truly unfortunate, for if death comes to take him outside of visiting hours, he is alone, without seeing around him his family and receiving the consolations that are such a joy in the last moments, but sees around him *only the cold or curious faces of the doctors who coldly examine the patient's last crises,* and sometimes hears scoffing, which adds to the horror of his agony, so that he draws his last breath cursing the society that has brought such a fate upon him" (Faure and Rancière, *La Parole ouvrière,* 362–63 [cited chap. 6, n.42]).

33. For France, see Y. Lemel and A. Villeneuve, *Les Consommations médicales des français: Quelques résultats de l'enquête santé 1970–71,* Collection de l'I.N.S.E.R.M, 57 (1977); for the United States, R. Anderson, O. Anderson and J. Lion, *Two Decades of Health Services* (Cambridge, Mass.: Ballinger, 1977).

34. A. Chauvenet, *Médecines au choix, médecine de classe,* Collection "Politiques" (Paris: P.U.F., 1978). For the differential use of the health-care system, see A. Letourmy and J. Pierret, *Inégalités sanitaires et inégalités sociales* (Paris: C.E.R.E.B.E., 1982), in particular pt. 1, chap. 1.

35. This interview was communicated to us by J. C. Guyot, Professor at the University of Bordeaux II.

36. Norman Cousins, *Anatomy of an Illness as Perceived by the Patient: Reflections on Healing and Regeneration* (New York: W. W. Norton, 1979).

37. This expression is taken from A. Van Gennep, *Manuel de folklore français contemporain* (Paris: Picard, 1972), 106.

12. From Self-help to the Duty to Be Healthy

1. Briche, *Furriculum Vitae*, 335 (cited chap. 11, n.25). There are several sociological studies on the problem of chronic illness in English, which reach similar conclusions as certain of our analyses. Cf. for example F. Davis, *Passages through Crisis: Polio Victims and Their Families* (Indianapolis: Bobbs-Merrill, 1963); M. Z. Davis, *Living with Multiple Sclerosis: A Socio-Psychological Analysis* (Springfield, Ill.: Charles C Thomas, 1973); A. Strauss, *Chronic Illness and the Quality of Life* (St. Louis: C. V. Mosby, 1975).

2. Cf., on this point, A. Hervouet, "Le Diabète insulino-dépendant; deux idéologies médicales, deux modalités thérapeutiques, deux attitudes du malade," Mémoire D.E.A. [Diplôme d'Etudes Approfondies], Ecole des Hautes Etudes en Sciences Sociales, Paris (1980).

3. At the time of the survey (1974), kidney patients underwent three dialysis sessions, lasting on the average eight hours each, per week. These sessions have become much shorter today.

4. In certain cases this refusal can be motivated by the wish to establish a clear separation between the illness and its treatment, which fall into the realm of medicine and are circumscribed in time (the duration of the session) and space (the dialysis center), and the patient's ongoing family and professional life. Leading a "normal life" demands this separation, which does not mean, however, that such persons refuse to care for themselves. Moreover, in the case of "self-dialysis" (which developed largely after 1974), that is, dialysis performed by the patients themselves in a center, the treatment is "in their hands" just as in the case of dialysis performed at home.

5. Montaigne, *Oeuvres complètes, Journal d'un voyage en Italie par la Suisse et l'Allemagne* (Paris: Pléiade Edition), 1267–68.

6. Briche, *Furriculum Vitae*, 299.

7. Ibid., 282.

8. Ibid., 285.

9. Ibid., 218.

10. Ibid., 289.

11. Ibid., 329.

12. Ibid., 258.

13. Renée Fox, "Red Carpet Treatment," in *Experiment Perilous: Physicians and Patients Facing the Unknown* (Glencoe, Ill.: Free Press, 1959).

14. The recipients of the first kidney and heart transplants are of course the very prototypes of these "medical superstars."

15. Briche, *Furriculum Vitae*, 337.

16. Ibid., 329.

17. Alf Trojan, a German scholar who has made the only existing systematic study of the French groups, notes that there is no French equivalent for the term *self-help*. He sees this as one of the reasons for their lesser development in France. See Alf Trojan, "Groupes de santé: The Users' Movement in France" (1982), 17 pp.

18. "Self-Help and Health: Report on a WHO Consultation," W.H.O., ICP HED O 14, 6484 B (1981), 19 pp.

19. A First National Epilepsy Self-help Workshop took place at Northwestern University in July 1980; and a seminar on the theme "Hospital and Self-help/Mutual Aid Groups: The Developing Relationships" was held there in November 1981.

20. *L'Impatient* in France, and in the United States such publications as *Medical Self-Care Magazine*.

21. The same woman told us how the group came into being. "This wonderful group was founded about three years ago by a young man who is diabetic and wrote to the Association Française des Diabétiques, asking that his letter be published . . . 'We are

planning to create a group to work with and investigate the diabetic's psychosociological problems—social integration, daily life, relations with family and friends, autonomy and dependence; the themes to be treated and the manner of proceeding will be decided collectively at the time of the first meetings. If you are interested, please get in touch with me; I would be grateful if you inserted this appeal in the publication of the A.F.D.' They did not do it right away, but finally the letter appeared. At the time I did not read this journal; it bored me. And one day—I did read the letters to the editor, because that was the most interesting part—I read that and immediately grabbed the telephone."

22. Cf. chap. 5 above.

23. In the sense given to this term by Alain Touraine in "Les Deux Faces de l'identité," in P. Tap, ed., *Identité collective et changements sociaux* (Paris: Privat, 1980), 25.

24. Cf. for example Martine Tourolle, "Cancer: Le langage de la dissidence," *Autrement: La Santé à bras le corps* 26 (September 1980): 103–10.

25. For the cleavage between childhood and adult diabetology, see Hervouet, "Le Diabète insulino-dependant."

26. In January 1982 the press reported a "strike" (a twenty-four-hour interruption of their treatment) by patients with chronic renal insufficiency treated by hemodialysis in a private clinic in Paris. This was a protest action against bad conditions in the clinic and the insufficient quality of the treatment they received.

27. Briche, *Furriculum Vitae*, 342.

28. Ibid., 340.

29. Ibid., 342.

30. Dr. H. Pradal, *Le Guide des médicaments les plus courants*, Collection "Points" (Paris: Seuil, 1974).

31. M. Dagnaud and D. Mehl, "Profil de la nouvelle gauche," *Revue française des sciences politiques* 2 (April 1982): 372–93.

32. M. Wieviorka, *L'Etat, le patronat et les consommateurs* (Paris: P.U.F., 1977), 245.

33. "Quand les patients s'impatientent" ["When Patients Get Impatient"], *L'Impatient*, editorial no. 1, November 1977, 3.

34. P. Clermont, " 'L'Impatient,' dénoncer l'O.P.A. sur les corps" ["No to Takeover Bids for Our Bodies"], *Autrement: La Santé à bras le corps* 26 (September 1980): 180.

35. This is the "Maternité des Lilas," one of the first places to practice first "childbirth without pain" and then the "childbirth without violence" developed by Dr. F. Leboyer. In 1976–77 the clinic threatened to close because of its financial deficit. The personnel and the "users" pooled their efforts to obtain the status of "private hospital," which has ensured the continued existence of "Les Lilas."

36. G. Briche, "Au Carrefour du solitaire du politique," *Autrement: La Santé à bras le corps* 26 (September 1980): 11–12.

37. Cf. Dagnaud and Mehl, "Profil de la nouvelle gauche."

38. It should be noted that these groups, usually without being aware of it, take up certain of the themes of the American libertarian movement, and especially those of the late nineteenth-century German *Lebensreform* groups. These movements hoped to achieve a reform of day-to-day private life, especially with respect to food, hygiene, and physical exercise, through the action of small decentralized groups, usually founded by middle-class individuals. The objective of these reforms was a return to nature, and a concomitant critique of industrial and urban society.

39. Briche, *Furriculum Vitae*, 344–45.

40. P. Coudray, M. Cerisé, and P. Fréour, *L'Information médicale du public, aspects psychosociaux*, introductory report of the Ninth International Congress of Medical Psychology (Paris, 1966).

41. Victor Fuchs, "Health Care and the United States Economic System: An Essay in Abnormal Physiology," *Milbank Memorial Fund Quarterly* 50 (1972): 211–37.

42. Bozzini et al., *Médecine et société*, 529 (cited chap. 4, n.5).
43. Robert Crawford, "You Are Dangerous to Your Health: The Ideology and Politics of Victim-Blaming," *International Journal of Health Services* 7 (1977): 663–80.

Conclusion

1. Louis Dumont, *Homo aequalis: Genèse et épanouissement de l'idéologie économique* (Paris: Gallimard, 1977). Cf. also Marcel Gauchet, "De l'Avènement de l'individu à la découverte de la société," *Annales, E.S.C.* 34 (1979): 451–63.
2. At the end of the eighteenth century this conception was held, as we pointed out, above all by physicians, especially by the authors of medical topographies.
3. Certain groups of sick persons, especially among cancer victims, have banded together precisely on the grounds of this rejection, but we have no example of this in our material. Another new and striking phenomenon today is the incidence of outright rejection of medical treatment, a behavior that was unthinkable a few years ago. In December 1982, for instance, there were press reports about a decision of the Court of Appeals at Nancy, which had permitted a 14-year-old girl to refuse the medical treatment indicated, in principle, for her case (idiopathic medullary aplasia). The head of the hospital department, through the intermediary of the children's judge, asked the court to order the resumption of the treatment, which the young girl had broken off as deleterious to the quality of life. She preferred a "less aggressive" treatment worked out by a general practitioner. By deciding in her favor, the Court of Appeals ratified the rejection of a medicine perceived as too aggressive and asserted the young girl's right to find her own way to survival, and indeed to decide whether she wanted to live or die.
4. This concern comes into play, for instance, in the practice of artificial insemination by anonymous donor.
5. In the United States these problems have led to the formation of a new discipline called "Bioethics," which sponsors numerous meetings, debates, and publications and has established specialized institutes. In practice, this new discipline usually brings together philosophers, jurists, and theologians, for whom the encounter with medical and biological issues has meant a renewal of their traditional concerns.

Index

Claudine Herzlich is senior researcher at Centre National de la Recherche Scientifique and teaches at the Ecole des Hautes Etudes en Sciences Sociales. She is the author of *Santé et Maladie* and *Médecins, Malades, et Société*.

Janine Pierret is a researcher at Centre National de la Recherche Scientifique and has served on the editorial board of Sciences Sociales et Santé.

Illness and Self in Society

Designed by Ann Walston.

Composed by Rosedale Printing Company, Inc., in Plantin with Plantin Bold Italic display type.

Printed by the Maple Press Company on 50-lb. S. D. Warren's Sebago Eggshell Cream Offset, and bound in Holliston Roxite A.